The Healing Nutrients Within

Facts, Findings, and New Research on Amino Acids

Eric R. Braverman, M.D.

with Carl C. Pfeiffer, M.D., Ph.D., Ken Blum, Ph.D., and Richard Smayda, D.O.

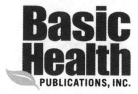

Basic Health
PUBLICATIONS, INC.

The information contained in this book is based upon the research and personal and professional experiences of the authors. It is not intended as a substitute for consulting with your physician or other healthcare provider. Any attempt to diagnose and treat an illness should be done under the direction of a healthcare professional.

The publisher does not advocate the use of any particular healthcare protocol but believes the information in this book should be available to the public. The publisher and authors are not responsible for any adverse effects or consequences resulting from the use of the suggestions, preparations, or procedures discussed in this book. Should the reader have any questions concerning the appropriateness of any procedures or preparation mentioned, the authors and the publisher strongly suggest consulting a professional healthcare advisor.

The Healing Nutrients Within is not intended as medical advice. Its intent is solely informational and educational. Please consult a health professional should the need for one be indicated.

Basic Health Publications, Inc.
8200 Boulevard East
North Bergen, NJ 07047
201-868-8336

Editor: Cheryl Hirsch
Typesetter/Book design: Gary A. Rosenberg
Cover design: Mike Stromberg

Library of Congress Cataloging-in-Publication Data
Braverman, Eric R.
    The healing nutrients within / Eric R. Braverman.—3rd ed.
        p. cm.
Includes bibliographical references and index.
    ISBN 1-59120-037-7
    1. Amino acids in human nutrition. 2. Amino acids—Physiological effect.
3. Amino acids—Therapeutic use.   I. Title.

QP561.B73 2003
613.2'82--dc21
                                                    2002156739

This book is a revised version of The Healing Nutrients Within published in 1987.

First Edition, Second Edition, Third Edition

Printed in the United States of America.

10   9   8   7   6   5   4   3   2

Contents

Section Six: Threonine Amino Acids

Section Seven: Branched-Chain Amino Acids

Section Eight: Amino Acids with Important Metabolites

Section Nine: Putting It All Together

My thanks to Tatiana Karikh, M.D.
for her valuable medical and editorial expertise
in the preparation of this book.

Preface to the Third Edition

The Healing Nutrients Within, now in its third edition, has been providing health professionals and interested general readers with the latest research available on amino acids for more than fifteen years. When *The Healing Nutrients Within* was first published, amino acid research was in its infancy. Amino acids and nutritional therapies were controversial and not readily practiced in conventional medicine, let alone found on the shelves of natural food stores.

Since then, doctors have continued to pioneer and change the face of medicine. Medical school programs like those at Columbia and Harvard are now teaching courses in nutrition. Major health and medical organizations, such as the American Heart Association, the Cancer Society, the Arthritis Foundation, and the American Diabetes Association, are all incorporating diet and nutrition into their medical protocols. And too, more individuals are now taking an active part with their healthcare providers in the maintenance of their health and in the treatment of their health problems.

Out of this changing environment, amino acids have arrived—big time. News about amino acids is even the stuff of headlines and best-sellers. Research and clinical use are booming worldwide. Amino acids are becoming part of everyday life—helping people sleep better, feel better, and overcome anxiety, depression, and substance abuse. They are in dietary sweeteners. They are part of new anti-aging compounds and weight-loss regimens. They are used in emergency rooms for treatment of medication overdose and liver detoxification. And they are now gaining repute in blood tests, as powerful indicators of mental and physical illnesses.

The quality and quantity of research and clinical applications have established hard proof that amino acid nutrition is an important element in many medical treatments. The revelations to date make it clear that we have only begun to tap into a vast, uncharted frontier that will surely continue to yield many medical bonanzas for years to come. After all, amino acids are the building blocks of protein, and protein is the building block of the brain. In that way, amino acids are human beings' most important nutritional building blocks— more critical than any other nutrient, including vitamins, essential fatty acids, and trace minerals—because amino acids help support brain function, which, in turn, runs the body. We are now learning that when the brain is functioning well, the body will follow suit.

There is growing understanding and acceptance of how imbalances of certain amino acids affect illness and wellness in body and mind. Supplementation with amino acids offers a new strategic medical dimension in the fight against chronic illness. Increasingly, amino acids are becoming not only part of the armamentarium of hospitals and physicians, but also of informed consumers everywhere.

At the Place for Achieving Total Health (PATH Medical) in New York City, we have been using amino acids in the treatment of many serious illnesses for years. Our continued success and the successes of other physicians new to amino acids show how nutritional science can make the practice of medicine more effective. We achieve our best results in most aggravated cases by combining nutritional supplements, such as amino acids, with medication. We are strong believers in complementary medicine—using the best that both medical and nutritional research has to offer.

This third edition has given The Healing Nutrients Within a face lift and reflects a comprehensive accumulation of new research and its future implications. As with previous editions, the fundamentals of amino acids are included to give the reader a foundation, as well as a synopsis of verified research findings, on the individual roles of amino acids. As the sheer volume of research on amino acids continues to accumulate, information that is now outdated has been eliminated. Material has been reorganized to make it easier to quickly reference and research, and scientific information has been translated into practical terms for all to understand. A section on guidelines for amino acid supplementation has been added.

We continue to cover new exciting developments in detail in this revised edition. The updates feature information on many new medically "hot" topics, including the following:

- Arginine has been shown to act similar to, and in some cases replace, Viagra for restoring erectile function and a sagging libido. It has also been found to increase sperm count.

- New research measuring the breakdown products of bone in hydroxyproline may prove more advantageous for assessing bone loss than the standard bone density test.

- Scientific evidence shows that boosting energy levels in the brain with phenylalanine and tyrosine is key to weight loss.

- Melatonin and tryptophan (which, unfortunately, is still available only by prescription) have established themselves as multipurpose nutrients to improve sleep, defuse anxiety, and slow down the aging process. Recent studies show promise for the use of tryptophan in the treatment of autism.

- Homocysteine has gained recognition as a major independent risk indicator for cardiovascular disease. New research suggests it may also portend neural tube defects, sickle cell disease, rectal polyps, and liver failure, and may contribute to depression, dementia, and loss of brain function in the elderly.

- Research shows how tyrosine can help cocaine and alcohol abusers kick their habits and combat the effects of stress, narcolepsy, chronic fatigue, and attention deficit disorders.

- Amino acid blood levels are increasingly serving as important indicators of physical and mental illnesses. They provide major nutritional and biochemical clues for more effective treatment.

- Carnitine has been shown to offer significant protection against the common side effects of Depakote, a popular drug used for seizures and psychotic disorders. Its derivative N-acetyl-carnitine may surpass the metabolic potency of carntine in the brain, where it has been found to slow the progression of Alzheimer's disease.

- Scientific evidence continues to mount showing N-acetyl cysteine, an amino acid compound, to be perhaps the most powerful detoxifier in the body. It is now found in every emergency room as an antidote to overdose cases and as well can render harmless everyday environmental toxins.

- New, modified GABA compounds such as gabapentin (Neurotin) and tiagabine (Gabitril) are producing improved uptake in the brain and appear to be important products in the control of seizures and anxiety disorders. Early studies indicate GABA may also be correlated to a decrease in benign prostatic hypertrophy.

- Research with serine compounds shows that blocking serine metabolism may serve to prevent autoimmune activity present in psychoses.

- Two amino acids—glutamic and aspartic acids—create additional neurotoxic damage in the brain following stroke. New drugs that block the action of the excitory amino acid transporters (EAATs) have recently been approved.

- For years, bodybuilders, weight lifters and athletes believed that branched-chain amino acids (BCAAs)—leucine, isoleucine, and valine—enabled them to create bigger and better muscles and improve performance. Accordingly, they led the world in consumption of BCAAs. Now, scientific research has confirmed that they were right. Not only do branched-chain amino acids aid athletes, they also offer promise for staving off muscle loss as we age.

- Cranial electrical stimulation (CES), an increasingly popular method of therapy for many conditions, has been found to promote the neurotransmitter functions of amino acids. This represents a major breakthrough in amino acid therapy.

At this point in time, so much research and clinical experience has occurred that medicine can no longer ignore or minimize the influence of amino acids. We believe that solid nutritional management involves the use of amino acids and offers substantial treatment benefits that can be applied by physicians and by any individual with the guidance of a healthcare professional. Amino acids for prevention of disease and obtainment of optimum health are proven. There is nothing here that is unbelievable.

The last fifteen years of research has shown that nutrition continues to represent the ultimate recognition that the body is the temple of the holy spirit. Every doctor, every person should be paying attention to their nutritional status or that of their patients because nutrition is a part of every disease and is certainly a vital part of any longer-term preventive course. It is our hope that this new edition will be of continued benefit in helping you understand that the best-stocked drugstore of all still remains in the human body.

How to Use
This Book

The twenty-four amino acids discussed in this book are divided into eight sections according to their chemical similarities. Amino acids with similar structures participate in the same or similar actions and perform the same or similar functions. Within these sections, each amino acid is discussed individually.

The information presented is intended to provide a comprehensive review of the uniqueness of each amino acid, its function and metabolism within the body, food sources for, therapeutic use in clinical syndromes, form and absorption, guidelines for supplementation, as well as its latest findings in research for more than fifteen years. Each section about an individual amino acid concludes with a summary where the most important information of the chapter is condensed.

The back of the book provides an extensive glossary of terms for the layperson and facilitates the use of the book as a textbook for high-school and college-level students. The book can also be referred to by physicians and nutritionists as a guide to using amino acids as therapy for various clinical conditions.

Lastly, a comprehensive index can be used to find selected topics. The numerous scientific references provided for each amino acid are grouped in a bibliography and can be used as a source tool for expanding your knowledge of amino acids. We believe this book will be a foundation of your library for years to come.

SECTION ONE

An Introduction to Amino Acids

STRUCTURE OF AN AMINO ACID

C = Carbon
O = Oxygen
N = Nitrogen
H = Hydrogen

CARBON (Hydrogen)
CHAIN

ACID (Vinegar)
CARBOXYL GROUP

$$CH_3 - CH - COOH$$
$$NH_2$$

AMINO GROUP (Ammonia)

CHAPTER ONE

Amino Acids: The Building Blocks of Life

*P*roteins are chains of amino acids linked together. The word "protein" comes from the Greek *protos,* meaning "first," deservedly enough, as it is the basic constituent of all living cells. Protos may also be the root of the name of Proteus, the Greek mythological sea-god who could change form; appropriately, food protein changes form to become human substance after being eaten. The body breaks down dietary protein into amino acids that are then used to build the very specific proteins the body needs.

Protein is the second most abundant substance in our bodies after water. It constitutes three-fourths of the dry weight of most body cells. It is involved in the biochemical structure of genes, blood, tissue, muscle, collagen, skin, hair, and nails, and is a major constituent of all the many hormones, enzymes, nutrient carriers, infection-fighting antibodies, neurotransmitters, and other chemical messengers in the body—just for starters. This continuous cell-building and regeneration necessary for life requires non-stop supplies of protein.

Simple proteins made up of two to three amino acids linked together are called *peptides.* The word "peptide" comes from the Greek *peptos,* meaning "cooked," a rather poetic way of referring to digestion. Peptides are often no more than digested proteins. Many short-chain peptides are absorbed directly into the bloodstream after eating. New roles for these very small proteins are being discovered daily. For example, many peptides work as neurotransmitters—chemical substances that send messages to and from the brain and help regulate the body—and as natural pain-relieving substances in the brain.

All protein is made up of different combinations of amino acids. Proteins vary from simple to complex depending on the number, variety, and order of amino acids in the structural chains. In one protein molecule, several to hundreds to thousands of amino acids can be linked together by peptide bonds in a variety of forms, including chains, helixes, spheres, and branched structures, that give the proteins their unique functions and characters. Each protein is designed for a specific purpose and cannot be interchanged. The instructions for making all those proteins are encoded in the DNA in the nucleus of every cell.

These essential proteins that make up the human body are not taken directly from our diet. The body first breaks down dietary protein into individual amino acids and then reassembles these amino acids to build the specific proteins it needs. Scientists now know that simple protein as peptides can be absorbed immediately, without digestion, into the bloodstream. However, the majority of proteins are composed of longer, more complex chains of amino acids that the digestive system has to break down into absorbable constituents before they can be absorbed. Twenty-four known amino acids are needed by the body to form more than 50,000 unique proteins it needs. It is these amino acids, the primary building blocks of human life, to which we devote this book.

WHAT IS AN AMINO ACID?

Like carbohydrates and fat, "protein" is composed of hydrogen, oxygen, and carbon. Yet, protein also contains nitrogen. It is because of this nitrogen that protein is able to repair and build tissue.

While protein is a well-recognized term, the term "amino acid" can be confusing. Amino acids are made up of a weak acid molecule group—a chemical fragment containing carbon, oxygen, and hydrogen—in conjunction with a strong basic amino molecule group—a chemical fragment containing nitrogen. The mild basicity or acidity of amino acids is too minimal to affect acid-base balance in the body, which is preserved by multitudes of protective buffer systems, and is a misnomer that we hope will cease to confuse our readers.

More accurately, amino acids can be thought of as useful ammoniated vinegars. Glycine, for example, has a more correct chemical name: *alpha aminoacetic acid.* Since "amino" also means ammonia and acetic acid is vinegar, we can call this amino acid "ammoniated vinegar." This basic structure found in glycine is common to all amino acids. Smelling salts are usually ammonium carbonate, which can restore sensibility to people who have become faint. When added to salads and other foods, vinegar makes the taste of food more palatable. Similarly, some amino acids can "improve flavor" by stimulating the mind, controlling depression, or invoking sleep.

When acid, or "vinegar," portions are removed from the amino acids, the basic amines become messengers in the nervous system. When the amine or ammonium portions are removed, the remaining "acid" can be used for fuel, detoxification, or in many processes throughout the body.

People often do not realize their need for amino acids, because they are not aware of how busy the human body is. Every second, the bone marrow makes 2.5 million red cells. Every four days, most of the lining of the gastrointestinal tract and the blood platelets are replaced. Most of the white cells are replaced in ten days. A person has the equivalent of new skin in twenty-four days and bone collagen in thirty years. All this continuous repair work requires amino acids.

ESSENTIAL AND NONESSENTIAL AMINO ACIDS

Amino acids fall into two basic categories: essential and nonessential. In the human body, the liver produces about 60 percent of the amino acids needed. The remaining 40 percent must be obtained from the diet. Essential amino acids are the nine to eleven amino acids that cannot be synthesized by the body and must be supplied by diet. The other amino acids are classified as nonessential amino acids. Although no less important, these amino acids can be synthesized by the body by combining two or more of the essential amino acids.

The list of the essential amino acids was begun by scientists in the early 1900s. The main essential amino acids are now known to be lysine, leucine, isoleucine, methionine, phenylalanine, threonine, tryptophan, tyrosine, and valine. A person would begin to die without ingesting these amino acids daily, although the gut flora (bacteria) provide small quantities of each of them. This actual continuous low level of synthesis is essential; otherwise, symptoms of their absence would be noticed often throughout the day.

Histidine and taurine are also essential amino acids for early growth and development in premature infants and possibly for all neonates (newborns one month or younger). Preterm babies are also known to require cysteine, because the fetal liver cannot convert methionine to cysteine.

There are many other amino acids besides the essential ones that the human body normally manufactures. These nonessential, or conditionally essential, amino acids may become essential to a particular individual through an inborn error of metabolism (genetic defect). If an enzyme necessary for the manufacture of a particular amino acid by the body is absent, that amino acid becomes an essential requirement of the diet.

Nonessential, or conditionally essential, amino acids can also become essential during disease states or stress when there is either increased need and/or increased breakdown of them. Virtually all stress states require more amino acids, some more than others; distinguishing the source of the increased amino acid requirements is often difficult. Burn patients require more amino acids because of oozing wounds, while a schizophrenic patient may have a recently expressed inborn error of metabolism that dictates the need for less wheat gluten or the amino acid serine. Certain cancers can be starved by withholding their "favorite" amino acids. For example, melanomas consume excessive phenylalanine and tyrosine; reducing these two amino acids in a cancer patient's diet can slow tumor growth. The understanding and manipulation of required amino acids in the diet are essential in maintaining health and controlling disease.

Table 1.1 lists the core essential and nonessential amino acids. Many other amino acids occur in humans in very small amounts, but as yet little is known about them. In the future, the list of essential and nonessential amino acids may well be expanded.

DIETARY REQUIREMENTS FOR AMINO ACIDS

The body's need for protein and amino acids in the diet is cruelly evident during great famines and throughout several Third World countries. Children suffering from *kwashiorkor* (malnutrition caused by protein deficiency) with their protruding abdomens, atrophied muscles, and mental retardation vividly demonstrate the essential nature of proteins and amino acids.

To determine the body's requirement for essential amino acids, first it is necessary to determine the body's protein needs. Minimum protein requirements for a healthy adult are based on the sum of the requirements for each of the eleven essential amino acids, plus a sufficient intake of nitrogen for protein synthesis and breakdown. Nitrogen is lost during protein metabolism and in urine, feces, skin, hair, nails, semen, and menstrual discharge. Proper protein metabolism requires that the body maintain a balance between the amount of nitrogen excreted and the amount assimilated.

There are no universally accepted dietary requirements for protein. However, the World Health Organization (WHO) recommends 0.3 to 0.4 grams (g) of protein per kilogram (2.2 pounds) of body weight per day, or about 30 to 40 g for

TABLE 1.1. THE AMINO ACIDS	
ESSENTIAL AMINO ACIDS	**NONESSENTIAL AMINO ACIDS**
Histidine	Alanine
Isoleucine	Arginine (essential for babies)
Leucine	Aspartic acid
Lysine	Carnitine (essential for babies)
Methionine	Cysteine
Phenylalanine	Gamma-amino-butyric acid (GABA)
Taurine	Glutamic acid
Threonine	Glutamine
Tryptophan	Glycine
Tyrosine	Homocysteine
Valine	Hydroxyproline
	Proline
	Serine

an average adult male weighing approximately 150 pounds. This number assumes a majority of the protein consumed is high-quality protein and contains all or most of the essential amino acids. The current recommendation for dietary intake of protein proposed by the National Academy of Science's Food and Nutrition Board, which sets the Recommended Dietary Allowances (RDAs), is 44 to 56 g per day. In America, most people eat two to three times the RDA for protein. Even vegetarian diets contain 80 to 100 g of protein per day.

Newborns and children have higher requirements for amino acids. In percentages, the World Health Organization (WHO) suggests that a newborn infant needs dietary protein that contains 37 percent of its weight in the form of essential amino acids, whereas for an adult, who has lower growth needs, the figure is less than half that, or about 15 percent.

As long as the body has a reliable source of dietary proteins containing the essential amino acids, it can adequately meet most of its needs for new protein production. Protein requirements are also determined by age group, the degree of stress, energy requirements, and one's state of health. Considering all these factors, Table 1.2 presents the minimum daily requirements for the essential amino acids for various age groups. Keep in mind that ideal intakes of these essential amino acids are more difficult to determine than their minimum daily requirements.

Many factors can influence the body's balance of amino acids and can contribute to deficiencies in one or more of the essential amino acids, even if you eat a well-balanced diet that contains adequate amounts of protein. Poor digestion, infection, trauma, stress, drug use, age, environmental pollution, processed foods, and personal habits such as smoking and drinking are factors that can influence the availability of essential amino acids. Deficiencies of vitamin and

TABLE 1.2. MINIMUM ESSENTIAL AMINO ACID REQUIREMENTS (mg/kg per day)			
AMINO ACID	INFANT (4–6 MONTHS)	CHILD (10–12 YEARS)	ADULT
Histidine	33	N.A.	N.A.
Isoleucine	83	28	12
Leucine	135	42	16
Lysine	99	44	12
Methionine plus cysteine	49	22	10
Phenylalanine plus tyrosine	141	22	16
Taurine	N.A.	N.A.	N.A.
Threonine	68	28	8
Tryptophan	21	4	3
Valine	92	25	14

minerals, especially of vitamin C and pyridoxine (vitamin B_6), which are important for the absorption and transport, respectively, of amino acids, can contribute
to deficiencies of essential amino acids in the body.

FOOD SOURCES FOR AMINO ACIDS

Adequate amounts of the essential amino acids should be consumed daily. In
order for the body to make the proteins it needs, it must have adequate supplies
of the amino acids. The removal of even one essential amino acid from the diet
leads rather rapidly to a lower level of protein synthesis in the body, which sooner
or later, will lead to some type of physical disorder, and eventually to death.

Both animal and plant proteins contain the known essential amino acids. The
proportion of these amino acids varies according to the characteristics of each
protein. Foods that are high in protein typically are high in amino acids. Protein
from animal sources—meat, chicken, fish, milk and milk products, and eggs—is
of greater nutritional value than protein from plant foods. Animal proteins are
considered "complete," or "high-quality" protein because they contain all the
essential amino acids, plus the nonessential ones.

The extent to which a food's amino acid pattern, that is, its digestibility and
composition, matches that which the body can use is expressed in the "biological value" of that food. The net protein utilization (NPU) reflects the biological
value and the digestibility of a protein—in other words, how much of the protein
a person eats is finally available to his body. No food corresponds exactly with
the body's required amino acid pattern, but the amino acid content in eggs
come closest to the combination required by healthy bodies. The protein in eggs
is such high-quality protein that eggs are used as the standard other proteins'
NPUs are rated by. (See "The Much Maligned Egg: The Best Amino Acid Food"
on page 7.)

Each of the following chapters gives a summary of the foods in which a particular amino acid is most concentrated. Plant foods are generally not considered
because of their negligible protein content. Protein from plant food is considered
"incomplete" because one or more of the essential amino acids is present in only
small amounts.

The essential amino acids most commonly lacking in plant foods are lysine,
tryptophan, and methionine. All cereals are deficient in lysine; corn and rice are
also low in tryptophan and threonine. Soybeans and oils are low in methionine.
Legumes are low in methionine and tryptophan; peanuts are deficient in methionine and lysine. Poor-quality meats seem to have higher concentrations of less
essential, and sometimes even toxic, amino acids, such as serine and proline. The
amino acid profiles for fermented foods, fungi, and other sources of protein are
being investigated. (See "The Optimal Amino Acid Diet" on page 8 for suggestions on how to obtain a well-balanced amino acid intake.)

The Much Maligned Egg:
The Best Amino Acid Food

Heart disease often involves obstruction of the coronary arteries by fatty plaques, which consist mainly of cholesterol. Cholesterol combines with calcium to become hard, hence the term "hardening of the arteries." The plaque that accumulates on the walls reduces arterial volume and results in higher blood pressure and harder work for the heart.

A well-proven strategy to prevent heart disease is to reduce dietary cholesterol intake. The overall rate of cholesterol intake in this country has dropped from 800 mg a day to less than 500 mg a day in the last ten years. At the same time, consumption of the "good" unsaturated fats and olive oil has increased by 60 percent. These changes in diet have done more to reduce heart disease than all medical procedures combined, according to Robert Levy of Columbia University.

Changes in cholesterol consumption have come mainly from reduction in meat intake, which is 40 percent less than fifteen years ago. Egg consumption has dropped only 12 percent, so it is apparent that the reduction in eggs has made little contribution to the decrease in heart attacks. In spite of the almost universal advice to limit the consumption of eggs because of their high cholesterol content, we think it is good to eat eggs, because the egg is a nearly perfect amino acid food. Furthermore, the egg, because of its high lecithin content and other nutrients, does not raise blood cholesterol levels by more than 2 percent.

Most foods are of lower quality as protein sources than the egg, which is proportionally the most balanced and best source of the essential amino acids. In each food, only one or two essential amino acids are deficient or totally lacking, and these are called the "limiting amino acids" for that food. The protein will be utilized by the body only to the extent that the limiting amino acid is present. The egg's superior balance makes its proteins more usable than those of most other foods.

Careful study of the effect of egg proteins on plasma amino acids shows that egg, like steak, raises lysine, valine, threonine, and leucine to extremely high levels. Yet the ratio to other amino acids is slightly better balanced in eggs than in steak. For example, steak increases the plasma valine to plasma methionine ratio to more than five to one, while for egg, it is only four to one. The egg is slightly better balanced, but not perfectly balanced. Amino acid formulas are now being studied, which may suggest ways to achieve a more balanced rise in plasma amino acids than food itself can provide.

The National Academy of Sciences has reviewed amino acid protein for high quality and recommends the amounts in Table 1.3.

The Optimal Amino Acid Diet

Many people throughout the world adopt a vegetarian diet for religious, ethical, and health reasons. It is beyond the compass of this book to address these issues, but we feel that some discussion is relevant here, as a vegetarian diet can present problems with respect to an adequately balanced intake of amino acids.

Vegetarians don't get enough of the core proteins that supply an adequately balanced intake of amino acids. Epidemiologists have suggested that true vegetarian societies cannot adapt to stress as well as meat eaters for lack of nutritional advantages. Most vegetable proteins have amino acid deficiencies and are thus unsatisfactory as a sole source of protein. These deficiencies can be overcome in part by the addition to the diet of other proteins rich in amino acids.

Part of the problem in a vegetarian diet is not in the toxins in the vegetables, but in the deficiencies they induce. Vitamin B_{12} deficiency and vitamin D deficiency rickets can occur with vegetarianism. Vegetarian children less than two years old may be shorter and lighter than other children. Vegan (pure vegetarian) diets are well below recommended calcium requirements for females. Lacto-ovo vegetarians, who eat eggs and milk, seem to have less deficiency in zinc, calcium, and vitamin D. Meat, fish, fowl, and liver are concentrated sources of vitamins E, A, and B complex. Furthermore, animal foods are loaded with iron, zinc, and other nutrients.

The advantages of a high-vegetable diet are increased fiber and beta-carotene, which protect against cancer, particularly colon cancer. A high-vegetable diet is undoubtedly healthy, but probably should not exclude meat and other proteins. We degrade fiber faster on high-meat diets. Beef protein in amounts as great as 55 percent of the diet will not raise cholesterol levels in normal men. The real danger of high-protein, high-meat diets is that they are frequently accompanied by a high consumption of refined carbohydrates. A diet high in vegetables, whole grains, and lean meats may be the best for optimal health. The great contribution of vegetarianism is that it has made us aware of the need to eat more vegetables and fruits and fewer refined carbohydrates and junk foods.

If sufficient vegetables, whole grains, and fish are eaten, the hazards of meat (produced organically) are lessened. Some meat is necessary for resistance to stress. But excess meat and fat are to be avoided since they are implicated in cancer and heart disease. The threats to our meat and fish supply such as steroids, PCBs, antibiotics, or hormones should be reduced or eliminated. The nutrients, such as cysteine, that protect us against those hazards should be increased. Meat diets should be high in vegetables, whole grains, fish, fowl, eggs, and supplemental nutrients. We believe that this combination is the one that leads to a well-balanced amino acid intake and optimum health for most people.

TABLE 1.3. AMINO ACID PATTERN FOR HIGH-QUALITY PROTEINS			
AMINO ACID	MILLIGRAMS/ GRAMS	AMINO ACID	MILLIGRAMS/ GRAMS
Histidine	17	Phenylalanine plus tyrosine	73
Isoleucine	42	Threonine	35
Leucine	70	Tryptophan	11
Lysine	51	Valine	48
Methionine plus cystine	26		

Kirschmann, J.D., and Dunne, L. J. *Nutrition Almanac.* New York: McGraw-Hill Book Co., 1984.

We believe the value shown for tryptophan is too low and the value shown for lysine is too high. The FDA has considered regulating the amino acid patterns of protein sources to insure proper quality of diet.

Another criterion for determining amino acid value is to calculate the percent of usable protein; that is, the proportion of usable protein in relation to the total weight of the food. Meats are 20 to 30 percent usable protein, ranging from lamb at the bottom to turkey at the top. Soybean flour is 40 percent protein; most cheeses are 30 to 35 percent protein; many nuts and seeds range between 20 and 30 percent protein; and peas, lentils, and dried beans are between 20 and 25 percent protein. Whole grains contain a fairly small quantity of protein (12 percent); but so do milk (4 percent) and eggs (13 percent). Thus, in evaluating the value of a protein source, both quality and quantity must be considered. Each of the following chapters in this book provides this information about a particular amino acid, enabling laypeople and dieticians to make sophisticated dietary choices to promote health and alleviate disease.

METABOLISM OF AMINO ACIDS

Protein and amino acid metabolism is combined with the body's metabolism of carbohydrates and fats. Digestion begins when food is in the stomach where hydrochloric acid and enzymes start to attack the peptide links that join amino acids together. This digestive breakdown of dietary protein continues throughout the small intestine. Once the amino acids are broken down into individual amino acids, they are absorbed into the bloodstream.

The liver is the primary site of amino acid metabolism. It serves as the primary storage center for amino acids derived from the diet and those recycled from other proteins.

Approximately 75 percent of the amino acids in the average adult are metabolized for the purpose of creating proteins and nonessential amino acids. The body breaks down excess amino acids into either fat or sugar to obtain energy.

Amino acids that are manufactured into sugar are called glycogenic; amino acids that are broken down into fat are called ketogenic. As Table 1.4 illustrates, all amino acids are valuable energy sources.

TABLE 1.4. GLYCOGENIC AND KETOGENIC AMINO ACIDS		
GLYCOGENIC	KETOGENIC	BOTH GLYCOGENIC AND KETOGENIC
Alanine	Leucine	Isoleucine
Arginine		Lysine
Aspartic acid		Phenylalanine
Glutamic acid		Tyrosine
Glycine		
Histidine		
Hydroxyproline		
Methionine		
Ornithine		
Proline		
Serine		
Threonine		
Tryptophan		
Valine		

Nutritional Interactions

Proper metabolism of amino acids is dependent upon many diverse interactions within the body. There are four families of essential nutrients: minerals and trace elements, including zinc, magnesium, calcium, and iron are associated with the dairy group; essential fatty acids such as linolenic and linoleic acids come from the fat group, vitamins come from carbohydrates; and amino acids come from protein. Amino acids interact with each of these groups. Total nutrition cannot be achieved without understanding the relationship among nutrients. In each chapter, these relationships are covered in detail.

Amino acids and vitamins interact in interesting and important ways (see Table 1.5 on page 11). Of all the vitamins, pyridoxine (vitamin B_6), is the most important for amino acid metabolism. Pyridoxine is the cofactor (a substance important for the activity of the enzyme) for the important enzymes called transaminases, which transfer amine groups from one amino acid to another. Pyridoxine helps build amino acids (amination) and remove amine groups (deamination). It also assists in the transport of amino acids from the intestines to the blood. A deficiency of pyridoxine in the body produces profound effects upon amino acid metabolism.

Riboflavin (vitamin B_2) and niacin (vitamin B_3) are the next most important vitamins required for amino acid metabolism. They contribute to the deamination of amino acids.

Amino Acid Interactions

Because many amino acids are absorbed and metabolized in a similar fashion, there is a great deal of competition between molecules. Sometimes, one amino acid can cancel the effect of others. This adds to the overall complexity of using amino acids to treat disease.

Typically amino acids compete for absorption with others in the same group. For example, the aromatic amino acid group (tryptophan, tyrosine, and phenylalanine) can inhibit one another's passage into the brain. This competition usually occurs among amino acids with similar structure. Amino acids in each group participate in the same or similar actions and perform the same or similar functions, while dissimilar amino acids are absorbed differently and perform different functions. For this reason, we have divided the twenty amino acids in this book into seven groups according to their chemical similarities. At the beginning of each of the following chapters, we include diagrams of the molecular structure of each amino acid described.

Table 1.5 lists the nutrients and fellow amino acids that support or hinder the breakdown of a particular amino acid. The details of these interactions are described in each chapter.

TABLE 1.5. SOME NUTRIENT INTERACTIONS		
AMINO ACID	COMPLEMENTARY RELATIONSHIP	ANTAGONISTIC RELATIONSHIP
Arginine	Aspartic acid, citrulline, ornithine	Lysine
Carnitine	Lysine, niacin, taurine	Tyrosine, vanadium
Cysteine	Methionine, taurine	Copper, lysine, zinc
Phenylalanine	Tyrosine, methionine, copper	Tryptophan
Taurine	Alanine, GABA, glycine	Aspartic acid, glutamic acid
Tryptophan	Niacin, vitamin B_6, zinc	Phenylalanine, tyrosine
Threonine	Arginine, glycine, proline	Copper

Drug Interactions

Some amino acids also have complementary or antagonistic relationships with drugs formed from amino acids that are structurally related to them as illustrated in Table 1.6. An example of this is the amino acid tyrosine, the metabolism of which is inhibited by the tranquilizer haloperidol (Haldol) and by the antihypertensive methyl dopa (Aldomet). In contrast, the metabolism of tyrosine is enhanced by the drug levodopa/carbidopa (Sinemet), whose constituents L-dopa and carbidopa are both amino acids. N-acetyl cysteine (NAC), an antitoxic and antimucous agent, is converted in the body to the amino acid cysteine. The anticlotting agent, aminocaproic acid (Amicar), useful in urology, is a normal breakdown product of the amino acid lysine.

Knowledge of amino acid metabolism has also been critical for the discovery of new drugs. Many analogs that change the structure of amino acids have led, and are leading to, the production of new and exciting drugs. Take, for example, cycloserine (Seromycin), an amino acid antibiotic; Thioproline, an amino acid cancer treatment; gabapentin (Neurotin), an amino acid calming agent; or thyroid hormone, an amino acid hormone.

TABLE 1.6. SOME DRUG-NUTRIENT INTERACTIONS

Drug	Nutrient with Similar Action	Nutrient with Antagonistic Action
Anabolic steroids	Alanine, branched-chain amino acids	Aspartic acid, glutamic acid
Anticoagulants (for example, aspirin)	Carnitine, eicosapentaenoic acid (MaxEPA), vitamin E	
Anticonvulsants	Alanine, GABA, glycine, taurine, tryptophan	Aspartic acid
Antidepressants	Methionine, tyrosine, tryptophan	Glycine, histidine
Antiheart failure (inotropes)	Carnitine, taurine, tyrosine	Niacin, tryptophan
Antimanias	Glycine, taurine, tryptophan	Methionine
Antipsychotics	Isoleucine, tryptophan	Leucine, serine
Antitoxins	Cysteine, glycine	
Antivirals	Lysine, zinc	Arginine

Inborn Errors of Metabolism

Many important clues about amino acid metabolism come from studies of patients with inborn errors of metabolism. All the amino acids discussed in this book are involved in thousands of metabolic pathways—the way in which energy is taken from protein, fat, or carbohydrate—which can malfunction due to genetic disease. Inborn errors of amino acid metabolism typically involve defects or deficiencies in the enzymes required to break down a particular amino acid. The inability to properly metabolize an amino acid often results in excessively high levels of the amino acid that can result in ill health. Two of the more common inborn errors of amino acid metabolism are Hartnup's disease, which is caused by ineffective absorption of tryptophan from the intestine, and phenylketonuria (PKU), a condition in which the body fails to produce the enzyme required to convert the amino acid phenylalanine into tyrosine.

Metabolism within the Brain

The most exciting area of amino acid research is the study of brain metabolism. Essentially, amino acids run the brain. The central nervous system is almost completely regulated by amino acids and their peptides. Communication within the brain and between the brain and the rest of the body's extensive nervous system occurs through chemical "languages" by which brain cells or neurons communicate. There are about fifty such languages that neurotransmitters use to transmit message from one neuron, or nerve cell, to a specific organ such as a muscle or gland that releases hormones. Neurotransmitters are powerful chemicals that can regulate numerous physical and behavioral processes, including the cognitive and mental performance, emotional states, and the pain response.

Many neurotransmitters are composed of amino acids. Amino acids in the form of precursors of neurotransmitters, neurotransmitters, and peptides form the majority of these languages as Tables 1.7 to 1.9 illustrate.

TABLE 1.7. AMINO ACIDS AS PRECURSORS OF NEUROTRANSMITTERS

AMINO ACID	NEUROTRANSMITTER(S)
Cysteine	Cysteic acid
Glutamine	GABA, glutamic acid
Histidine	Histamine
Lysine	Pipecolic acid
Phenylalanine	Phenylethylamine plus dopamine, norepinephrine, epinephrine, tyramine
Tyrosine	Dopamine, norepinephrine, epinephrine, tyramine
Tryptophan	Serotonin, melatonin, tryptamines

The brain's amino acids are now being recognized for their importance, and amino acid therapies are revolutionizing the treatment of psychiatric disease. In each of the following chapters, we describe a particular amino acid's therapeutic potential in psychiatry and the regulation of brain function.

Metabolism throughout the Body

Apart from the brain, amino acids are present and important throughout the

TABLE 1.8. AMINO ACIDS AS NEUROTRANSMITTERS

AMINO ACID	FUNCTION
Alanine	Inhibitory or calming
Aspartic acid	Excitatory
GABA	Inhibitory or calming
Glutamic acid	Excitatory
Glycine	Inhibitory or calming
Taurine	Inhibitory or calming

TABLE 1.9. PEPTIDES AS NEUROTRANSMITTERS

GUT-BRAIN PEPTIDES	HYPOTHALAMIC-RELEASING HORMONES	OTHERS
• Cholecystokinin octapeptide (CCK-8)	• Luteinizing hormone-releasing hormone (LHRH)	• Angiotensin II
• Glucagon	• Pituitary peptides	• Bombesin
• Insulin	– Adrenocorticotropin (ACTH)	• Bradykinin
• Leucine enkephalin	– Endorphin	• Carnosine
• Methionine enkephalin	– Melanocyte-stimulating hormone (MSH)	• Oxytocin
• Neurotensin	• Somatostatin (growth hormone release-inhibiting factor, SRIF)	
• Substance P	• Thyrotropin-releasing hormone (TRH)	
• Vasoactive intestinal polypeptide (VIP)		

body. Muscle, for example, is very high in protein and amino acids. The heart muscles and other organs derive their structure and function primarily from amino acids. When the brain and other organs such as muscles "talk" to each other, amino–acid-related neurotransmitters are again the primary language. Throughout the body, the amino acids have important functions themselves and serve as precursors for the manufacture of other important substances listed in Table 1.10.

THE HEALTH AND HEALING BENEFITS OF AMINO ACIDS

Table 1.11 on page 16 shows the impact amino acid therapies have on maintaining health and treating disease conditions. Each chapter of this book explains the unique metabolism of a particular amino acid and its therapeutic role in improving health and alleviating disease.

Amino Acid Therapy

There are many theories and anecdotal reports on the use of amino acids. We believe that we are the first to document with scientific data the effects of amino

TABLE 1.10. PRECURSOR FUNCTIONS OF SOME AMINO ACIDS

AMINO ACID	PRECURSOR FOR
Arginine	Spermine, spermidine, putrescine
Aspartic acid	Pyrimidines
Glutamic acid	Glutathione
Glycine	Purines, glutathione, creatine, phosphocreatine, tetrapyrroles
Histidine	Histamine, erothioneine
Lysine	Cadaverine, carnitine, amino-caproic acid
Ornithine	Polyamines
Serine	Sphingosine, phosphoserine
Tyrosine	Epinephrine, norepinephrine, melanin, thyroxine, mescaline, tyramine, morphine (bacteria), codeine (bacteria), papaverine (bacteria)
Tryptophan	Nicotinic acid, serotonin, kynurenic acid, indole, skatole, indoleacetic acid
Methionine	Cysteine, taurine

acid supplementation on the amino acid profile in plasma or serum (fluid portion of the blood). We have measured plasma amino acids in hundreds of people treated with amino acid supplementation and have studied the changes in blood levels that occur with amino acid therapy and amino acid loading (an experimental process in which one nutrient is given in extremely large doses to overload the system and then to study its effect).

Amino acids are found in small amounts in plasma and urine. It is their detection in plasma that allows us to correlate the concentration of a specific amino acid in certain diseases where it is deficient, as well as to monitor therapy. This scientific advancement is an extremely important tool for physicians treating metabolic and medical diseases, as well as for those practicing general preventive medicine. Levels of amino acids increase after therapy. High levels of certain amino acids may correlate to successful therapy and may need to be monitored like drug levels are monitored. Hence, therapeutic ranges can be established for treatment of specific conditions.

Debate continues about which media—plasma or urine—is most useful for studying amino acids. We feel strongly that plasma is best. Studies of twenty-four-hour urinary amino acids tend to show abnormalities in unimportant amino acids that are very difficult to interpret. Moreover, urine is less tightly regulated by the body than blood. We have found that plasma levels are more likely to provide useful information about abnormalities in the major amino acids. We have watched the increase in serum amino acid levels correlate frequently to improve-

TABLE 1.11. THERAPEUTIC ROLE OF AMINO ACIDS IN GENERAL MEDICINE

AMINO ACID	THERAPEUTIC ROLE
Alanine, aspartic acid, cysteine, glycine, lysine, threonine	Help build immune system
Alanine, carnitine, isoleucine, leucine, valine	Build muscle tissue
Alanine, cysteine, tryptophan	Help control diabetes
Alanine, GABA	Help control hypoglycemia
Arginine, carnitine, GABA, phenylalanine, tryptophan	Help curb appetite
Arginine, carnitine, glycine, methionine, taurine	Lower serum cholesterol and triglycerides
Arginine, glycine, ornithine, tryptophan, valine	Cause the release of growth hormone, prolactin, and other hormones
Arginine, methionine, cysteine, proline, glycine	Speed wound healing
Carnitine, dimethylglycine (DMG)	Promote stamina
Cysteine, glutamine, glycine, methionine, taurine, tyrosine	Promote detoxification
Cysteine, glycine, methionine, dimethylglycine, taurine	Help resist effects of radiation
GABA, glycine, tryptophan	Help prevent insomnia
GABA, isoleucine, leucine, valine	Relieve chorea and tardive dyskinesia
GABA, taurine, tryptophan	Reduce blood pressure
GABA, taurine, tryptophan	Calm aggressiveness
Glycine, isoleucine, leucine, methionine, taurine, valine	Provide relief for ailing gallbladders
Isoleucine, leucine, valine	Benefit liver disease patients
Isoleucine, leucine, valine	Counter stress of surgery
L-Dopa, GABA, methionine, tryptophan, tyrosine, threonine	Control Parkinson's disease
Lysine	May be useful in osteoporosis and some viral illnesses
Methionine (heroin addiction), tyrosine (cocaine addiction), glutamine/GABA (alcohol addiction)	Fight drug addiction
Methionine, tryptophan	Relieve pain

ment in clinical syndromes, and blood levels have been useful in monitoring therapy with amino acid supplements.

Determining the normal plasma levels for amino acids is now easy. We usually test fasting values but some clinicians recommend two- to four-hour post-meal values. Amino acid levels are affected by diet, geography, sex, and diurnal rhythms. In addition, higher plasma amino acids are found in youth than in adulthood.

Form and Absorption

Some amino acids are more easily absorbed from the diet and in supplements than others. Some are better absorbed by the body, and others by the brain.

Amino acids are water-soluble and most can occur in two different forms: L-form or D-form. The "L" and "D" simply refer to the direction of light rotation by the molecules of the amino acid. The L-form of an amino acid (from the word "levorotary") rotates light to the left and the D-form (from the word "dextrorotary") rotates light to the right. Amino acids in the L-form are the natural form of amino acids found in living plant and animals tissues (dietary sources of protein), and are considered to be more compatible to human biochemistry. D-form amino acids, unlike the L-form, are absorbed very slowly into the bloodstream because they must be converted by the body to the L-form before being used and are not normally used. In some amino acids, the D-form has been suspected of inhibiting antibiotic function and suppressing the immune system. Occasionally, an amino acid also appears in the DL-form. The DL-form amino acid contains a 50/50 mix of both D- and L-form amino acids. For some amino acids, such as such as phenylalanine or methionine, this DL-combination is better.

Generally, we advocate use of the L-form amino acid supplements. This form of amino acid is also called *free-form,* which means the amino acid supplement is already in its simplest form, and contains just that particular amino acid in its pure form, and not as part of a larger protein. Free-form amino acids are generally the best form for absorption throughout the body and brain.

All the amino acids can enter the brain; however, some amino acids cross the blood-brain barrier—a physiological mechanism that alters the permeability of small brain vessels and prevents the passage of some substances from the blood to the brain—more easily than others. Phenylalanine enters the most easily, followed by leucine, tyrosine, isoleucine, methionine, tryptophan, histidine, arginine, valine, lysine, threonine, serine, alanine, citrulline, proline, glutamic acid, and aspartic acid respectively. The essential amino acids in general are better absorbed into the brain than the nonessential.

In each chapter to follow, we discuss the toxicity and therapeutic dose range for a particular amino acid. Toxicity of amino acids often occurs only at doses 50 to 500 times the therapeutic dose range.

Supplementation with Individual Amino Acids

Early in the use of B vitamin supplements, physicians thought that the entire B family of vitamins had to be given together. We have since discovered that taking multi–B vitamins are not always a good idea. For example, thiamine can raise blood pressure; pantothenic acid can cause joint pain; and too much folic acid can't be tolerated by patients with epilepsy or allergies.

The same is true for amino acid supplementation. Biochemical individuality (unique needs) demands the selective use of amino acid supplements for each person. Individuals have different amino acid needs; even the amino acid structure of common proteins within individuals is absorbed differently. Multi–amino-acid formulas are rarely useful except for treating generalized amino acid deficiencies.

As we mentioned earlier, scientific testing is a necessary part of amino acid therapy in order to monitor changes in plasma. Changes often do not occur in people during low-dose individual amino acid therapy because of homeostasis, the body's tendency to keep equilibrium among its parts. High doses of amino acids, like drug therapies, result in changes in health; the orchestra of the body is sensitive to the addition of new instruments. People on amino acid therapy often notice changes in their own dietary selections. Some individuals report that refined foods with additives no longer are pleasing to them. The healthy body prefers that which is good for it.

Natural Healers

Amino acids are making a significant contribution to the treatment of disease. Nutritional assessment without measuring plasma amino acids is incomplete, and marginal deficiencies caused by an imbalance of amino acids are significant. We have begun to outline amino acid patterns and deficiencies found in many diseases.

We have developed amino acid therapies that arrest herpes, improve memory, erase depression, relieve arthritis and stress, prevent aging and heart disease, control allergies and improve sleep, arrest alcoholism, restore hair growth, and alleviate many other conditions. The study of amino acids is particularly relevant to all disease, because the body normally uses amino acids to promote health and fight disease. By using amino acid therapies, we are imitating the body's natural medicines and thereby are following two important principles of medicine:

1. *Imitatio Corporis* (Imitation of the Body). In the practice of medicine, it is wise to imitate the body's natural healing mechanisms. For example, when we can't sleep, we need to initiate the body's usual biochemical mechanism of falling asleep by giving more of the dietary substances the body normally uses to put itself to sleep. Every nutrient has at least one therapeutic use in the

treatment of disease. Respect for God's mysterious harmonies is the foundation of good health and of a "physical morality."

2. ***Pfeiffer's Law.*** We have learned that if a drug can be found to do the job of medical healing, a nutrient can be found to do the same job. When we understand how a drug works, we can imitate its action with an amino acid. For example, antidepressants usually enhance the effect of serotonin and epinephrines. We now know that if the amino acids tryptophan or tyrosine are taken, the body can synthesize these neurotransmitters, thereby achieving the same effect and imitating, or adding to, the net effect of these drugs.

Amino acids have fewer and milder side effects, and the challenge of the future is to replace or sometimes combine drugs with these natural healers. At present, less than 20 percent of the current drugs administered by a physician are effective. All the healers a physician needs are there in the body for harvesting by future generations of physicians and scientists. Amino acids are an example of this harvest.

We echo the rabbi doctor Maimonides, who wrote a thousand years ago, "The knowledge of nutrition is the most helpful thing in the field of medicine because of the constant need for food during health as well as illness." Because of their fundamental contributions to body constituents and biochemical functioning, amino acids, particularly the essential ones, may prove even more valuable in the treatment of human disease than minerals, fats, or carbohydrates. Amino acids are indeed on the new frontier in medicine. Our clinical experience, described throughout this book in case histories rich with interesting reports of the benefits of amino acid therapy, document this belief.

SECTION TWO

Aromatic Amino Acids

PHENYLALANINE
The Pain Reliever

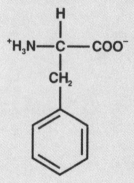

TYROSINE
The Addiction Fighter

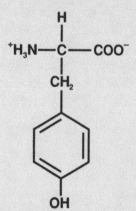

TRYPTOPHAN
The Sleep Promoter

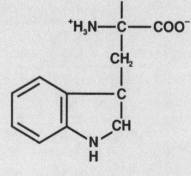

CHAPTER TWO

Phenylalanine: The Pain Reliever

Phenylalanine is an essential amino acid best known for supplying the raw material for many potent substances in the brain. It is recognized as being the precursor for many proteins, but most important, for the amino acid tyrosine, which in turn, is the precursor for dopamine, tyramine, epinephrine, and norepinephrine, critical neurotransmitters that promote alertness in the brain. Because phenylalanine can cross the blood-brain barrier easily, it has a direct effect on brain chemistry. The psychotropic drugs mescaline, morphine, codeine, and papaverine also have phenylalanine as a constituent.

FUNCTION

Phenylalanine is highly concentrated in the human brain and plasma. Early studies suggest that phenylalanine crosses the blood-brain barrier faster than any other amino acid. It is present in significant amounts in brain proteins (although less so than some other amino acids) and is distributed equally in both white and gray matter. The cerebral cortex—the furrowed gray matter covering the cerebral hemispheres—is composed of nerve cell bodies and their dendrites. White matter is a nerve tissue of the brain and spinal cord, consisting mostly of myelinated nerve fibers (axons) that connect the parts of the brain and spinal cord, cortical regions of the same hemisphere, and the two hemispheres with each other.

Phenylalanine is a constituent of numerous substances in the brain that affect mood, pain, memory and learning, and appetite. It supplies the raw material for important brain neuropeptides, including somatostatin, vasopressin, melanotropin, adrenocorticotropin (ACTH), substance P, enkephalin, vasoactive intestinal peptide, angiotensin II, and cholecystokinin. Many peptides contain mixtures of amino acids in which phenylalanine, like the amino acid methionine, is commonly found. Phenylalanine, like tyrosine, is converted into the neurotransmitters epinephrine, norepinephrine, and dopamine, adrenalinelike substances. Unlike tyrosine, however, phenylalanine is also converted to the important brain compound phenylethylamine, a substance that is also found in chocolate that may trigger the release of endorphins.

Phenylalanine occurs in below-average amino acid quantities in muscle. Alanine, arginine, aspartic acid, glutamic acid, lysine, threonine, serine, tyrosine, valine, leucine, and isoleucine all exceed phenylalanine concentrations in muscle. Only tryptophan and histidine are significantly less present in muscle than phenylalanine.

METABOLISM

Phenylalanine is metabolized primarily in the liver by phenylalanine hydroxylase, an enzyme that is present in large quantities in the liver and in other cells such as fibroblasts (large cells found often in newly formed tissue or tissue in the process of being repaired). Phenylalanine hydroxylase also occurs in small concentration in the brain where it has limited activity.

Phenylalanine hydroxylase is made up of several components that are relevant to a full understanding of the disease phenylketonuria (PKU), a condition in which the body fails to produce the enzyme required to convert the amino acid phenylalanine into tyrosine, which is part of the process of normal protein metabolism. PKU is an inherited, metabolic disorder that has the potential to cause varying amounts of mental retardation and is the most prevalent form of aminoaciduria, an excess excretion of amino acids in urine. (People with this disorder must severely limit their ingestion of phenylalanine.) Its incidence in the United States is reportedly one in every 15,000 births. Phenylalanine is converted directly to tyrosine, except in those with PKU and in the synthesis of the unusual metabolite tyramine.

Normal metabolism of phenylalanine requires biopterin (a form of folic acid), iron, copper, niacin (vitamin B_3), pyridoxine (vitamin B_6), and vitamin C.

REQUIREMENTS

Phenylalanine is an essential amino acid and cannot be manufactured in the body. It is therefore imperative that adequate amounts be included in the diet.

The National Academy of Sciences has not yet established RDAs for amino acids, thus there is no RDA for phenylalanine. However, they have published estimated human amino acid requirements for both phenylalanine and tyrosine to be 16 mg/kg (milligrams per kilogram) or about 1 g daily for a normal, average, male adult.

Some scientists and healthcare professionals think phenylalanine and tyrosine are interchangeable because 16 mg/kg of either one satisfies the requirement. This is true of phenylalanine, but not of tyrosine. For example, if sufficient phenylalanine is in the diet, there is no need for tyrosine. However, since phenylalanine also produces other important byproducts, tyrosine cannot satisfy the body's requirements for this amino acid.

Cheraskin and colleagues have reported that a healthy person consumes a daily average of 5 g of phenylalanine and may need up to 8 g per day. They recommend that the ideal daily requirement of phenylalanine plus tyrosine may be as great as 16 g.

FOOD SOURCES

Phenylalanine can be found in almost all natural foods. Banana, avocado, almonds, fish, cheese, corn, eggs, lima beans, peanuts, soy products, brown rice, and sesame seeds are all known to be good sources of this important amino acid in addition to the foods listed in Table 2.1. Like most amino acids, phenylalanine is highly concentrated in high-protein foods such as meat and dairy products.

TABLE 2.1. PHENYLALANINE LEVELS IN FOOD		
FOOD	AMOUNT	CONTENT (GRAMS)
Avocado	1	0.15
Cheese	1 ounce	0.35
Chicken	1 pound	1.00
Chocolate	1 cup	0.40
Cottage cheese	1 cup	1.70
Duck	1 pound	1.30
Egg	1	0.35
Granola	1 cup	0.65
Luncheon meat	1 pound	2.10
Oatmeal	1 cup	0.50
Pork	1 pound	2.90
Ricotta	1 cup	1.35
Sausage meat	1 pound	1.00
Turkey	1 pound	1.30
Wheat germ	1 cup	1.35
Whole milk	1 cup	0.40
Wild game	1 pound	3.30
Yogurt	1 cup	0.40

Artificial Sweeteners

Small contributions of phenylalanine in the diet may occur from foods that contain synthetic sweeteners made with aspartame (L-aspartylphenylalanylmethylester). When phenylalanine is combined with aspartic acid, it forms aspartame, commercially known as Nutrasweet, a synthetic sweetener added to diet drinks and foods. Ingesting aspartame is similar to supplementing with phenylalanine and aspartic acid.

According to the Center of Science in the Public Interest (CSPI), hundreds of consumers have reported symptoms ranging from headaches to seizures after using aspartame. Yet documentation of these effects occurred only in people with PKU who lack the ability to break down phenylalanine.

Studies conducted by Wurtman of the Massachusetts Institute of Technology (MIT) suggests that aspartame in large doses may cause mood changes in laboratory rats. In such studies, rats given a large dosage (200 mg/kg) of aspartame increased their plasma levels of phenylalanine and tyrosine. In addition, the administration of glucose (3 gm/kg) was enough to cause insulin-mediated reduction of large neutral (non-acidic) amino acids such as leucine, isoleucine, and valine, doubling the brain phenylalanine and tyrosine levels by twice enhancing the aspartame effect. The aspartame-glucose combination also reduced brain levels of leucine, isoleucine, and valine significantly compared with aspartame or glucose alone. However, the dose used in these experiments is so great that it cannot be applied to normal humans, except possibly to people with cirrhosis (liver disease), who do better with less phenylalanine.

Olney, a scientist at Washington University, disagreed with the FDA's choice to market the "synthetic nutrient." One concern was with the phenylalanine portion of the molecule, particularly with regard to use during pregnancy. However, a normal pregnant woman would have to consume six and a half gallons of diet soft drink, or take 600 packets of aspartame, to raise blood levels to toxic levels for the fetus *in utero.* Yet, there are several women each year that reach childbearing age whose natural blood levels of phenylalanine fluctuate, and for them, a smaller dose of aspartame could theoretically be dangerous. Prudence and knowledge of case histories dictate our recommendation that pregnant women not use artificial sweeteners.

A newer study on aspartame has been conducted by a team of researchers at the University of California at San Diego. Bada and colleagues warn against the use of the low-calorie sweeteners containing aspartame in cooking and in hot beverages. The study showed that heat causes structural changes in aspartame's two primary amino acids. At present, the potential health consequences, if any, of ingesting the altered form of sweetener are unknown.

At our clinic, we do not recommend the sweetener in hot beverages such as tea and coffee, but we do recommend its use in general and herald aspartame as an advance in food additives because of its basic nutritional value. Used in low doses, it could theoretically even be used by individuals with PKU.

FORM AND ABSORPTION

Phenylalanine is available in all three amino acid forms: D-, L-, and DL-. The L-form is the most common structure in which phenylalanine occurs in dietary protein and supplements. D-phenylalanine and D-methionine are the only known D-form amino acids that can be converted to their natural L-forms by enzymes in the liver, and therefore, humans can potentially use both D- and L-forms of phenylalanine.

Competition for absorption by the body exists among phenylalanine, tryptophan, tyrosine, leucine, and valine in experimental models, but our loading studies in humans, an experimental process in which one element or nutrient is given in extremely large doses to overload the system and then to study its effect, do not confirm significant antagonism in most cases. Phenylalanine absorption may be increased when it is given in dipeptide form (the combination of two amino acids) with glycine. But other studies have also suggested that superior amino acid absorption can be achieved with peptides. Trials using pure phenylalanine or di- or tripeptides (the joining of three amino acids) would be interesting. Such trials have been done for other amino acids, resulting in recommendations that can improve absorption.

CLINICAL USES

Aromatic amino acids are similar in structure and function to amphetamines. They work in the body as natural stimulants.

Athletic Performance

Athletes have been reported to use 0.15 g to 2 g of L-phenylalanine on an empty stomach for the purpose of stimulation and increasing alertness. We have not yet confirmed a role for phenylalanine in athletic performance.

Attention Deficit Disorder

Children with attention deficit disorder (ADD) and hyperactivity have been found to have elevated levels of plasma phenylalanine. These children respond to L-tryptophan therapy, which lowers the phenylalanine level and improves their ability to concentrate. Phenylalanine enhances the effects of methylphenidate (Ritalin), a common medication used to treat ADD.

Cancer

Low-phenylalanine diets have been recommended for various cancers. Melanomas, or skin cancers, and papillary and serous cyst adenocarcinomas seem to require more phenylalanine. There are a few reported successful treatments with phenylalanine-restricted diets, but some unsuccessful results as well.

Another strategy for lowering phenylalanine in the brain is mega amino acid therapy using large neutral amino acids; for example, tyrosine, tryptophan, leucine, isoleucine, and valine, which compete with phenylalanine for uptake into the brain.

A phenylalanine derivative, L-phenylalanine mustard, is an anticancer agent that works by inhibiting phenylalanine metabolism.

Depression

We have found low plasma phenylalanine levels in some 10 to 15 percent of depressed patients. (These patients often have low plasma tyrosine as well.) The catecholamine hypothesis, or biochemical basis, of depression has been accepted in medicine for more than twenty years. This theory postulates that there is a deficiency of norepinephrine transmission at specific locations in the brain cortex and hippocampus, an important area of the brain where much of our new learning takes place. A practical method for correcting this catecholamine deficiency has been precursor loading with the well-known amino acid precursors of catecholamines, L-dopa, L-tyrosine, and L-phenylalanine. (Phenylalanine is the precursor of the precursor of the precursor!)

D-phenylalanine has been evaluated for use in depression in several studies with a reported efficacy comparable to the antidepressant imipramine (Tofranil) when an average dose of 200 mg a day is used. Mann and colleagues from the Cornell University School of Medicine found that 200 mg/daily of DL-phenylalanine had no effect on blood tyrosine and phenylalanine levels or on depression. We believe that adequate levels of blood phenylalanine may require as much as 6 g daily of supplemental phenylalanine.

Reduced urinary excretion rates of phenylethylanine (the decarboxylated amino breakdown product of phenylalanine) have been found in depression. This excretion normalizes with antidepressant treatment; similarly, phenylalanine metabolism also increases phenylethylanine concentration. This may point to a

Case History of Depression

A twenty-year-old, unenthusiastic, withdrawn woman with hair loss came to our clinic for help. Supplements and antidepressants had no effect. Yet her normal personality returned with 2 g of phenylalanine taken daily in the morning. Her mood changed, and she developed once again a full range of emotions. Later, her hair loss responded to cysteine therapy, as we'll describe in Chapter 7.

mechanism whereby phenylalanine is effective in treating depression and is more useful than tyrosine.

Both tyrosine and phenylalanine elevate norepinephrine, which is found to be low in some depressed patients. Phenylalanine may be a better choice for treating this condition than tyrosine because it is better absorbed. Taking 15 g of phenylalanine raised plasma levels seventeen times above baseline, while the same dose of tyrosine raises plasma levels only three times above normal.

Phenylalanine has also been shown to enhance the effects of the commonly used antidepressants selegiline (Eldepryl), bupropion (Wellbutrin), venlafaxine (Effexor) and modafinil (Provigil).

Infections and Stress States

Infections or inflammatory states often cause significant increases in serum phenylalanine and in the ratio of phenylalanine to tyrosine. Generally, the increase in the ratio is a result of evaluations in the phenylalanine concentration in the presence of unaltered tyrosine. In contrast to the increase in free phenylalanine concentration, most other serum amino acids are decreased as a consequence of the infectious process.

An increased phenylalanine-tyrosine ratio also occurs in inflammatory diseases such as arthritis. Fox also found an increase in this ratio in monkeys with induced Rocky Mountain spotted fever, viral encephalitis, yellow fever, or pneumococcal and/or salmonella infections.

Infection-related increases in serum phenylalanine cannot be explained by decreased hydroxylation or oxidation (the chemical reaction in which a substance combines with oxygen). Rather, the data are consistent with an increased influx of phenylalanine into serum, most likely as the result of increased skeletal muscle catabolism (the breakdown of chemical compounds into simpler ones). Elevations in the serum phenylalanine to tyrosine ratio have potential value for estimating the presence of an inflammatory disease and the catabolic state of a patient.

Elevated levels of phenylalanine combined with low serum zinc and iron levels indicate the presence of infection. The significance of these findings is not clear. Zinc is useful during colds and other viral illnesses.

Liver Disease

Phenylalanine levels are relatively increased in hepatic cirrhosis (a long-term disease in which the liver becomes scarred with fibrous tissues, which prevents it from functioning normally), primary biliary cirrhosis, and portal hypertension. In particular, the blood ratio of the branched-chain amino acids (BCAAs)—valine, leucine, and isoleucine—to phenylalanine and tyrosine is altered. Lowering the plasma phenylalanine with BCAAs improves these conditions.

Migraine Headache

Migraine headaches cause an intense or throbbing pain, often accompanied by nausea, vomiting, and visual disturbances. People who suffer from migraines have been found to have elevated levels of plasma phenylalanine. These patients respond to L-tryptophan therapy, which lowers the phenylalanine level.

Carbohydrate and fat ingestion can elevate concentrations of the aromatic amino acids (AAA)—phenylalanine, tyrosine, and tryptophan—in the brain and decrease the branched-chain amino acids (BCAA)—valine, leucine, and iso-leucine. In contrast, phenylalanine in plasma is decreased by drinking caffeine.

Note: Both phenylalanine and tyrosine form tyramine, a substance that can trigger migraine headaches and hypertensive crisis in patients on monoamine oxidase inhibitor (MAOI) antidepressants. Some tyramines occur through the transformation of phenylalanine from either dopa or dopamine; other tyramines are synthesized directly from L-tyrosine. People who get migraines may want to avoid taking supplements of phenylalanine and tyrosine and avoid foods that are naturally high in tyramine (see "Foods High in Tyramine" on page 31). In general, all aged, dried, pickled, preserved, fermented, cured, or cultured foods should be avoided, as they contain bacteria with enzymes that can convert tyrosine to tyramine.

Pain

DL-phenylalanine may have the unique ability to block certain enzymes known as enkephalinase in the central nervous system that are normally responsible for breaking down natural morphinelike peptide hormones called endorphins and polypeptides called enkephalins. Endorphins and enkephalins act as mild mood elevators and are potent analgesics, that is, substances that alleviate pain. Studies suggest that DL-phenylalanine is effective against the chronic pain of osteoarthritis, rheumatoid arthritis, low back pain, joint pains, menstrual cramps, whiplash, and migraine headache. In one study, a seventy-year-old man was suffering from severe bone pain due to metastatic prostate cancer, which was eating away at his bones. His pain was resistant to analgesics and diethylstilbesterol (DES), an estrogen used for cancer bone pain, the usual treatments for this problem. Supplementation with 1.5 g of phenylalanine in the morning and in the evening brought this man's terrible pain under complete control.

Parkinson's Disease

Phenylalanine is the precursor of L-dopa, the most common modified amino acid used to treat Parkinson's disease. It is believed to be potentially beneficial for people that are taking the anti-Parkinson medication levodopa/carbidopa (Sinemet).

Foods High in Tyramine

The following foods contain significant amounts of tyramine and are sometimes banned from diets of headache sufferers and people with hypertension. The tyramine content of foods is not entirely predictable.

- Aged cheese (general rule of thumb, all cheeses, except cottage cheese and cream cheese)
- Bananas and any food product made with bananas
- Beer and ales
- Broad beans and pods (lima beans, Italian broad beans, lentils, snow peas)
- Chocolate in any form
- Cultured dairy products (buttermilk, yogurt, sour cream)
- Figs (canned)
- Legumes
- Livers
- Monosodium glutamate or MSG (additive in Chinese food, soy sauce, hydrolyzed vegetable protein, and some packaged and snack foods)
- Nuts and any food product containing nuts
- Pickled herring and salted dry fish
- Pineapple and any food product containing pineapple
- Prunes
- Raisins and any food product containing raisins
- Soy sauce
- Vanilla extracts and any food product containing vanilla
- Wine (especially Chianti) and any food product made from wine
- Yeast extracts

Premenstrual Syndrome

Phenylalanine has been shown to alleviate a variety of emotional and physiological symptoms prior to the onset of menstruation.

Substance Addictions

DL-phenylalanine has been shown to curb cravings for carbohydrates, tobacco, cocaine, and other addictive substances.

Stimulant Enhancer

Phenylalanine enhances the effects of caffeine and herbal stimulants such as ephedra (Ma Huang), rhodiola rosea, and guarana. It also been shown to augment dopaminergic agents and commonly used antidepressants such as selegiline, bupropion, venlafaxine, and modafinil.

PHENYLALANINE LOADING

The interest in oral dosing with aspartame also sparked research trials with L-phenylalanine loading. These trials found that doses as low as 4 g could produce headache side effects. Doses of 15 g or even more could be tolerated well in some individuals, while others experienced slight headaches. Dosing with 15 g raised phenylalanine levels to six to seven times normal after two hours. BCAA levels decreased significantly, as did threonine and proline. This high load of phenylalanine did not acutely alter aromatic amino acids.

SUPPLEMENTATION

Phenylalanine is unique among amino acids in that it is available in three different forms: L-, D-, and DL-form. Typically D-form amino acids, unlike the L-form, are absorbed very slowly into the bloodstream; however, this is not true of D-phenylalanine. Typically, L-phenylalanine is used to increase alertness and to treat conditions that can benefit from increased production of catecholamines (adrenalinelike substances) such as appetite control problems, Parkinson's disease, or PMS. The D-form helps increase pain tolerance; and DL-phenylalanine acts as a combination of the two.

Deficiency Symptoms

Symptoms and signs of deficiency include muscle deterioration, decreased growth, apathy, and generalized weakness.

Availability

Free-form L-phenylalanine, D-phenylalanine, and DL-phenylalanine (DLPA) are each available in 500 mg capsules. Absorption of DL-phenylalanine is inhibited if it must first be released from solid tablet form. Therefore, according to manufacturers of amino acid supplements, pure capsules of DL-phenylalanine, with their quick and efficient release of the amino acid into the stomach, offer greater bioavailability and are the best dosage form.

Therapeutic Daily Amount

The normal range of supplemental L-, D-, or DL-phenylalanine may vary widely from 0.5 g to 4 g a day, depending upon the condition being treated.

Maximum Safe Level

Not established.

Side Effects and Contraindications

For the general public, phenylalanine toxicity is rare but has been seen with excessive ingestion, resulting in migraine headaches and hypertension. People who suffer from the metabolic disease PKU should avoid all forms of phenylalanine (L-, D-, and DL-forms). Phenylalanine can cause hypertension when taken with monoamine oxidase inhibitors (MAOIs).

PHENYLALANINE: A SUMMARY

Phenylalanine is an essential amino acid and a precursor of the neurotransmitters called catecholamines; these are adrenalinelike substances. Normal metabolism of phenylalanine requires biopterin, iron, niacin, pyridoxine, copper, and vitamin C. Phenylalanine is highly concentrated in the human brain and plasma. An average adult ingests 5 g of phenylalanine per day and may optimally need up to 8 g daily.

Phenylalanine is concentrated in high-protein foods, such as meat, cottage cheese, and wheat germ. A new dietary source of phenylalanine is Nutrasweet, which is safe and nutritious except in hot beverages. However, it should be avoided entirely by people with PKU and pregnant women.

We have found that about 10 to 50 percent of depressed patients have low plasma phenylalanine, and supplemental phenylalanine is an effective treatment. Elevated phenylalanine levels occur during infection. Phenylalanine levels are lowered by caffeine ingestion as the brain takes in more phenylalanine. Phenylalanine is probably most effective in treating mild depression, particularly in countering fatigue.

DL-phenylalanine can be an effective pain reliever. Its use in premenstrual syndrome and Parkinson's enhances the effects of acupuncture and electric transcutaneous nerve stimulation (TENS). Phenylalanine and tyrosine, like L-dopa, produce a catecholamine effect. Phenylalanine is better absorbed than tyrosine and may cause fewer headaches. Low phenylalanine diets have been prescribed for certain cancers with mixed results. Some skin tumors (primarily melanomas) can have increased phenylalanine requirements, and the approach most likely to succeed is not dietary restriction, but medication to reduce the absorption of phenylalanine.

In sum, phenylalanine is an antidepressant and a pain reliever with many potential therapeutic roles. L- or DL-phenylalanine supplements are widely available and have an important role in general medicine and health.

CHAPTER THREE

Tyrosine:
The Addiction Fighter

Tyrosine is an essential amino acid that readily passes the blood-brain barrier, although it is the least water-soluble of the amino acids. Once in the brain, it is a precursor of the neurotransmitters dopamine, norepinephrine, and epinephrine, better known as adrenaline. These neurotransmitters are an important part of the body's sympathetic nervous system, and their concentrations in the body and brain are directly dependent upon dietary tyrosine.

Tyrosine's ability to critically impact brain chemistry balance has attracted much attention in recent years, particularly for its use in reducing the symptoms and cravings in people undergoing withdrawal from alcohol and drugs.

FUNCTION

Tyrosine is thought to be primarily concentrated in brain tubulin, an intracellular protein that is important for the structure of neurons. Neurons are nerve cells that transmit electrical impulses, causing the release of neurotransmitters. Its content in the cerebrum (white matter) in the brain is small. Amino acids such as glutamic acid, glutamine, aspartic acid, cystathione, alanine, serine, and taurine are much more concentrated in the human brain than tyrosine. It should be noted that the artificial sweetener aspartame, which contains phenylalanine, increases brain levels of tyrosine.

In contrast to in the brain, tyrosine concentration in muscle is high. Only glutamic acid, lysine, aspartic acid, alanine, valine, threonine, and leucine are more concentrated in muscle tissue than tyrosine.

Tyrosine is also only minimally concentrated in cerebrospinal fluid (CSF). Under stress of infection in a newborn, tyrosine, like many other amino acids, increases in concentration.

Tyrosine is also the precursor for hormones such as thyroid and catecholestrogens (chemicals that are both estrogens and catecholamines) and for the major human pigment, melanin. Synthesis of these hormones may also be dependent on dietary tyrosine. Tyrosine is also an important part of peptides, such as enkephalins, which serve as pain relievers in the brain. Furthermore, tyrosine is a constituent of protein amino sugars and amino lipids, which have important roles throughout the body.

METABOLISM

Tyrosine is manufactured from the amino acid phenylalanine. It is not found in large concentration throughout the body, probably because it is rapidly metabolized. Metabolism of tyrosine requires several nutrients, such as biopterin, NADPH and NADH (forms of niacin), copper, and vitamin C. The folic acid-like derivative seems to be the most important of the nutrients, all of which work with tyrosine hydroxylase, the enzyme primarily responsible for the breakdown of tyrosine.

REQUIREMENTS

No RDA has been established for tyrosine. However, the National Academy of Sciences estimates minimum requirements for both tyrosine and phenylalanine to be 16 mg/kg or about 1 g daily for a normal, average, male adult.

FOOD SOURCES

Tyrosine is primarily found in almonds, avocados, meats, dairy products, fish, beans, and pumpkin and sesame seeds. Table 3.1 on page 37 lists other foods naturally high in tyrosine. Very little tyrosine is found in cereals and grains, and it is difficult to find significant amounts of tyrosine in vegetables, fruits, and oils.

FORM AND ABSORPTION

Dietary and supplemental tyrosine is available in L-form only. D-tyrosine, in contrast, can be toxic and has suppressed growth and weight gain in experimental animals.

The uptake of tyrosine by the brain is quite competitive, that is, limited by other amino acids. When administered along with tryptophan, leucine, isoleucine, and fluoro-phenylalanine (a form of phenylalanine), all markedly inhibit uptake of the tyrosine by the brain. Conversely, glutamic acid, glutamine, and many other amino acids (valine, cysteine, histidine, alanine, serine, threonine, arginine, lysine, glutamate, and glutamine) do not.

Tyrosine may interact with tryptophan, phenylalanine, and especially the branched-chain amino acids. Because these amino acids may compete with tyrosine for absorption and beneficial effects, each of these amino acids may have to be taken at a different time of day.

TABLE 3.1. TYROSINE LEVELS IN FOOD		
FOOD	AMOUNT	CONTENT (GRAMS)
Avocado	1	0.10
Cheese	1 ounce	0.30
Chicken	1 pound	0.80
Chocolate	1 cup	0.40
Cottage cheese	1 cup	1.70
Duck	1 pound	1.10
Egg	1	0.25
Granola	1 cup	0.40
Luncheon meat	1 pound	0.10
Oatmeal	1 cup	0.35
Pork	1 pound	2.50
Ricotta	1 cup	1.50
Sausage meat	1 pound	0.05
Turkey	1 pound	1.30
Wheat germ	1 cup	1.00
Whole milk	1 cup	0.40
Wild game	1 pound	3.00
Yogurt	1 cup	0.40

CLINICAL USES

Aromatic amino acids are similar in structure and function to amphetamines. They work in the body as natural stimulants.

Appetite Suppression

Tyrosine in extremely large doses—greater than 20 g a day—reduces appetite. It may be used as an alternative to using phenylpropanolamine or amphetamines, two stimulants used for controlling appetite. Moreover, phenylpropanolamine can cause hypertensive crisis in predisposed individuals. A low dietary intake of tyrosine combined with zinc deficiency increases food intake, according to Reeves and O'Dell of the Missouri Agricultural Experiment Station. It has been found that tyrosine deficiency can increase appetite, while tyrosine excess may decrease appetite. We have not had consistent results, and these effects seem to be very dependent on a particular patient's situation.

Diet pills that stimulate tyrosine metabolism in the brain, such as the phentermine family of weight-loss drugs (Adipex, Fastin, and Ionamin) and mazindol (Sanorex) should be accompanied by tyrosine supplementation for maximum effect. For such drugs to work, a high tyrosine pool is required to create the adrenaline necessary to speed up metabolism and turn down the brain's appetite center. We have seen people of all ages experience faster weight loss while taking tyrosine.

Attention Deficit Disorder

Tyrosine is effective as an alternative treatment in attention deficit disorder (ADD). We recommend it in all cases where an identified adrenaline and dopamine metabolism problem exists. We have had numerous youngsters attain substantial improvement using our Brain Energy Formula, a formula we designed for individuals with stress and fatigue, or for people who are otherwise healthy and want more energy (see "Energy in a Capsule" on page 43). We believe that this approach may work well with approximately 5 to 10 percent of cases. The percentage of significant responders is greatly increased when such modalities as cranial electrical stimulation (CES), a therapy involving gentle, low-voltage stimulation (see "Cranial Electrical Stimulation" on page 63), and/or the antidepressant bupropion (Wellbutrin) are used; the latter helps increase tyrosine metabolism. Dosages of tyrosine may be as high as 10 g in older persons and 5 g in younger individuals. For some patients with ADD, only drug therapy is effective.

Cancer

A recent approach to tumor therapy has been selective amino acid starvation. Some tumors, like malignant melanoma (melanin is made from tyrosine) or glioblastoma multiforme, a form of brain cancer, have been found to have an extraordinary need for tyrosine as demonstrated when these tumors are cultured. By withholding tyrosine, some of these tumors can be starved. The antinutrient may be supplemented instead by giving the patient large amounts of competing amino acids, such as tryptophan and possibly the branched-chain amino acids. Tyrosine (and phenylalanine) starvation in melanomas is a wise idea.

Cognitive Performance

Deficiencies in the tyrosine-derived neurotransmitters L-dopamine, epinephrine, and norepinephrine are found in people with Alzheimer's disease. In general, tyrosine levels decrease in the body with age. The brain's voltage decreases causing decreases in memory and concentration. Two major neurotransmitter systems are fundamentally damaged in many of these patients—the tyrosine and choline systems. Thus, as supplemental precursors, tyrosine and choline offer considerable promise in the prevention of Alzheimer's disease.

L-tyrosine may offer significant benefits for individuals with symptoms associated with Alzheimer's disease. In our clinic, we have had a number of cases of individuals experiencing poor cognitive performance who improved dramatically after taking our Brain Energy Formula. Medications can frequently aid this improvement as well.

Depression

Clinical depression usually does not respond to tyrosine alone. In such cases, the potential for significant results is greater when tyrosine is administered in combination with medication. Some dysthymia, mild depression, may benefit from tyrosine exclusively.

L-tyrosine was first used in psychiatry for medication-resistant depression. Physicians at Harvard Medical School pioneered the use of 1 to 6 g of L-tyrosine for the effective treatment of medication-resistant depression with good results. Several other studies, notably by Goldberg of the Psychopharmacological Institute, New York, found similar results in two patients with electroconvulsive therapy (ECT) and drug-resistant depression. We have found L-tyrosine effective in lower doses and begin supplementation at 1 to 2 g per day. Quirce and Odio have suggested that as little as 0.5 mg/kg will increase the brain catecholamines, norepinephrine, epinephrine, and dopamine in the rat. For an average adult man weighing approximately 150 pounds, this would be a 350-mg dose per day.

Research suggests that an individual's blood levels of tyrosine can help indicate which antidepressant should be used and which antidepressant a person will respond to best. We believe that low levels of tyrosine call for medications such as methylphenidate, bupropion and venlafaxine (Effexor). Studies also suggest that precursor levels of both tryptophan and tyrosine are useful in determining the most effective drug. When a patient's tyrosine level is low, we recommend using bupropion. If the level of tryptophan is low, our preference is to use fluoxetine (Prozac), a selective serotonin reuptake inhibitor (SSRI). MAO inhibitors may also be helpful when tyrosine is low.

The amino acid tyrosine is a precursor of the thyroid hormones thyroxine and triiodothyronine. Tyrosine supplementation may increase thyroid hormone levels when health and iodide intake are adequate. Thyroid is a useful adjunct in treatment of depression, and this may be another therapeutic mechanism of tyrosine in depression. There may be a relationship between dietary tyrosine and thyroid hormone synthesis under the same circumstances. A slightly increased tyrosine plasma level is found in hyperthyroidism, a condition in which the thyroid gland becomes overactive and secretes excessive amounts of thyroid hormone; a slightly reduced level is found in hypothyroidism, which is caused by low activity of the thyroid gland, resulting in underproduction of thyroid hormones. Thyroid hormones influence tyrosine level, but it is unclear if the reverse is also true.

Tyrosine Restores Well-Being

A twenty-two-year-old woman from Princeton came to our clinic suffering from sleepiness, lethargy, and loss of appetite; her weight had fallen to ninety-two pounds. She had regressed into such a deep depression that she was forced to leave Princeton University. She was started on tyrosine therapy—up to 6 g per day, which gradually began to lift her out of her depression. Eventually, she was left on a maintenance dose of 1,500 mg three times daily. Gradually her depression subsided, and she was able to resume her studies in nursing.

We are fascinated by the fact that while this patient was on tyrosine, her levels went from low to high. Her tyrosine level went as high as 16—roughly two times normal. Concurrently, her phenylalanine level went from normal range to 22—levels three times normal. The phenylalanine buildup was due to the high-tyrosine intake. This high level seemed necessary for this person to stay out of depression.

Tyrosine's ability to elevate mood and promote well-being suggests that it may benefit the cardiovascular system in depressed individuals. For some people, tyrosine improves the pumping action of the heart. The same effect is attributed to other dopamine-related biochemicals. With the increasing prevalence of side effects from antidepressants, tyrosine has become a very attractive alternative.

Dysthymia

Twenty-five to 50 percent of the population experiences dysthymia (mild depression) sometime during their lives. Tyrosine benefits dysthymias of both the primary type or secondary to borderline personality disorders.

Long-term use of tyrosine appears to be highly effective in promoting well-being among people who are generally healthy, yet suffer from stress and a loss of energy. Many individuals over age fifty tend to experience more chronic fatigue or "blah" days when they're just not feeling good. Some people try to counteract these feelings with antidepressants. In our experience, many of these individuals do extremely well on a high dose of tyrosine, regardless of whether these symptoms are the result of a general slowdown from aging or whether the person is experiencing menopause or andropause (male menopause). As one example, we treated a fifty-five-year-old man who was complaining of fatigue and feeling worn down with a multivitamin and mineral formula, antioxidants, fish oil, borage oil, niacin (vitamin B_3), and our Brain Energy Formula. Within four weeks, he reported that his energy level was back up where it used to be when he was younger.

In many cases, we also use dehydroepiandrosterone (DHEA), an adrenal steroid hormone found abundantly in the brain and bloodstream. DHEA concentrations decline sharply with age, and low levels are believed to be associated with many symptoms related to aging, including senility. We now know that just as the ovaries and testicles become dormant as people enter menopause and andropause, the activity of the adrenal glands also slows down. Tyrosine stimulates the adrenal hormone. When an individual has a low blood level of DHEA, we add the adrenal hormone supplementally to the combination of nutritional factors. In our clinical experience, these patients seem to have better results when the adrenal hormone DHEA is added.

We take this same combined approach for menopausal women, often adding a natural estrogen. The strategy works either with or without the estrogen.

For both older male and female patients, we often see a turnaround within a month. Even for those fifty and younger, this approach works well.

Tyrosine Relieves Marathon Twelve-Year Depression

C.W., a sixty-one-year-old active bulldozer operator, first saw us in February 1970, when he was seeking relief from a constant depression that was much worse in the winter months when he had less work.

Zinc, manganese, and adequate pyridoxine gave him more energy, but over the years he still had his depression in winter in spite of lithium, MAO inhibitors, antidepressants, and a vacation in Florida. He was not intoxicated by lead, aluminum, or copper as shown by normal blood levels. Cyanocobalamin (vitamin B_{12}) given intravenously in 2-mg doses would clear his depression for half a day, but the next day he always had a severe rebound depression. Six tablets of the MAO inhibitor isocarboxazid (Marplan) would modify the depression slightly, but the side effects were severe and included an inability to urinate, elevated blood pressure, and severe back pain.

After thirteen years of trials with vitamins, trace elements, and every new antidepressant, he was given L-tyrosine in 500-mg capsules with directions to take as many as six tablets per day. Within days of a dose of two tablets, three times per day, his depression was completely relieved and he was able to stop taking the isocarboxazid. This relief from depression was maintained with only four 500-mg tablets per day. A trial of phenylalanine at the tyrosine dosage produced less relief of his depression. Both he and his wife proclaim the L-tyrosine cure as a modern nutritional miracle.

Heart Conditions

A striking study was conducted on tyrosine administration during ventricular fib-rillation (a life-threatening heart arrhythmia) in dogs. Intravenous infusion with 1 to 4 mg of tyrosine reduced the susceptibility of dogs to ventricular fibrillation.

Rats made acutely hypotensive (having low blood pressure) by blood loss (hemorrhage) had a 30 to 50 percent rise in blood pressure when 100 mg/kg of tyrosine was injected intravenously. A significant increase in blood pressure also occurred with doses as low as 25 mg/kg and 50 mg/kg. Another study found that tyrosine lowers blood pressure and increases the concentration of norepi-nephrine metabolites in the brain stem of hypertensive rats. These studies sug-gest that tyrosine has a useful regulatory function when given in certain types of hypertension.

All these data suggest that tyrosine might be added to the physician's "code cart" for cardiac emergencies. and even possibly hypertensive crisis—although tyrosine's role in hypertensive crisis is still doubtful since drugs like methyldopa (Aldomet), a commonly prescribed drug for hypertension, block the full effect of tyrosine.

Hypoglycemia

Increased insulin output associated with a hypoglycemic (low blood sugar) reac-tion may elevate various amino acids, including tyrosine. Therefore, tyrosine may actually benefit individuals with hypoglycemia. However, it is still generally unclear as to what role amino acids have in the metabolism of insulin.

Steroids such as prednisone that raise blood sugar may decrease the avail-ability of tyrosine in depressed patients. As the sugar level rises, the plasma level of tyrosine falls.

Narcolepsy and Dopamine-Dependent Depression

Research conducted in France suggests that people with narcolepsy, a condition marked by an uncontrollable desire to sleep or sudden attacks of sleep occurring at intervals, or Parkinson's disease, or certain patients with depression, have sim-ilar amino acid abnormalities indicating a deficiency in dopamine. These findings suggest a promising role for tyrosine among depressive individuals who have dopamine-dependent depression (DDD) and patients with narcolepsy. The researchers coined the term DDD to describe a subset of depressed individuals who experience rapid eye movement (REM) sleep disturbances along with a dis-interest and lack of emotions unaccompanied by moral pain or culpability feel-ings. Piribedil rapidly reduced the depression and sleep abnormalities; however, the patients relapsed after a few months of treatment.

The researchers then tried oral tyrosine. They hypothesized that if DDD was

Energy in a Capsule

At our clinic, we use supplemental tyrosine as part of two multinutrient combinations. We believe that tyrosine in combination with other nutrients, particularly phenylalanine, methionine, and octacosanol (a naturally-derived wheat germ oil concentrate), increases its absorption and efficacy. The first, our "Brain Energy Formula," is designed for individuals with stress and fatigue, or for people who are otherwise healthy and want more energy. Generally, we recommend one to three tablets daily.

Brain Energy Formula

L-phenylalanine: 300 mg	Rhodiola rosea, 75 mg	Octacosanol: 2 mg
L-tyrosine: 200 mg	L-methionine: 60 mg	

The second tyrosine combination is the "Save Formula." Here, we have added multivitamins and minerals to our Brain Energy Formula for individuals who prefer not to take many different capsules and tablets. Two to three capsules are taken twice a day.

Save Formula

DL-phenylalanine: 133 mg	Pantothenic acid (vitamin B_5): 1 mg	Magnesium chelate: 26 mg
L-tyrosine: 133 mg	Pyridoxine (vitamin B_6): 6 mg	Manganese chelate: 133 mcg
DL-methionine: 50 mg	Folate: 13 mcg	Selenium (sodium selenite): 14 mcg
Octacosanol: 0.67 mg	Biotin: 20 mcg	Zinc chelate: 3 mg
Vitamin A: 1,110 IU	Cyanocobalamin (vitamin B_{12}): 2 mcg	Molybdenum chelate: 33 mcg
Thiamine (vitamin B_1): 1 mg	Vitamin E: 6 IU	Chromium chloride: 13 mg
Riboflavin (vitamin B_2): 1 mg	Iron chelate: 3 mg	
Niacin (vitamin B_3): 1 mg		

due to loss or decreased activity of some dopaminergic neurons (nerve cells that transmit electrical impulses to release dopamine), the surviving neurons would be hyperactive, and therefore tyrosine hydroxylase (the primary enzyme that converts tyrosine to dopamine) might not be saturated by its substrate (a substance acted upon by an enzyme). The use of 3.2 g of tyrosine twice a day—once in the morning and again either at noon or evening—achieved long-term remission of depression, improved sleep patterns, and corrected polysomnographic abnormalities observed using an EEG during sleep.

Having been successful, the researchers turned their attention to narcolepsy, which exhibits the same polysomnographic abnormalities as in DDD. Narcoleptic patients, most of whom were depressed, were given 64 to 120 mg/kg of body weight daily, equivalent to 4.8 to 8.4 g per 150-pound person. After six months of treatment, all patients were free of cataplexy (a sudden loss of muscle tone), sleep attacks, sleep paralysis, hypnogogic hallucinations, insomnia, and depression during the one-month control.

In a follow-up trial involving nondepressed narcoleptic patients, similar positive results were obtained. The researchers commented that the symptom that responds most quickly (within days) is cataplexy. Some degree of daytime sleepiness may persist for many months, they added, especially in patients who have been treated with antidepressants, amphetamines, or neuroleptics.

In our experience, anyone with narcolepsy can benefit from tyrosine to some extent. In cases of mild narcolepsy, improvement may be 50 to 75 percent with tyrosine alone. People with severe narcolepsy may experience 10 to 25 percent improvement; generally, these individuals require amphetamines as well.

In our clinic, we once treated a severely narcoleptic patient who slept ten to sixteen hours a day with dramatic results. After daily supplementation with our Brain Energy Formula, he reported 50 percent reduction in his excessive sleep. Then we added bupropion and he improved further. On this combined regime for several years, this patient now sleeps seven to eight hours a day and has excellent energy.

Neonatal Growth

Tyrosine is thought to be essential for neonates (newborns less than one month old). It is also a component of total parenteral nutrition, a complete nutritional supplement administered intravenously to premature neonates. When provided to premature neonates during the first weeks of life, it may reduce necrotizing enterocolitis, an inflammation that can cause injury to the bowel, due to their inability to digest and their immature and fragile bowels.

Medication Side Effects

Tyrosine exerts an antidotal influence against some side effects created by antipsychotic medication. Occasionally some individuals need a minor antidepressant effect because while their antipsychotic medication suppresses hallucinations, the intensity of withdrawal worsens; in these instances, tyrosine can help a patient by taking lessening the side effects of haloperidol (Haldol) and related medications.

Parkinson's Disease

Parkinson's disease is marked by decreased movement, rigidity, disturbed postural reflexes, and tremor. It is primarily caused by a dopamine deficiency in the striatal regions of the brain's basal ganglia—islands of gray matter located in the lobes of the cerebrum. L-dopa, the primary treatment for Parkinson's disease, is made from tyrosine. The nutrient tyrosine can be used as an adjunct or sole treatment for very early stages of this disorder.

Tyrosine's usefulness alone in treating advanced stage Parkinson's has been somewhat of a disappointment. However, we have had considerable success combining tyrosine with levodopa/carbidopa (Sinemet), a medication for Parkinson's patients, which prevents the breakdown of L-dopa in the body so that more L-dopa may enter the brain. Typical is the case of a seventy-year-old man who experienced a total loss of tremors in two months on tyrosine and levodopa/carbidopa. Happily, he was able to resume the fine dexterity work called for in his professional engineering activities.

Plasma Levels and Clinical Syndromes

Elevated tyrosine levels in blood are found in patients with abnormal reactions to chloral hydrate (Notec), a sedative used as a sleeping pill. Low–birth-weight infants have elevated levels of tyrosine in the first days of life. Some patients with liver diseases such as hepatitis and portacaval shunt show abnormal tyrosine levels, which may be increased as much as tenfold. High tyrosine levels also occur in patients who are hyperthyroid and are taking doses of thyroid, which is made from tyrosine. (Hypothyroid patients have low tyrosine levels and may benefit from tyrosine.) Elevated levels can also be found in chronic schizophrenic patients, migraine sufferers, those with high blood pressure, and depressed patients who are also taking tryptophan.

A decrease in tyrosine levels occurs in kwashiorkor (protein-calorie malnutrition), and low plasma tyrosine is found in patients with chronic renal disease. Low plasma tyrosine is common in patients with depression and/or sexual dysfunction. We have been impressed by the fact that as little as 2 g of tyrosine a day can raise plasma tyrosine levels to nearly twice normal. This appears to correlate with relief from depression. Furthermore, long-term phenylalanine therapy—a precursor of tyrosine—seems to raise tyrosine levels the same amount.

We have treated seventeen patients with low tyrosine out of 100 amino acid profiles: nine with depression, two who had been institutionalized chronically in mental hospitals, two with severe kidney disease, one with hypertension, one with impotence, one with folliculitis (a bacterial infection of the hair follicle), and one patient who was healthy. These low levels have been useful guidelines to therapy. Several of these patients have responded to tyrosine therapy. When several amino acids are low, then a multi–amino acid supplement is used.

Other researchers, such as Goodnick and colleagues of Wayne State University, have found low tyrosine levels in cerebrospinal fluid of various adults with bipolar and unipolar depression. Although in acute doses tyrosine is not well absorbed, chronic therapy can result in tyrosine levels as much as two or three times normal.

On average, 2 to 3 g of tyrosine will gradually raise tyrosine levels in most individuals. This may occur more frequently in depressed patients.

Caffeine intake can lower plasma tyrosine levels. Patients with migraine headache often have high tyrosine levels, treatable with caffeine or better yet, with tryptophan, which can have the same effect.

Schizophrenia

It has long been postulated that dopamine, a tyrosine metabolite, is increased in certain types of schizophrenia. Haloperidol and other powerful antipsychotic drugs block conversion of tyrosine to dopamine. Although antipsychotic medications are not well understood, studies show tyrosine hydroxylase (the enzyme that converts tyrosine to dopamine) to be inhibited by them. The slowing or blocking of tyrosine metabolism to dopamine is one mechanism by which antipsychotic medications work.

Risperidone (Risperdal) and clozapine (Clozaril), medications used in treating schizophrenia, as well as the older drugs such as haloperidol and fluphenazine (Prolixin) often cause side effects of fatigue and drowsiness. Typically, people will attempt to counteract their sluggishness with caffeine and nicotine. We have found that tyrosine, in the range of 1 to 3 g, is a useful antidote that helps eliminate some of the side effects of the medication.

Sex Drive

The herbal aphrodisiac yohimbine acts by prolonging the dopamine effects of tyrosine. Large doses of 4 g or more of tyrosine supplements may stimulate sex drive (and may raise blood pressure) by raising dopamine in the brain.

A thirty-five-year-old man came to our clinic with a seven-year history of reduced sex drive and gradual progression toward impotence. We found him to be rather intense. He was tense, yet was able to express a wide range of emotions. His blood pressure was slightly on the low side. His plasma amino acids were strikingly abnormal for tyrosine, the lowest we had seen—50 percent of normal. He was started on 1 g of tyrosine in the morning and in the evening and a month later was increased to 2 g in the morning and in the evening. Gradually, his sex drive returned.

Stress

MIT scientists reported that rats receiving tyrosine-enriched diets displayed neither stress-induced depletion of norepinephrine nor behavioral depression. These preventive effects of tyrosine on stress were countered by co-administration of valine, a large neutral amino acid that competes with tyrosine for transport across

Tyrosine for Smoking Cessation

A fifty-year-old woman with depression and a ten-year smoking addiction came to us after failing a trial of nicotine chewing gum. One gram of tyrosine in the morning and in the evening broke her habit. She was amazed because she had tried many methods always unsuccessfully. The drug clonidine (Catapres) has also been reported to be effective for smoking cessation. This drug works like tyrosine by influencing catecholamine metabolism.

the blood-brain barrier. The authors concluded that supplementary tyrosine may be useful therapeutically in some people exposed to some forms of stress.

Because of its role in assisting the body to cope physiologically with stress and building the body's natural store of adrenaline, tyrosine could well be the "stress" amino acid. Stress exhaustion needs tyrosine, which is converted to dopamine, norepinephrine, epinephrine, and tryptamine. Most supplemented tyrosine is converted to these adrenalinelike products, according to Agharanya and colleagues of MIT. This increased utilization of tyrosine often results in extreme reduction of brain tyrosine. Tyrosine is needed during stress to continue coping with stress physiologically.

In recent years, the U.S. military has taken an interest in the potential of tyrosine to counteract decreased performance caused by stress and fatigue during sustained operations. Most recently, a stimulant in the tyrosine family called modafinil (Provigil) was used by pilots who were flying direct from the United States to Afghanistan to deliver troops to fight in the war against terrorism. In past conflicts, the buildup of stress and fatigue has often generated serious losses of manpower from critical activities. Shell shock, combat fatigue, or battle stress are various terms used to describe a string of symptoms that render individual troops ineffective and unable to carry out duties. Individuals become either nervous, withdrawn, and dazed, or scared, excited, and loud.

Tyrosine supplementation may offer a practical means of both preventing and treating combat stress, which is predicted to accelerate in the future due to intensified weapon lethality and increased battlefield complexity. First, it offers potential as a replacement for other more powerful stimulants such as amphetamine dexedrine, whose effectiveness is offset by side effects. Second, tyrosine would appear to increase an individual's natural ability to maintain high performance even under prolonged mental and physical strain.

Both animal and human research has linked stress-induced decrease in performance to depletion of brain stores of norepinephrine. Evidence strongly suggests that norepinephrine is involved in the neurochemical manifestations of acute stress and related behavioral deficits. We know there is a major reduction in norepinephrine and dopamine levels in the rat brain after exposure to sleep deprivation and other types of stress such as immobilization and cold exposure. The stress-induced depletion of norepinephrine is intimately related to reduced performance. We also know that sleep deprivation in humans leads to decreased mood and performance. In the laboratory, tyrosine administration has been shown to alleviate a loss in both neural norepinephrine and performance.

Lastly, a controlled study was conducted with a double-blind crossover design among military personnel who were given 100 mg of L-tyrosine/kg of body weight. Individuals given tyrosine scored markedly higher on cognitive performance and mood measures, as well as on a reaction time task. There was also a significant increase in plasma tyrosine. Overall, tyrosine lessened stress-related declines in mood and performance.

Substance Abuse

A substantial body of research on using tyrosine and other amino acids to reduce cocaine and alcohol cravings has been conducted by coauthor Blum of the Department of Pharmacology of the University of Texas at San Antonio. Studies suggest that multinutrient supplements containing tyrosine or tyrosine-building amino acids such as phenylalanine can effectively help many addicted individuals when used either by themselves or in conjunction with medication. These formulas mimic the action of opiates, thus reducing alcohol or cocaine consumption. Subsequent to the original research conducted by Blum, many major medical centers have adopted these supplements in their substance abuse programs.

In our clinic, we have found amino acid–containing supplements to be very useful in early intervention and in preventing or delaying relapse. In crisis, the amino acids and other nutrients usually need to be used along with medication. Once out of crisis, many individuals do well with the supplements alone. Halikas of the Department of Psychiatry at the University of Minnesota has described the effectiveness of preventing relapses with long-term supplementation using amino acids.

One dramatic case involved an alcoholic who had failed to find any means—medical or otherwise—to beat a twenty-year habit. Now he is off alcohol and says he never felt better in his life. The magic for him was our Brain Energy Formula along with bromocriptine (Parlodel), a drug that cuts cravings for alcohol. Unfortunately, for many substance abusers, relapse remains a common pattern until brain chemical imbalances and psychosocial factors are addressed. In such cases, individuals with this condition will often return for more medication and many may need to use medication permanently.

As a precursor to dopamine and norepinephrine, tyrosine supplies a reward, anticraving effect, and antistress influence, and should always be utilized for a high-risk population. If introduced early enough, it may prevent substance abuse. We believe this was achieved in the case of a sixteen-year-old son of an alcoholic father. The boy was extremely fatigued, withdrawn, given to antisocial behavior, and had an attention deficit problem. He was clearly heading in the direction of drug addiction. On our Brain Energy Formula, his energy improved and his constant fatigue lifted. Time will tell whether supplements alone will suffice or whether he will need medication. Sometimes such individuals need to combine tyrosine with methylphidate or one of methylphidate's alternatives.

Either alone, or in conjunction with medication, tyrosine appears to be an intriguing addiction-stopping potentiator.

TYROSINE LOADING

Agharanya and colleagues at MIT were among the first to study tyrosine loading. They made the remarkable discovery that even when large doses (approximately 7 g) of tyrosine are loaded, only a fraction of less than 1 percent is not metabolized. Urinary tyrosine increased by 138 percent. Furthermore, they showed that tyrosine can be used for disease characterized by a deficiency of catecholamines (dopamine, epinephrine, norepinephrine) in the brain. Other amino acids were not significantly changed. Blood histamine, copper, zinc, iron, and cholesterol were not affected.

SUPPLEMENTATION

For transporting tyrosine across the blood-brain barrier, evidence suggests that it is most effective to take a tyrosine supplement along with a protein-rich meal. When 100 mg of L-tyrosine was given orally to subjects as a supplement along with a protein-containing meal, the tyrosine ratio in the brain rose from 0.10 to 0.35, with a concomitant increase in plasma levels. A tyrosine supplement alone at a higher dosage will also do the job.

When supplementing with tyrosine, keep in mind that the quantity of tyrosine that can enter the brain is proportional to the sum of other neutral amino acids (valine, isoleucine, tryptophan, leucine, methionine, and phenylalanine), which compete for transport with tyrosine. Because so many other amino acids interfere with tyrosine's absorption, more L-tyrosine to protein should be used. Tyrosine enters the brain more readily when the quantity—and ergo the ratio— of tyrosine increases. When there is less tyrosine, the ratio is decreased and less enters the brain. Therefore, L-tyrosine should be taken with a high-carbohydrate meal so it does not have to compete for absorption with amino acids in a meal high in protein.

People who cannot tolerate tyrosine should use N-acetyl tyrosine (Norival). This amino acid modifier will likely be absorbed better. Adding an acetyl group to an amino acid appears to increase absorption.

Deficiency Symptoms

Signs and symptoms of tyrosine deficiency include apathy, blood sugar imbalances, depression, edema, fat loss, fatigue, liver damage, mood disorders, muscle loss, and slowed growth in children.

Availability

Free-form L-tyrosine is available in 500-mg capsules and tablets.

Therapeutic Daily Amount

The normal range of supplemental tyrosine is 7 to 30 g daily, depending upon the condition being treated.

Maximum Safe Level

Not established.

Side Effects and Contraindications

Toxicity with tyrosine may occur when it is given in conjunction with MAO inhibitors, causing sweats and mild elevation in blood pressure. Toxicity is rare or almost nonexistent in tyrosine therapy. Tyrosine is generally recognized as one of the safe substances. D-tyrosine, in contrast, can be toxic and has suppressed growth and weight gain in experimental animals.

TYROSINE: A SUMMARY

Tyrosine is an essential amino acid that readily passes the blood-brain barrier. Once in the brain, it is a precursor for the neurotransmitters dopamine, norepinephrine, and epinephrine, better known as adrenaline. These neurotransmitters are an important part of the body's sympathetic nervous system, and their concentrations in the body and brain are directly dependent upon dietary tyrosine.

Tyrosine is not found in large concentrations throughout the body, probably because it is rapidly metabolized. Folic acid, copper, and vitamin C are cofactor nutrients of these reactions. Tyrosine is also the precursor for hormones, thyroid, catecholestrogens and the major human pigment, melanin. Tyrosine is an important amino acid in many proteins, peptides, and even enkephalins, the body's natural pain reliever. Valine and other branched-chain amino acids, and possibly tryptophan and pheylalanine may reduce tyrosine absorption.

More tyrosine is needed under stress, and tyrosine supplements prevent the stress-induced depletion of norepinephrine and can cure biochemical depression. However, tyrosine may not be good for those with psychosis. Many antipsychotic medications apparently function by inhibiting tyrosine metabolism.

L-dopa, which is directly used in Parkinson's disease, is made from tyrosine.

Tyrosine, the nutrient, can be used as an adjunct in the treatment of this disorder. Peripheral metabolism of tyrosine necessitates large doses of tyrosine, however, compared to L-dopa. When combined with the drug Sinemet, tyrosine's effectiveness is increased.

Drugs like yohimbine that prolong the effects of tyrosine products have been used as aphrodisiacs. Tyrosine supplements in large doses may stimulate sex drive by raising blood pressure and catecholamine levels.

Tyrosine, like amphetamines, in large doses will reduce appetite, but in low doses it stimulates appetite. Tyrosine therapy may be useful in drug addiction, temporarily replacing codeine and amphetamines as methadone does for heroin addicts.

Physicians at Harvard Medical School have pioneered the use of 1 to 6 g of tyrosine for the effective treatment of medication-resistant depression. Many antidepressants work by prolonging the action of tyrosine metabolites. Tyrosine is safer, although the results may be less dramatic in the short term than the antidepressants. Lower doses, as little as 1,000 to 2,000 mg have been found to be effective clinically, as well as experimentally in animals. The minimum daily requirement for adults of tyrosine and its precursor, phenylalanine, is 16 mg/kg a day or about 1,000 mg total. Hence, 6 g is at least six times the minimum daily requirement.

Tyrosine can be used as a safe and lasting therapy, useful in a variety of clinical situations—depression, hypertension, Parkinson's disease, low sex drive, appetite suppression, and therapy for substance abusers. Tyrosine, like the branched-chain amino acids, fights all kinds of stress because it is the precursor of adrenaline, which is used during times of stress.

CHAPTER FOUR

Tryptophan:
The Sleep Promoter

Tryptophan is an essential amino acid that works primarily in the central nervous system. It is converted into serotonin, a necessary neurotransmitter that transfers nerve impulses from one cell to another, and is directly linked to feelings of well-being. As such, tryptophan works to control sleeping patterns, hunger patterns, depression and anxiety, aggressive behavior, sexual behavior, pain and temperature interpretation, and appetite regulation. Niacin (vitamin B_3), 5-hydroxytryptophan (5-HTP), and melatonin are important metabolites of tryptophan.

Due to a number of deaths in 1989 caused by a contaminated batch of tryptophan, the amino acid was banned from the market (see "The Tryptophan Controversy" below). It became available again in 1996 but only by prescription. During the six years tryptophan was off the market, physicians began achieving similar results with the use of such popular antidepressants as paroxetine (Paxil) and fluoxetine (Prozac), among others. However, tryptophan produces an antidepressant effect without the side effects of those drugs. Because it's a natural substance, tryptophan can produce its effects without distortion or disruption of normal body physiology.

THE TRYPTOPHAN CONTROVERSY

Tryptophan was implicated in the fatal 1989 outbreak of eosinophilia myalgia syndrome (EMS), a rare autoimmune disease marked by severe muscle pain, spasms, and weakness; swelling of the arms and legs; numbness; fever; and rashes; and in severe cases death. The evidence trail pointed squarely to major contamination in a new processing method developed by one Japanese manufacturer.

Prior to this development, tryptophan had been used safely for many years worldwide without incident by consumers and physicians alike. The medical literature contains no record of tryptophan consumers having developed symptoms of EMS, other than some individuals who ingested the contaminated amino acid in 1989. The bibliography of this book is filled with important research showing that tryptophan is safe and effective.

Many people who developed EMS in 1989 initiated lawsuits against the Japanese manufacturer. Among them were individuals who attempted to bolster their claims by contending that their illness and pain persisted even after symptoms disappeared. Regretfully, most of the studies of these EMS cases failed to carefully screen individuals for preexisting myalgic, or muscle-aching, disorders, which are quite common in the population. In addition, some people may have had medical conditions that made them more vulnerable. Some may perhaps have had abnormalities in tryptophan metabolism.

Recent research has uncovered a number of disorders associated with defective tryptophan metabolism and elevated tryptophan blood levels. Among them are myopia, speech impediment, muscular skeletal abnormalities, and perception hypersensitivity. Interestingly, no patient with a genetic tryptophan abnormality or inherently high blood level was diagnosed with EMS—more evidence that tryptophan is not the cause of EMS.

Abnormal cerebral spinal fluid, 5-hydroxyindole acetic acid, and serum iron levels may occur in some EMS patients. Nonetheless, without specific blood tests for inflammation such as erythrocyte sedimentation rate and C reactive protein markers, EMS is not always easy to diagnose. Testing for T-helper and T-suppressor ratios, an indication of immune response, also figure in a diagnosis.

The prohibition of tryptophan is all the more remarkable in the light of a study on the safety of amino acid supplementation prepared by the Center for Food Safety and Applied Nutrition at the FDA. PATH Medical provided FDA researchers with extensive documentation, including this book, on the use of tryptophan and other amino acids in clinical medicine. The report concluded that amino acids *are* safe. (A copy of the FDA report can be obtained from the Life Sciences Research Office, Federation of American Society for Experimental Biology, 9650 Rockville Pike, Bethesda, MD 20814-3998; refer to FDA contract no. 223-882124, task order no. 8.) Recent data makes it even more clear that tryptophan in particular is also safe.

In the flood of media that followed the 1989 EMS outbreak and the regulatory ban against the sale of tryptophan by the U.S. Food and Drug Administration (FDA), reporters and commentators by and large failed to point out tryptophan's safety record over the years. A *New York Times* article said the incident showed that taking dietary supplements was "chancy." However, the chanciness of dietary supplements is trivial. Chanciness, in our opinion, is paying attention to the media attitude toward nutritional supplementation, which is typically colored by mainstream medicine. Perhaps this will change as the massive volume of positive research emerges on the role of supplements for health.

In our opinion, if there is any risk at all to amino acid therapy it is taking imbalanced amino acids that do not contain tryptophan. Without tryptophan, some individuals experience increased achiness and inability to sleep. Researchers and clinicians alike have commented on this. As long as tryptophan is banned, these symptoms are possible. In our clinic, we have confirmed a number of cases where individuals using new amino acid combinations without tryptophan have developed muscle aches or myalgia.

But now we will leave politics aside and express our excitement that trypto-phan has once again been made available for the therapeutic treatment of depression, insomnia, and weight loss. As of late 1996, tryptophan can be read-ily prescribed by your physician, who should be familiar with your particular bio-chemical needs. To achieve optimal results, he or she should know that there is a distinct dosage range. Since tryptophan is a nonpatentable natural substance, it cannot be claimed by any one pharmaceutical company. Your physician's best source is any pharmacy that specializes in custom compounding.

FUNCTION

Tryptophan is the single most studied nutrient in the research oriented psychi-atric community today. Researchers into mental illness became interested in tryp-tophan therapy in 1971, when Wurtman and colleagues from MIT discovered that the concentration of the brain neurotransmitter serotonin was dependent upon dietary intake of tryptophan.

Further Wurtman studies showed that serotonin concentration in the brain is directly proportional to the concentration of brain and plasma tryptophan. Dietary intake of tryptophan directly influences the amount of serotonin in the plasma and brain and throughout the entire body. This was the first accepted demonstration of the direct dietary control of a brain neurotransmitter by a sin-gle amino acid.

It is probably tryptophan's building of serotonin that allows it to function so effectively as a sleep-inducing agent and to yield such positive benefits in obese patients by helping to dampen the craving for carbohydrates that increase body fat.

METABOLISM

Tryptophan metabolism is complex and has many metabolic pathways. The pri-mary enzyme involved in metabolism of tryptophan is hydroxylase. This enzyme starts the conversion of all the aromatic amino acids to neurotransmitters. It requires adequate biopterin, pyridoxine (vitamin B_6), and magnesium to per-form this function. Pyridoxine is involved in the conversion of tryptophan to serotonin and in metabolism of other tryptophan metabolites. Adequate utilization of tryptophan is especially dependent upon the amount of pyridoxine available.

Normal tryptophan metabolism also requires niacin and the amino acid glutamine, which supply the cofactor nicotinamide adenine dinucleotide (NAD), for normal tryptophan metabolism. The relationship between niacin and tryptophan is particularly interesting because niacin can be made from dietary tryptophan; in such instances, tryptophan acts as the vitamin and niacin becomes a metabolite.

Two other important metabolites of tryptophan covered later in this chapter are 5-HTP and melatonin. Interest in 5-HTP and melatonin skyrocketed after the ban on tryptophan—5-HTP for its ability to manufacture serotonin and melatonin for its antiaging and sleep-promoting properties.

Another metabolite derived from tryptophan is picolinic acid. Picolinic acid is important as it may increase zinc absorption. Tryptophan- or pyridoxine-deficient animals cannot absorb zinc, according to G. W. Evans of the USDA. People who have pyroluria, and thus zinc and pyridoxine deficiency, often experience severe inner tension, anxiety, and phobias. These individuals do well with L-tryptophan supplementation. Many require the nutrient combination of zinc and pyridoxine as well.

Inborn errors of tryptophan metabolism can produce psychiatric symptoms such as hallucinations, depression, anxiety, delerium, dementia, and hysteria. Carcinoid syndrome is a disease wherein small (carcinoid) tumors of the intestine make increased amounts of the tryptophan metabolite serotonin. Hartnup's disease is a condition in which tryptophan, and possibly other amino acids, are not absorbed properly. It leads to a disease similar to pellagra, a niacin-tryptophan deficiency disease caused by high corn or other tryptophan-deficient diets, with symptoms of dermatitis, diarrhea, and dementia. Tryptophan supplements may be useful in each condition—in carcinoid, replacing the over-metabolized nutrient, and in Hartnup's, supplementing a malabsorbed nutrient. Some disorders of excess tryptophan in the blood may contribute to mental retardation.

REQUIREMENTS

No RDA has been established for tryptophan, but an intake of 3 mg a day is assumed adequate for healthy adults. Because tryptophan is an essential amino acid, and so cannot be manufactured in the body from other amino acids, it is therefore important that adequate amounts be included in the diet. Like the requirements for most essential amino acids, however, requirements for tryptophan appear to decrease with age. Infants four to six months old require 21 g a day, while children aged four to twelve need only 4 g, and adults seem to require just 3 g per day.

FOOD SOURCES

Tryptophan is the least abundant essential amino acid in foods. It is not typically found in any significant amount in the normal diet, and most dietary proteins are deficient in this amino acid. Ham, meat, and beef extract contain relatively large amounts of tryptophan, as do salted anchovies, Parmesan and Swiss cheeses, eggs, and almonds. Therefore, L-tryptophan supplementation (1 to 2 g) can create a significant increase in tryptophan blood levels. In contrast, other amino acids, like glutamine, glutamic acid, and aspartic acid, must be given in megadoses (5 to 10 g) to affect blood levels.

TOXICITY

Tryptophan derivatives in broiled and burnt foods are some of the most powerful carcinogens known to man. Abnormal amounts of tryptophan metabolites have been found in various cancers, primarily in breast and bladder.

TABLE 4.1. TRYPTOPHAN LEVELS IN FOOD		
FOOD	AMOUNT	CONTENT (GRAMS)
Avocado	1	0.40
Cheese	1 ounce	0.09
Chicken	1 pound	0.28
Chocolate	1 cup	0.11
Cottage cheese	1 cup	0.40
Duck	1 pound	0.40
Egg	1	0.10
Granola	1 cup	0.20
Luncheon meat	1 pound	0.50
Oatmeal	1 cup	0.20
Pork	1 pound	1.00
Ricotta	1 cup	—
Sausage meat	1 pound	0.30
Turkey	1 pound	0.37
Wheat germ	1 cup	0.40
Whole milk	1 cup	0.11
Wild game	1 pound	1.15
Yogurt	1 cup	0.05

FORM AND ABSORPTION

L-tryptophan is the desired therapeutic form. All other metabolites of tryptophan, except niacin, have significant side effects. D-tryptophan is barely metabolized in humans or dogs and is excreted largely unchanged.

Tryptophan's transport in plasma, the brain, and throughout the body is unique among amino acids in that it exists "free" in a small plasma pool and is bound to albumin (a water-soluble protein and the principal protein in blood) in a larger pool. Other amino acids are not carried by albumin.

As many as five other dietary amino acids—tyrosine, phenylalanine, valine, leucine, and isoleucine—may share with tryptophan a common transport system from blood to brain, thus competing for its uptake by the brain. Brain tryptophan availability depends on this active uptake mechanism. Changes in serum tryptophan levels result in parallel changes of tryptophan and serotonin concentrations in the brain.

At our clinic, we use brain mapping (see the box "Brain Electrical Activity Mapping" on page 59), which we believe can identify serotonin metabolism through a balanced spectral analysis. When all four brain waves—alpha, beta, theta, and delta—are balanced, it is believed that tryptophan or serotonin metabolism is properly balanced.

CLINICAL USES

Tryptophan is similar in its chemical structure to the other aromatic amino acids, which behave as stimulants; however, it acts as a "modified antiamphetamine" and therefore is able to control the brain's adrenaline.

Aging

At our clinic, a comparison of chronic (long-term or frequently recurring) and acute (a rapid, short course) tryptophan-loaded patients showed significant elevations of several amino acids in the chronic group compared to the acute. Our studies show that prolonged tryptophan supplementation raises many other plasma amino acids beside tryptophan. This is significant because many plasma amino acids decrease with age.

Aggressive Behavior

Biochemical mechanisms underlying aggression are just beginning to be explored. Evidence suggests that serotonin and tryptophan may inhibit aggressive behavior in experimental animals and humans.

Tryptophan-free diets for four to six days reduced mice-killing in rats. Twenty-five to 30 percent reduction in brain tryptophan metabolites was identified as the primary cause of the decreased aggressive behavior.

Brain Electrical Activity Mapping

Amino acids run the brain. Every serious biochemical disorder is associated with a brain chemical imbalance that amino acids can help restore. For this reason, we conduct a test called Brain Electrical Activity Mapping (BEAM) on most patients. This technique is a huge boon in evaluating mental illness, degenerative aging of the brain, and the effectiveness of exciting, restorative nutritional treatments. BEAM is a simple office procedure that provides reliable spectral analysis of alpha and theta waves, evoked potentials, visual evoked response, auditory evoked response, and positive brain wave (P300) voltage. This technique evaluates electrophysiological function of the brain and tells us if imbalances are mild or severe.

P300 is a particularly outstanding marker for understanding degenerative processes in the brain. P300 refers to a positive brain wave, occurring at 300 milliseconds, that is generated during BEAM testing. Abnormally low waves are seen in individuals with such conditions as attention deficit disorder, schizophrenia, drug craving, alcohol or cocaine abuse, chronic organic depression from biochemical imbalance, Alzheimer's disease, and Parkinson's disease. Low P300s are also seen as risk factors for developing Alzheimer's disease, depression, anxiety, and possibly other conditions such as cancer. With age, P300 readings decrease as well.

Cranial electrical stimulation (CES)—gentle, low-voltage stimulation—improves P300 voltage as do androgenic hormones such as DHEA, and levodopa/carbidopa (Sinemet) and dopaminergic compounds that act like dopamine.

Amino acids, in specific, and nutrition, in general, make a powerful impact on P300. Tyrosine, in particular, as well as phenylalanine, and N-acetyl cysteine are the amino acids we have found improve the P300 marker most. We believe that a patient with a P300 voltage reading under 10 should receive 1 to 6 g of tyrosine supplementally.

Tryptophan-free diets have also produced specific increases in shock-induced irritable fighting and pain sensitivity in animals. Depressed levels of the tryptophan metabolite 5-hydroxyindole acetic acid have been found in hyperactive and aggressive mentally retarded children, suggesting again a dysfunction of serotonin metabolism. Retarded patients who tend to be aggressive have been found to have significantly low tryptophan levels.

A large percentage of mentally retarded children have abnormal tryptophan metabolism, as shown by studies that monitored tryptophan-loading doses and subsequent production of tryptophan metabolites. Oral supplementation with 30 mg of pyridoxine corrected this defect, which reduced aggressive behavior. Tryptophan and pyridoxine deficiency often paint the same clinical picture. This is not surprising since pyroluria patients (who need more pyridoxine and zinc) may also have abnormal tryptophan metabolism as determined by loading studies.

Physicians at the North Nassau Mental Health Center found tryptophan to be useful in treating obsessive-compulsive disorders, although they remarked that they did have a few cases where aggressive behavior was aggravated.

Epidemiologic studies suggest that in areas where corn is a major dietary staple—and thus tryptophan levels are low—rates of homicide have increased. Periods of protein malnutrition have been marked by increased criminality according to Mawson.

The data is quite convincing that disordered tryptophan metabolism is involved in many forms of aggressive behavior. We have found that clinically low-histamine, paranoid, aggressive people can benefit from tryptophan supplementation. Therapy can be evaluated by monitoring plasma tryptophan levels.

Alcoholism

Studies utilizing plasma amino acid assays indicate a deficiency of tryptophan in alcoholics. At present, more research studies are needed.

Anorexia

Low plasma and serum tryptophan levels are common in anorexic patients. The significance of this finding is unclear since many plasma amino acids are often low in this condition. We have found that multi–amino acid formulas are frequently necessary in treating anorexic patients.

Brain Disorders

Studies have fortified the reputation of tryptophan as an adjunctive therapy in many brain disorders. Tryptophan's benefits have been documented in treating

Tryptophan Restores Emotional Equilibrium

A thirty-one-year-old female entered my office with her two-year-old baby and promptly declared, "I'm going to hurt my baby and myself." She continued her story by saying that she wanted to hit everyone who spoke to her. She had been suffering from uncontrolled aggression for months. We started the patient on 3 g of L-tryptophan daily and increased it to 6 g daily (3 g in the morning and in the evening). The patient noticed slight but tolerable nausea with her morning dose. Her fear that she would hurt her baby had previously driven her to put her child up for adoption. After one month, her abnormal aggression disappeared and she withdrew that application.

many brain disorders, including affective disorder, obsessive compulsive disorder, eating and sleeping disorders, panic disorder, seasonal affective disorder (SAD), and attention deficit disorder (ADD), and in such illnesses as hypokinetic and psychotic syndromes, phenylketonuria (PKU), Alzheimer's disease, migraines and pain, suicidal behavior, alcohol and drug addiction, and sexual dysfunction.

Measuring the tryptophan plasma level for individuals with these conditions can provide valuable information. One can measure neurotransmitters in platelets and in cerebral spinal fluid, as well as tryptophan breakdown products in the urine. Hormonal states also provide clues to tryptophan levels in the body. For example, estrogen raises dopamine and progesterone raises tryptophan. In addition, low blood flow due to poor carotid circulation can cause tryptophan deficiency. Individuals with brain disorders, particularly the elderly, should undergo a carotid Doppler procedure to determine .whether circulation is involved. Among other things, decreased blood flow affects the transportation of neurotransmitters through the blood and impairs the normal ability of the brain and body to communicate. These are all techniques for determining tryptophan status.

Delgado and colleagues revealed that a rapid dietary depletion of tryptophan caused a transient return of depression in 67 percent of patients who were responding well to antidepressant medication. Five hours after the administration of tryptophan-deficient amino acids, subjects were found to have low plasma amino acid levels and signs of depression associated with depletion of tryptophan. The bottom line is that protein formulations without tryptophan exacerbate depression. Even while taking the best drugs, such individuals do better with tryptophan. We believe that tryptophan plasma levels can also help pinpoint people who are vulnerable to depression.

Tryptophan has been used effectively in the past with the antidepressant medications fluoxetine (Prozac), sertraline (Zoloft), and paroxetine (Paxil), a group of medications known as selective serotonin reuptake inhibitors (SSRIs). These medications keep tryptophan from being depleted. From research on depression, anxiety disorders and obsessive-compulsive disorders, it has been identified that many of these people are serotonin depleted to the point that some psychiatric journals have come to call these conditions "tryptophan-depletion disorders," especially social phobia disorders.

Since then, numerous tryptophan or serotonin receptors have been discovered that enable medications to target specific sites.

- Fenfluramine (pondimin) can have an effect on the appetite receptor.

- Paroxetine seems to hit the receptor for social phobia.

- Sertraline affects the receptor for obsessive-compulsive disorders.

- Fluoxetine works best on the receptor for depression.

- Receptors for nausea may respond to ondansetron (Zofran).

- Other serotonergic agents like ergoloid mesylates (Hydergine) may affect memory receptors and serotonin control.

- Carbamazepine (Tegretol) may hit the receptor associated with mood.

Today, tryptophan has been replaced by the use of trazodone (Desyrel) or nefazodone (Serzone), a unique class of medications that have serotonergic actions and may affect sleep receptors.

Many borderline patients with personality disorders, including narcissistic individuals and those with aggressive impulse disorders, have mild depression and respond positively when administered with tryptophan or SSRI and other tryptophan-inducing medications.

Tryptophan is low in people with dysthymia. Cranial electrotherapy stimulation can enhance the effect of tryptophan for this condition (see "Cranial Electrical Stimulation" on page 63). Many people with this condition may also have dependent, histrionic, or dissociative personalities as well as some anxiety. They are all good candidates for L-tryptophan therapy.

Tryptophan and other brain chemicals are depleted in drug addiction. Drug addicts on methamphetamine drugs and their derivatives may respond to trazodone and tryptophan. A combination of 50 mg of trazodone with 1 g of tryptophan may be useful for addicts who exhibit aggressive behavior.

There is increasing data on the relationship between tryptophan and suicide. The newest research confirms our original findings that abnormalities of serotonin and tryptophan metabolism are associated with impulsive acts of suicide.

For more information on tryptophan's role in these brain disorders, refer to the specific disorder in this section.

Note: Tryptophan may strengthen or weaken the effect of a MAO-inhibiting medication such as phenelzine (Nardil). The antiaging benefits attributed to tryptophan may be enhanced when used in combination with MAO-B inhibitors such as selegiline. More research is needed.

Depression

Once called melancholia, depression has long plagued humankind. Sages thought the condition was caused by bad thoughts or evil spirits; psychiatrists reworded these ideas into the concept of depression as "aggression turned inward." Today we know that biochemistry is imbalanced in the depressed person, and we augment our understanding with the knowledge provided by these earlier psychiatrists and sages.

Cranial Electrical Stimulation

At our clinic, we find that cranial electrical stimulation (CES) substantially improves results when combined with amino acid therapy. We use it, for instance, in our treatment programs for drug abuse. Electrophysiological abnormalities are hallmarks of the drug abuser and the individual at high risk for drug abuse. The need to modify these electrophysiological parameters is of critical importance in treatment and prevention. Numerous reports documenting the benefits of CES have been published, including a study conducted in our clinic showing beneficial changes to abnormal patterns of electrophysiology in drug abuse and other organic brain disorders. This technique generates a gentle, minute low-voltage electrical stimulation to the brain. CES can be used in the clinic or at home by the patient who has purchased a CES device that is simple to operate.

We regard CES as a major breakthrough for augmenting neurotransmitter production. We believe it drives the neurons to utilize precursor amino acids more effectively. In our protocol, the precursors are first supplied supplementally. CES is then administered to stimulate the neurotransmitter synthesis.

The medical literature is replete with studies documenting the success of electrotherapy in the treatment of numerous conditions, such as depression, anxiety, alcoholism and substance abuse, withdrawal syndrome, insomnia, schizophrenia, learning disorders, hyperactivity, and even hyperacidity. Clinically, we have seen excellent results combining our fatigue and stress supplement Brain Energy Formula and CES for control of long-term anxiety and depression. This approach effectively enables patients to reduce their medication.

Electricity is widely and safely used throughout medicine to revive depressed brains and hearts, and fading muscles. Thousands of Americans are treated with CES each year, and more than 10,000 own CES devices prescribed for home use. A device costs about $500.

Depression that is caused by a chemical imbalance has been subcategorized into unipolar/bipolar, high histamine/low histamine, serotoninergic or catecholamine excess/deficiency. Unipolar, high histamine, and serotoninergic excess depression (catecholamine deficiency) is a flat-affect or low-energy depression. Bipolar, low histamine, catecholamine excess depression is an agitated form of depression. L-tryptophan is thought to be more effective in the agitated form, although the data paint less than a clear picture.

Tricyclic antidepressants such as imipramine (Tofranil) and nortriptyline (Aventyl, Pamelor) work by inhibiting uptake of various neurotransmitters, thereby prolonging the life of serotonin, dopamine, and other catecholamines. The excretion of the metabolites of tryptophan is decreased by tricyclic antidepressants. Six grams of L-tryptophan have been found to be as effective as 150 to 225 mg of imipramine in acute depression.

L-tryptophan (1.5 g twice a day) plus nicotinamide (250 mg four times a day) have been shown to be as effective as biweekly electroconvulsive therapy (ECT) for unipolar depression. D'Elia and colleagues found that L-tryptophan did not add to the antidepressant effect of ECT when both modalities were used.

Farkas and colleagues actually found L-tryptophan to be more effective in patients with bipolar depression. Other studies suggest that newly depressed patients, probably bipolar, respond well to 3 to 6 g of L-tryptophan and 1.5 g of nicotinamide. In general, newly depressed patients respond better to all methods of therapy used.

Lehman of Copenhagen suggests that symptoms of depression resulting from tryptophan deficiency occur when the amino acid has decreased to 0.5 mg percent or less. We measured plasma amino acid levels in eighteen patients with a primary diagnosis of depression. These eighteen patients were compared to healthy control subjects. The depressed group had tryptophan levels ranging from 5.3 plus or minus 2.3, while the range in the control group was 7.9 plus or minus 1.4, an extremely significant difference. Changes in thirty other amino acids were not significant. Other amino acid abnormalities, such as changes in threonine, arginine, and asparagine, showed up but only when the group was subdivided into low and extremely low tryptophan levels.

Study of plasma levels of tryptophan, particularly in ratio with other neutral amino acids, has been shown to be useful in treating depression. We have found many patients low in plasma tryptophan, and these patients respond well to therapy. Even small doses of 500 mg of tryptophan in the morning and in the evening can, on occasion, significantly elevate blood tryptophan levels up to two times normal when taken for long periods of time. Most individuals require 3 g of tryptophan to obtain significant antidepressive effects and elevations of 100 percent or more of plasma tryptophan. There are probably diurnal rhythms as well that alter the need for and the effect of tryptophan, depending on the time of day.

Tryptophan Lifts Depression

Recently, a forty-five-year-old man came in with severe chronic depression. His plasma tryptophan was half of normal. He was initially treated with 1 g of L-tryptophan that barely elevated his plasma levels and produced only slight improvement. Increasing his treatment to 3 g daily helped to stop the early morning waking, provided a more restful sleep, and gradually lifted his depression.

Down's Syndrome

Children with Down's syndrome, a genetic abnormality that causes varying degrees of physical and mental disability, who were supplemented for the first three years of life with a combination of pyridoxine and 5-HTP, a tryptophan metabolite, improved in social maturity and accomplishment. This preliminary study noted that use of either pyridoxine or 5-HTP alone raises serum serotonin levels. Low urinary metabolites of tryptophan have also been found in Down's syndrome, yet there is great variation in urinary metabolites in this disease, as well as in other psychiatric conditions. We have had many cases where mentally retarded individuals benefit from increased doses of pyridoxine. This effect may occur because of improved tryptophan metabolism.

Epilepsy

The similarity of manic episodes to epilepsy prompted a study of tryptophan in epilepsy. Since phenytoin (Dilantin) lowers tryptophan, while carbamazepine raises tryptophan, it is conceivable that a significant percentage of people with epilepsy may respond to tryptophan therapy.

Exercise

Studies suggest that tryptophan supplementation can prolong exercise time. Tryptophan probably contributes to muscle relaxation. An article in the *International Journal of Sports Medicine* describes tryptophan as increasing tolerance to exercise pain. The amount suggested is 1,200 mg daily in the morning plus 300 mg at night.

Female Conditions

Supplemental tryptophan has been found effective in the following conditions.

Premenstrual Syndrome. Recent studies have shown major benefits with fluoxetine in the treatment of premenstrual syndrome (PMS). We have seen similar results with tryptophan. Benefits include improved vigor, work performance, and interactions, as well as less depression, tension, irritability, pain, stress, food cravings, mood swings, anxiety, and edema. There is no question that progesterone (a female hormone made in the ovaries), L-tryptophan, and fluoxetine all can be beneficial. Dosages as high as 3 g of tryptophan are helpful with 20 mg of fluoxetine. Diet has also been found to have a significant impact on PMS.

Postpartum and Postmenopausal Depression. Bender has suggested a hormonal control of the synthesis of niacin from tryptophan. Estrogens increase the amount of tryptophan converted to niacin while progesterone and hydrocortisone, a steroid, decrease it. Postpartum women, whose estrogen levels are relatively high, have decreased serum tryptophan. Postmenopausal women on estrogen may become depressed because of lowered tryptophan levels.

Contraception. Women on birth control pills do not develop elevated serum tryptophan levels when given pyridoxine and tryptophan as do healthy individuals. Users of birth control pills need a minimum of 20 mg of pyridoxine to metabolize tryptophan normally.

Growth Hormone and Prolactin

Two g of tryptophan administered intravenously increase serum growth hormone and prolactin, a natural hormone that stimulates milk production in new mothers. Deficiency of pyridoxine and tryptophan may lead to a deficiency of growth hormone and possibly to prolactin deficiency. Tryptophan supplements may prove useful in treating growth hormone and prolactin deficiency. However, we have tested oral L-tryptophan for its effect on increasing plasma growth hormone and found this effect to be insignificant even at the dose of 5 g.

Heart Disease

Lehnart and colleagues report a major impact of tryptophan on the heart. Numerous studies indicate a higher risk of heart attack with low tryptophan levels.

Human Immunodeficiency Virus

Low plasma tryptophan levels along with low levels of methionine and cysteine are found in human immunodeficiency virus (HIV) patients. HIV exhausts the brain's storage of neurotransmitters and thereby contributes to break down the immune system. High levels of tryptophan have been found to reduce immune disorders. Lower levels of tryptophan are associated with poor immune function.

When tryptophan levels are built up in HIV patients, their ability to fight infections and to maintain musculature is enhanced. We have had a number of patients who we felt were near death from wasting syndromes related to immune disorders. Instead, they rebounded after starting on antidepressants, tryptophan, and other amino acids.

Infertility

Elevated serotonin and estrogen sensitivity have been linked to sterility secondary to tubal spasms, dysmenorrhea, and habitual abortion. Tryptophan theoretically should be used with caution in patients with infertility. Yet, tryptophan has been shown to have positive effects on human sperm viability.

Insomnia

Tryptophan promotes sleep. This is well documented and accepted throughout medicine. Although tryptophan has been available by prescription only since

1996, we continue to believe that tryptophan is the most reliable natural sleeping compound ever. The effectiveness of melatonin, an important tryptophan metabolite, (see "Important Metabolites" on page 74) to promote sleep has recently received considerable attention. However, careful attention should be given to melatonin dosing to avoid the sedation effect an excess produces in some individuals.

Hartmann, from Boston State Hospital, Tufts University found that the time it took people to fall asleep (sleep latency) could be significantly reduced by bedtime administration of tryptophan. The reduction in sleep latency by approximately 50 percent is significant even at a dose of 1 g of L-tryptophan, the approximate equivalent of the tryptophan content in 500 g of meat. The electroencephalographic stages of sleep and the cycle of sleep are not significantly affected by 1 to 5 g of L-tryptophan, but, at one or more of the higher doses (10 to 15 g), there is a decrease in desynchronized sleep and an increase in deep, slow-wave, rapid-eye movement (REM) sleep. Further studies by Hartmann and Spinweber at the Sleep and Dream Laboratory in Boston found doses of 25 g to be effective for people with insomnia. Patients with mild insomnia experienced significant reduction in the time they needed to fall asleep with 1 to 2 g of L-tryptophan. This is significant because 1 to 2 g of L-tryptophan is the minimal amount needed to raise blood levels of tryptophan. The effects of tryptophan seem to be directly proportionate to tryptophan levels in plasma.

Hartmann reviewed data from nine studies. He found that tryptophan, unlike hypnotics, produces no distortions in sleep physiology when first administered, on a long-term administration basis, or after withdrawal. He states that hypnotic drugs, in general, have many problems and dangers associated with the fact that they bear little or no relationship to the natural biochemistry of sleep.

Tryptophan Lengthens and Deepens Sleep

A seventy-year-old woman plagued by severe insomnia, who was resistant to barbiturate (Darvon), antihistamines, thioridazine (Mellaril), and diazepam (Valium), came to us for help. She had used 500 to 1,000 mg of L-tryptophan in the past with no side effects. We started her at 3 g of L-tryptophan, taken a half-hour to an hour before bed. This kept her asleep about four hours, which is about half the time it takes for plasma tryptophan levels to normalize. She would then take another 3 g of L-tryptophan. Six grams taken at one time lengthened her sleep time but again not through the whole night. Eventually, the pattern of midnight or late-night waking stopped. Relief may occur when the level of tryptophan builds up. Eventually, the dose was cut back to eliminate excessive sleeping and daytime drowsiness.

It has been noted by Cooper that the sedative action of tryptophan appears to be related to the time of administration. At night, levels of metabolites and 5-HTP are at a peak. Serotoninergic mechanisms are involved in the normal sleep process and may be the critical blood determinants of sleep.

Other researchers, Christian and Pegram, found the tryptophan metabolite niacin or niacinamide (a derivative of niacin that reduces "niacin flush"), to be effective for insomniacs and also to increase REM or dream sleep. We have found clinically that pyridoxine also increases REM or dream sleep. This may be a synergistic mechanism because tryptophan and niacin metabolism require pyridoxine for their production. Studies of L-tryptophan by Hartmann and Spinweber in a case of posttraumatic insomnia without REM sleep found that 3 g of 5-HTP were associated with the return of normal REM sleep. Hartmann noted that stage IV (REM) sleep could be increased by tryptophan.

The effect of tryptophan on all the stages of sleep remains unclear. Its effect on insomnia may be enhanced by eating a carbohydrate-rich snack, approximately one hour before bedtime. We have given tryptophan to several hundred patients to induce sleep. A common complaint is that it does not keep people asleep. Some individuals may also require niacin or niacinamide in addition. In most cases where tryptophan has not been helpful in inducing sleep, the dose was inadequate.

Kidney Failure

Modlinger and colleagues from the VA Hospital in East Orange, New Jersey, showed that 2 to 10 mg of L-tryptophan daily could stimulate aldosterone, renin, and cortisol, steroid hormones produced by the adrenal gland. Low doses of 25 mg to 100 mg/kg of L-tryptophan can lower blood pressure by ten to fifteen points in animals with normal blood pressure. This hypotensive effect may be one mechanism by which tryptophan prevents complete kidney failure in partially nephrectomized (kidney-removed) rats. Furthermore, patients whose kidneys are injured by uremia, a toxic condition caused by the accumulation of waste products in the blood, need more tryptophan because of poor absorption. Both hypertensive and/or uremic individuals may benefit from L-tryptophan supplements.

We have used tryptophan successfully as an adjunct nutrient in patients with hypertension. A twenty-seven-year-old, five-pack-a-day smoker with nutrient resistant hypertension had low plasma tryptophan. L-tryptophan therapy with 1 g in the morning and in the evening reduced the smoker's blood pressure from 140/100 to 130/80. Further studies are indicated.

Mania

In treating mania, a manifestation of bipolar disorder, Chouinard from McGill University considers L-tryptophan to be as effective as lithium and even more effective than the antipsychotic chlorpromazine (Thorazine). One mechanism by which lithium works is by promoting serotoninergic neuron transmission. We have often combined our nighttime lithium therapy with 1 to 3 g of L-tryptophan. Patients subjectively tell us that this dosage of tryptophan enhances the benefit of the lithium. A recent study using 12 g of L-tryptophan alone for mania found tryptophan extremely effective in treating this condition.

Pain

Tryptophan can alleviate or reduce pain associated with certain headaches, dental work, and cancer. The basis for this effect of tryptophan on pain lies in the area of the brain called the nucleus raphus magnus, a primary pain-inhibiting center. The nucleus raphus magnus is the brain's major serotoninergic structure; thus, it depends upon serotonin and its precursor, tryptophan, for optimal functioning.

Seltzer and colleagues from Temple University studied the effects on headaches caused by chronic maxillofacial pain associated with the sinuses with daily administration of 3 g of L-tryptophan in conjunction with a high-carbohydrate, low-fat, low-protein diet. After four weeks, the tryptophan group reported a greater reduction in pain and a greater increase in pain tolerance threshold than the placebo group.

Electrical pain inhibitors used in dentistry are reported to work by converting tryptophan to serotonin. These instruments cease to be effective after prolonged use unless the patient is given large doses of L-tryptophan supplementation.

Rats with reduced tryptophan intake demonstrate increased sensitivity to painful stimulation, as well as mouse-killing behavior. Tryptophan may be necessary for the release of beta-endorphin, a natural pain reliever in human and animals. Apparently, tryptophan-deficient diets can lead to increased aggressiveness and greater pain sensitivity.

A double-blind study by Lieberman and colleagues of the Wurtman group at MIT found that 50 mg/kg (equivalent to 3.5 g in an 150 lb adult male) decreased pain sensitivity and increased subjective drowsiness and fatigue but, unlike many hypnotics, did not impair sensorimotor performance. This hypnotic action probably accounts for the success of tryptophan therapy in insomnia. Tryptophan apparently had no effect on anxiety.

Parkinson's Disease and Movement Disorders

The metabolite 5-HTP has been used to augment carbidopa treatment of intention myoclonus (muscle spasms associated with numerous neurological conditions). L-tryptophan has been found to decrease tremor in Parkinson's disease patients. Both facts are consistent with serotonin's role as an inhibitor of neurotransmitters. Furthermore, according to Lehmann and colleagues, Parkinson's individuals with dementia showed improved mental behavior following supplementation with 5-HTP.

Progressive myoclonus epilepsy (PME) is a rare inherited disease. Patients are found to have excess metabolites of tryptophan in their urine and low free tryptophan in their blood. Typically, PME appears in adolescence or early adulthood, beginning with generalized convulsive seizures, followed by an interval of years with myoclonic jerks of increasing frequency and severity, and eventually progressing to dementia. The sedative sodium valproate (Epilim) has been used with some success in PME. Tryptophan may be a useful adjunct.

Anecdotal reports using 10 g of L-tryptophan to treat Parkinson's disease tremor successfully have not been scientifically evaluated.

Protein Intake

Rats fed 50 mg/kg of L-tryptophan, the equivalent of 3.5 g in an average 150 lb adult male, eat more protein to balance the tyrosine elevation in serum histidine and threonine. As we have said previously, a balance of amino acids is very important and can be affected by L-tryptophan supplementation. Excess tryptophan may require more protein intake because of decreased absorption of other amino acids. Tryptophan-free diets cause normal individuals to reduce protein intake. While there are contradictory studies concerning tryptophan and consumption of less protein, dietary compensation of protein intake undoubtedly occurs in tryptophan-supplemented patients.

Psychosis

The tryptophan metabolites methyl tryptamines are psychopharmacologically active hallucinogens, naturally formed in the brain, with similar effects to the psychotropic drug LSD. LSD affects serotoninergic mechanisms. Methyl tryptamines have been found in the urine of schizophrenics. Tryptophan metabolism is now the subject of much study and controversy in the area of schizophrenia.

Serum tryptophan levels increase in people with schizophrenia following insulin coma therapy (a once common therapy that used insulin to restrict glucose to the brain, thereby causing shock, which was later replaced by electroconvulsive therapy). The tryptophan inhibitor benserazine, a medication frequently prescribed for schizophrenics, is a weak antipsychotic. Yet, several studies have found no change in schizophrenic behavior with large doses of L-tryptophan and its metabolite 5-HTP. Limited systemic conversion of tryptophan and entrance into the brain are postulated causes of failure.

Various studies have found no correlation between tryptophan in cerebrospinal fluid and schizophrenia. Electroencephalograpy (EEG) studies found tryptophan to cause decreased amplitude of all evoked response components.

The debate continues and is fostered by the lack of recognition of the multiple biochemical defects that result in schizophrenia. As reviewed by Bender of Middlesex Hospital Medical School, London, there are controversies over whether schizophrenia is due to overactivity or underactivity of serotoninergic mechanisms that contribute to psychotic behavior. We have found that schizophrenia is a group of diseases with many causes.

Gilka reviewed schizophrenia as a disorder of tryptophan metabolism and took into account subtypes of schizophrenia. He identified tryptophan-niacin deficient schizophrenics in cases of starvation, pellagra, and nicotinic acid encephalopathy. It has been suggested that tryptophan-niacin deficiency may be due to impaired intestinal absorption and may cause occasional secondary psychotic symptoms in malabsorption syndromes such as sprue and celiac disease. Gilka identified metabolic factors that could lead to psychosis; for example, pyridoxine and riboflavin deficiencies, copper excess, liver disease, porphyria, and Wilson's disease, a genetic disorder characterized by increased intestinal absorption of copper and its accumulation in the brain and other organs. Individuals with tryptophan malabsorption identified by tryptophan loading have been associated with confusion, dementia, and depression.

Stress situations are factors in schizophrenia that can produce increased metabolism and depletion of niacin and tryptophan. These stresses include stimulants, caffeine, amphetamines, fever, hyperthyroidism, environmental stress, lactation, pregnancy, and puberty. Gilka reviewed the role of tryptophan excess in cirrhosis, and as a contributing cause of hepatic coma and encephalopathy.

Exploring tryptophan excess in schizophrenia, he identified that excess tryptophan in the gut is converted by bacteria to methyl tryptamines. This can occur when there is enhanced activity of bacterial flora, constipation, diverticulosis (tiny sacs in weakened areas of the intestines), malabsorption syndrome, Hartnup's disease, and celiac sprue—all of which occasionally produce psychotic symptoms. Increased levels of tryptophan metabolites also have been found in the serum and brain of patients with liver failure; tryptophan metabolites also may be a factor in hepatic encephalopathy.

Undoubtedly, altered tryptophan metabolism is involved in some forms of schizophrenia. Tryptophan loading with 2 g of L-tryptophan in schizophrenics has helped identify many psychotic patients with abnormal tryptophan metabolism. The defect shows a pattern similar to that in patients with acrosclerosis, a disease signaled by stiff and tight skin on the hands and feet and osteoporosis of the hands. The significance of these findings demonstrates abnormal tryptophan metabolism in some people with schizophrenia.

Ironically, we have found tryptophan supplementation useful in cases of low-histamine schizophrenia and possibly in pyroluric schizophrenia, for example, in patients who have an excess of dopamine and/or altered perceptions.

Tryptophan Replaces Antipsychotic Drug

A thirty-two-year-old, obese, chronic schizophrenic woman came to us after ten years of unsuccessful treatment with antipsychotic drugs. We started her on 2 g of tryptophan daily, and later increased the dose to 4 g daily when her plasma tryptophan levels were measured and found to be almost undetectable. On this dose of tryptophan, the hallucinations and voices she had been experiencing disappeared and her weight decreased by twenty pounds in two months. She eventually stopped taking trifluoperazine (Stelazine) and is approaching full recovery. Megatryptophan therapy undoubtedly has a role in the treatment of some chronic schizophrenics.

Suicide

Several studies have found low levels of the serotonin metabolite 5-hydroxyindole acetic acid (5-HIAA) in cerebrospinal fluid and of serotonin in the brain of suicidal patients indicating that some of these patients have impaired serotonin metabolism.

Tryptophan as a therapy in suicidal patients has been utilized by us only for impulsive patients. A sixteen-year-old boy came to the clinic with a history of vandalism, violence, and aggression. We started him on 2 g of L-tryptophan in the morning and in the evening. The results of his tests showed significantly low plasma tryptophan. He returned in two weeks slightly improved, with a few bursts of temper still occurring. One month later, the patient returned, having been transformed from a wolf to a lamb. Slowly, for the next two months, we tapered his dose to 2 g daily, without reappearance of symptoms.

Weight Control

DL-fenfluramine, a serotonin-imitating medication, is excellent for weight control. DL-fenfluramine's effect can be augmented by pyridoxine and chromium. Fluoxetine, sertraline, paroxetine, and nefazodone are milder serotonergic compounds that can also help with weight loss. However, these medications are not as good as the adrenaline-stimulating drugs, namely phentermines, mazindol, and diethylpropion (Tenuate). According to studies, the combination of DL-fenfluramine and diethylpropion is particularly effective.

Although not as effective as these drugs, L-tryptophan is useful in appetite control. Dosages ranging from 1 to 15 g have been found helpful as part of a weight-loss program. Melatonin with tryptophan may also be useful because melatonin appears to indirectly raise tryptophan levels.

For now, 5-HTP offers a natural, over-the-counter alternative to serotoninergic drugs. Dosages of 300 mg, three times daily, have been found to reduce appetite. Studies show that many patients previously unable to lose weight have achieved excellent results on a fenfluramine and 5-HTP regimen. This combination was sometimes bolstered with phentermine (Fastin), sometimes with diethylpropion. Normal weight was attained in a period of from one to six months, depending on how much weight loss was involved. Some of these individuals have used the medication for years and sustained their normal weight level. Relatively few side effects were experienced, particularly when antioxidants, fish oils, and niacin were added to the program. If these nutrients were not included, there was some concern that fenfluramine may be toxic to the brain and possibly increase the risk of stroke.

Both tryptophan and 5-HTP can aid against the depression associated with binge eating. Binge eating depletes tryptophan by using up serotonin. In another study, rats with hypothalamic hyperphagia (binge eating associated with a abnormality in the hypothalamus gland) and obesity stopped eating excessively when tryptophan and serotonin were elevated.

Because tryptophan may inhibit insulin release, raise blood sugar, and decrease appetite, Wurtman and colleagues from MIT applied for a patent using 0.5 to 15 g of L-tryptophan as an appetite suppressant with an adjunct use of tyrosine. Carbohydrate appetite is reduced by increasing protein calorie sources. We have found adolescents to have completely lost their appetites for carbohydrates on L-tryptophan doses of as little as 1 g. Higher doses are necessary in adults, and response is variable. When evaluating the effects of tryptophan, it is helpful to be aware of anorexia-causing substances that may augment tryptophan's effect. A partial list of these substances includes the following:

- Alpha-adrenergic antagonists

- Beta-adrenergic agonists (amphetamines)

- Bombesin

- Calcitonin (thyrocalcitonin)

- Cerulein

- Cholecystokinin

- Enterogastrone

- Estrogen

- Gastrin-releasing peptide

- Glucagon

- Glycerol

- Lactate

- Naloxone

Furthermore, tryptophan administration has been associated with a reduction of appetite in depressed patients. Tryptophan supplements can inhibit gluconeogenesis, raise blood sugar, increase delivery of sugar to the brain, and decrease appetite. Thus, it may be a useful adjunct to therapy of hypoglycemia.

IMPORTANT METABOLITES

Among the substances produced as a result of tryptophan's metabolic process, 5-hydroxytryptophan (5-HTP) and melatonin are two of the most important.

5-Hydroxytryptophan

Interest in the tryptophan metabolite 5-hydroxytryptophan (5-HTP) exploded after tryptophan was banned from the market. 5-HTP is a substance that is created naturally in the body from the tryptophan. The body uses 5-HTP to manufacture the neurotransmitter serotonin. Due to its effects on serotonin levels, supplemental 5-HTP is often used as an antidepressant—although studies show it may not benefit everyone who takes it. 5-HTP is also an extremely expensive source of tryptophan. Supplemental 5-HTP is manufactured from the seeds of *Griffonia simplicifolia,* a plant native to western Africa.

The effects of this precursor of serotonin, administered intravenously, have been extensively studied. Doses of 150 to 200 mg of 5-HTP produce an elevation of serotonin in serum in depressed patients over a three-hour period with some psychomotor agitation and altered perception. Some depressed patients are nonresponders; many did not respond to this dose, nor did healthy control subjects. The greater the agitation with depression, the more likely the response.

5-HTP (100 mg three times a day) in combination with a peripheral decarboxylase inhibitor such as carbidopa (approximately 150 mg a day) has been found to be superior to placebo in the treatment of depression. The therapeutic potency of 5-HTP is comparable to the drug clomipramine (Anafranil). The therapeutic efficacy of 5-HTP combined with clomipramine is superior to that of either compound given separately.

Note: Studies in men have shown that 100 mg/kg of 5-HTP given orally can cause gastric irritation, vomiting, and head twitching. Women may have fewer side effects than men from 5-HTP, according to Lacoste and colleagues.

Melatonin

Melatonin (N-acetyl-5 methoxytryptamine) is both an amino acid and a hormone. It is derived from tryptophan by the action of two enzymes in the pineal gland. The pineal gland is a small, light-sensitive structure located in the center of the brain that is sometimes referred to as the "third eye." Dietary tryptophan is converted in the body to serotonin, which is then converted to melatonin by the enzymes N-acetyl-transferase and hydroxyindole-o-methyl transferase, which characterizes melatonin as a modified amino acid. In essence, melatonin is an amino acid that wears two hats.

Melatonin is one of the principal neurotransmitters and neurohormones in the body involved in regulating mood and sleep. The fact that it is a modified amino acid does not mean it cannot function as a hormone. Fatty acids such as fish-oil derivatives and prostaglandins work as neurohormones. Vitamin D, a steroid vitamin, works as a hormone. A neurotransmitter functions from neuron to neuron. A hormone operates from gland to gland.

Melatonin became big news overnight when its antiaging and sleep-promoting properties were ecstatically discovered by legions of older Americans and those with insomnia.

Melatonin production exerts a master regulatory role in the body's circadian rhythm—the body's twenty-four-hour internal clock, which controls sleep-wake cycles. The level of melatonin in the body rises and falls in a twenty-five-hour biological rhythm influenced by environmental lightness and darkness. Production begins in the evening, sometimes after dusk, sometimes around 8 P.M., and peaks at about midnight. Another peak occurs at around 4 A.M. and wanes in about two hours. Morning melatonin levels are low. Its most important contributions involve body temperature, hormone secretion, the onset of puberty, the sleep cycle, and the body's repair and rejuvenation activities when we sleep.

Abnormalities in melatonin occur in many low tryptophan diseases, such as low melatonin in anorexia (low nocturnal levels), hypertension, manic depression (in depressive phase), schizophrenia , and psoriasis (pre-pellagra). The long list of melatonin's therapeutic benefits—which we touch on briefly with the following—establishes this substance as an important amino acid metabolite in the ranks of nutritional supplementation. We believe there is even greater potential for this amino acid when used in combination with tryptophan.

Aging. Melatonin production declines as we age. By boosting the melatonin level with supplementation to quantities existing, say, at age thirty or forty, we may be able to increase our repair processes and coax our bodies into a younger mode. It appears that supplementation can reinvigorate the pineal gland and help maintain the function and weight of the thymus, thus deterring atrophy with age. Melatonin also acts to mildly stimulate growth hormone secretion from the pancreas.

The most dramatic scientific research on melatonin involved the animal studies of Regelson with Pierpaoli. In one such study, Regelson added melatonin to the drinking water of mice. The result was healthier and longer-living rodents. Translated into human years, they lived the equivalent of what would be thirty additional years for us.

There is always a danger in comparing laboratory animals in carefully controlled conditions with humans, who live widely variable lives enveloped in stress and increasingly toxic surroundings and who tend to make poor lifestyle choices. Can melatonin alone compensate for all the self-inflicted errors of living that tend to shorten our lives?

We don't think so. We believe that melatonin represents another important component discovered by medical science that can aid the rejuvenation process, another key piece in the puzzle of aging. In this respect, it holds the promise of benefits, just as many other factors do. It may eventually rank along with other nutrients and hormonal replacements: vitamin E for the heart, estrogen for the ovaries, DHEA for the adrenals, growth hormone for the pancreas, thyroid hormone for the thyroid gland, and antioxidants for the whole body. When we put all these and other techniques together, as we do in our clinic, we help rejuvenate many people.

Cancer. There is increasing evidence that melatonin may slow cancerous growths. Studies with both animals and humans suggest that a low dose of interleukin 2, (a white cell responsible for mobilizing neutrophils and lymphocytes in the immune system) when combined with high doses of 40 to 200 mg of melatonin may be beneficial even in advanced cases. Melatonin has an antiestrogen effect that may suppress growth of breast tumor cells. It may add to the potency of tamoxifen (Nolvadex)—a commonly used breast cancer drug that blocks the effects of naturally produced estrogen—and improve the regulation of antioxidant metabolism.

Depression. Light suppresses melatonin production in humans. In winter, when natural light is diminished, melatonin production increases. As a result, some individuals develop a seasonal depression called seasonal affective disorder (SAD). Interestingly, melatonin can be used to improve sleep, which in turn may relieve the depression. But it should be used cautiously. Too much melatonin may possibly worsen seasonal depression. We have seen this effect in some cases.

Exposure to early morning light, or to 2,500 to 10,000 lux under a full-spectrum light, may be another way to prevent or alleviate SAD.

During a winter depression, patients may appear to be bipolar type II, or to have temporal lobe disorder or atypical depression. This situation represents brain-chemical imbalance, similar to that seen in the elderly with low urinary melatonin metabolite secretion.

People taking serotonin antidepressants (such as fluoxetine, paroxetine, and sertraline) may experience better results from medication by taking supplements of a small amount of melatonin such as 3 mg. We have seen improvement after melatonin supplementation with numerous patients. However, it's best to be alert for possible sedation effect. If it occurs, cut back the amount of melatonin to 1 or 1.5 mg.

Electromagnetic Field Exposure. Increasing scientific evidence is pointing to a link between extremely low-frequency electromagnetic fields (ELF-EMF) and a variety of health problems. Greater exposure to magnetic fields is believed to heighten the risk of myeloid leukemia, brain cancer in children, altered hormonal production, and effects on the central nervous system, immune system, and the pineal gland.

Surrounded as we are by computer screens, electrical wires, and electronic appliances and devices, we are constantly exposed to various levels of ELF-EMF. It is advisable and prudent that as much as possible, individuals should restructure the placement of equipment in their offices, homes, and classrooms to minimize exposure. Through brain mapping (BEAM) and subsequent cranial electrotherapy stimulation (CES) treatment, we can correct abnormal brain rhythms that may be created by ELF-EMF.

Studies also suggest that electromagnetic fields damage the pineal gland and consequently affect melatonin secretion. For treatment, we recommend CES, antioxidants, and 500 mg of N-acetyl cysteine as a minimum program to reduce the effects of ELF-EMF radiation. After age forty, we suggest adding melatonin.

High Blood Pressure. Melatonin may have a role in lowering blood pressure, although we are not yet sure of the biochemical mechanism involved. An antihypertensive effect may result from melatonin's ability to promote relaxation, reduce stress, and help improve sleep. The same properties may be helpful in preventing stroke; however, more research is needed.

Insomnia. Melatonin is a natural, nonaddictive sleeping agent that can help many people with insomnia or individuals who want to enjoy deeper sleep. A study in the *British Medical Journal* identified sleep disorders in the elderly with abnormal melatonin rhythms. Melatonin deficiency appears to be a key element in this problem.

We recommend taking melatonin one half hour to two hours before bedtime. For many people, melatonin may take a while to start working. Keep in mind that the body's own melatonin production starts increasing around 8 P.M. If possible, you want to work in sync with nature so you are more likely to fall asleep and experience a deeper sleep. If you take melatonin much later, you might find yourself sleep-drunk in the morning as though it were 4 A.M. Supplemental melatonin can shift the entire sleep phase.

People with severe insomnia who have refused medication have found the solution in melatonin. One example is a seventy-year-old woman who stopped taking tranquilizers because they caused muscular weakness. With 10 mg of melatonin, she reported "sleeping like a baby." Many such cases are successfully resolved with 10 to 20 mg of melatonin. Others with severe anxiety or depression, personality disorders, and brain-mapping abnormalities usually require much larger doses.

Many patients also sleep "deeper" after taking melatonin. With 3 mg before bedtime, a fifty-year-old patient told me melatonin restored her "deep, beautiful sleep." Many patients report they feel invigorated in the morning upon arising.

The twenty-four-hour-sleep-rotating-cycle syndrome is the way we describe the situation where an individual's bedtime hour is progressively later each night. Such a person may go to bed one night at midnight, the next night at 2 A.M., the next at 4 A.M., and so on. An individual who falls into this errant pattern often develops a schizoid personality. It is believed that melatonin may help normalize sleep patterns in such cases and assist in reducing symptoms.

Melatonin is a generally safe and readily available supplement. We recommend doses of approximately 1 mg, starting at age forty, and then adding another 1 mg every ten years. A dose of 1 to 5 mg is usually effective for individuals without mental disorders. However, patients with serious disease, with chronic and severe sleeping disorders, anxiety, depression, or other psychiatric problems will require higher amounts. Some studies have utilized as much as 200 mg and more. In our clinic, we have seen substantial improvement only when higher doses in the range of 200 mg were used.

Jet Lag. When traveling across time zones, taking 3 to 5 mg of melatonin prior to bedtime after arrival may be helpful to minimize jet lag and associated symptoms. If nighttime waking occurs, another 3 to 5 mg can be taken to promote drowsiness. This approach can be used for several days to assist the body in resetting the biological clock. One young patient who took melatonin after arriving at a distant location reported sleeping eighteen hours the first night. He said his jet lag was minimal. We believe more research is needed on jet lag. Some individuals have reported feeling overly sedated after using 3 to 5 mg of melatonin.

Menstruation. Melatonin levels may be related to menstrual migraine. In one study, a low level of melatonin was found when headaches occurred. This suggests that some individuals who suffer from migraines associated with their menstrual cycles may benefit from supplementation. Melatonin has been found to be lower in women with symptoms of premenstrual syndrome (PMS). It may offer benefits for individuals seeking natural solutions to PMS.

Neurologically Disabled Children. In a study with fifteen neurologically disabled children, supplementation with 1 to 6 g of melatonin resulted in health, behavior, and social skill improvements. Although the results were preliminary, melatonin may be useful in treating brain-injured or disabled children.

Psychiatric Disorders. The use of melatonin treatment in psychiatry has been comprehensively reviewed; it has been found that some conditions respond with doses of melatonin as low as 1 mg. All patients on any of the serotonin antidepressants (such as fluoxetine, Zoloft and paroxetine) can be placed on melatonin.

Supplementation. We recommend using melatonin under the supervision of a health professional. Melatonin has a time-dependent hypnotic effect. By that we mean this substance can make you drowsy depending on when you take it. The time it takes to work varies among different people. Caution should be taken inasmuch as melatonin, if taken at the wrong time, sometimes can worsen depression, headaches, and sleeping problems.

Melatonin is available in various forms. We are opposed to using melatonin derived from animal pineal glands. We believe that all glandulars from animals contain microorganisms and impurities and are potentially toxic. Our recommendation is to use the pure synthetic form purchased at a reliable pharmacy. (We obtain melatonin from Hopewell Pharmacy in northern New Jersey at 800-792-6670, which guarantees purity. There are many compounding pharmacies around the country able to provide high-quality nutritional ingredients.)

Along with melatonin, we generally recommend that patients take 30 to 90 mg of zinc daily. Zinc may be necessary to maximize the production and benefits of melatonin, although this is not yet proven. Studies show that the enzymes that metabolize and store melatonin in the pineal gland are zinc-dependent.

We often use melatonin supplementation with cranial electrical stimulation (CES), a safe and gentle low-voltage electrical stimulation of the brain. CES enhances amino acid production and neurotransmitter activity. We apply the CES device over the third eye (the middle of the forehead) area to stimulate natural melatonin secretion. We believe this can assist in extending the active life of the pineal gland. CES and melatonin supplementation maximize benefits. We have used the two quite successfully for insomnia, anxiety, and depression.

TRYPTOPHAN LOADING

Infusions of tryptophan can raise serum tryptophan six to ten times in healthy people without apparent side effects. Oral loading healthy control subjects with 4 g of L-tryptophan can increase plasma levels up to four times normal within two hours. Twelve grams daily to manic patients can maintain plasma levels at three times normal. In one study, we loaded five healthy control subjects with 5 g (per 150 pounds) of L-tryptophan and measured plasma amino acids, trace metals, polyamines, and growth hormone. L-tryptophan levels in plasma nearly doubled at two hours and increased to four times normal at four hours—a significant change. In another study, seven patients were loaded with 2 g (per 150 pounds) of L-tryptophan for an average of six weeks. The mean tryptophan level for these patients was nearly double that of a control group of ninety-six patients—once again a significant difference.

SUPPLEMENTATION

Supplemental tryptophan is an important medical therapeutic agent but should not be taken without advice and/or biomedical testing by a physician. All other metabolites of tryptophan, except niacin, have significant side effects.

Deficiency Symptoms

Signs and symptoms of tryptophan deficiency include: apathy, liver damage, muscle loss, skin lesions, weakness, and slowed growth in children.

Availability

Tryptophan is currently available only by prescription; although an expensive substitute, 5-HTP, is available in 50 mg capsules.

Therapeutic Daily Amount

Typical dosages for tryptophan range from 50 mg to 3 g depending upon the symptoms being treated. Nutrients like pyridoxine and niacin can increase tryptophan's therapeutic action. For 5-HTP, a typical dose ranges from 300 mg to 600 mg, depending upon the condition being treated.

Maximum Safe Level

Not established.

Side Effects and Contraindications

Occasionally nausea can be experienced at doses higher than 3 g of L-tryptophan, but is usually resolved by gradually increasing the dose over a few days. People taking monoamine oxidase inhibitors (MAOIs) and selective serotonin reuptake inhibitors (SSRIs) should be cautious when taking L-tryptophan or 5-HTP, as they can increase the risk of central nervous system excitation.

TRYPTOPHAN: A SUMMARY

Tryptophan is an essential amino acid and the precursor of serotonin. Serotonin is a brain neurotransmitter, platelet-clotting factor, and neurohormone found in organs throughout the body. Metabolism of tryptophan to serotonin requires nutrients such as pyridoxine, niacin, and glutathione. Niacin is an important metabolite of tryptophan. High-corn or other tryptophan-deficient diets can cause pellagra, which is a niacin-tryptophan deficiency disease with symptoms of dermatitis, diarrhea, and dementia.

Inborn errors of tryptophan metabolism exist where a tumor (carcinoid) makes excess serotonin. Hartnup's disease is a disorder in which tryptophan and other amino acids are not absorbed properly. Tryptophan supplements may be useful in each condition, in carcinoid replacing the over-metabolized nutrient and in Hartnup's supplementing a malabsorbed nutrient. Some disorders of excess tryptophan in the blood may contribute to mental retardation.

Assessment of tryptophan deficiency is done through studying excretion of tryptophan metabolites in the urine or blood. Blood may be the most sensitive test because the amino acid tryptophan is transported in a unique way. Increased urination of tryptophan fragments correlates with increased tryptophan degradation, which occurs with oral contraception, depression, mental retardation, hypertension, and anxiety states.

The requirement for tryptophan and protein decreases with age. The minimum daily requirement for adults is 3 mg/kg per day or about 200 mg of L-tryptophan a day. This may be an underestimation, for there are 400 mg of L-tryptophan in just a cup of wheat germ. A cup of low-fat cottage cheese contains 300 mg of L-tryptophan and chicken and turkey contain up to 600 mg per pound.

Tryptophan supplements of up to 3 g a day have been used to control intractable pain in various conditions. Furthermore, tryptophan supplements decrease aggressive behavior. Abnormalities in tryptophan metabolism occur in aggressive mentally retarded patients. Increased violent crimes occur in areas where tryptophan-deficient corn is a major dietary staple. Pyridoxine and tryptophan supplements can correct some of the biochemical disorders related to aggression. Drugs that increase the opposite neurotransmitter, dopamine—that is, phenelzine or bromocriptine—can produce rage reactions, as do drugs that inhibit pyridoxine, for example, isoniazid, which inhibits metabolism of tryptophan to niacin.

Tryptophan is also a useful treatment for insomnia, significantly reducing the time needed to fall asleep. Effective doses range from 500 to 2,000 mg. Disorders of REM sleep may require doses of 3 to 15 g.

Suicidal patients show a significant decrease in serotonin levels. These patients, as well as agitated, depressed patients, do well with tryptophan supplements. Most antidepressants prolong the effects of serotonin by preventing reuptake of this neurotransmitter, as well as the reuptake of catecholamine. Tryptophan at night and tyrosine in the morning can probably mimic the effects of most antidepressants. Levels of the neurotransmitters are directly dependent on dietary tryptophan and other amino acids.

Tryptophan has many other reported desirable effects. Appetite for carbohydrates is decreased and blood sugar is raised by tryptophan supplements. It stimulates growth hormone and prolactin, which is the basis of some of tryptophan's therapeutic effects.

Tryptophan is also beneficial in some forms of schizophrenia; it probably acts by balancing dopamine excess. In Parkinson's disease, it inhibits tremor, and possibly also in progressive myoclonic epilepsy. Patients with kidney failure, on birth control pills, or with Down's syndrome may need more tryptophan.

Chronic tryptophan supplementation (minimum 2 g daily), like supplementation with other amino acids, raises many plasma amino acids besides tryptophan itself. This is positive and exciting because many amino acids tend to decrease with age.

SECTION THREE

Sulfur Amino Acids

CYSTEINE
The Detoxifier

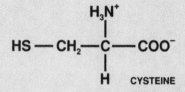

$$HS - CH_2 - \overset{\overset{\displaystyle H_3N^+}{|}}{\underset{\underset{\displaystyle H}{|}}{C}} - COO^-$$

CYSTEINE

HOMOCYSTEINE
The Predictor of Heart Disease

$$^-OOC - \overset{}{\underset{\underset{\displaystyle H_3N^+}{|}}{CH}} - CH_2 - CH_2$$

TAURINE
The Seizure Fighter

$$NH_3 - CH_2 - CH_2SO_3H$$

METHIONINE
The Antidepressant

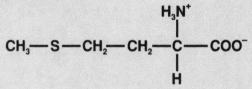

$$CH_3 - S - CH_2 - CH_2 - \overset{\overset{\displaystyle H_3N^+}{|}}{\underset{\underset{\displaystyle H}{|}}{C}} - COO^-$$

CHAPTER FIVE

Methionine: The Antidepressant

Methionine is a crucial essential amino acid that brings methyl groups and sulfur into the body, and as such is the first amino acid incorporated into proteins. It acts as a code breaker, initiating translation of the genetic blueprint sent by deoxyribonucleic acid (DNA) via the messenger ribonucleic acid (RNA), which carries instructions for making new body protein. It is required for the formation of body tissues and amino acids and for antioxidant and detoxification processes.

Methionine, like its sulfur derivative glutathione, is thought to be among the first organic substances on Earth. In early experiments on the origin of life, methionine was found to be a product of the action of a spark discharge in a simulated primitive earth atmosphere containing (CH_4), (N_2), (NH_3), oxygen (H_2O), (H_2S), and (CH_3SH). More proof of methionine's primitive ancestry has been gleaned from studies of methyl groups and bacteria, also one of the earliest representatives of life. Methionine is thought to donate a methyl group to dozens of substances in bacteria.

Unfortunately, human beings unlike bacteria, cannot make methionine from aspartic acid. As organisms living in harmony with bacteria, we are able to absorb some methionine—but not enough—from our bacterial flora, and therefore must rely on diet for our source of this important amino acid.

FUNCTION

Despite methionine's critical role as a catalyst for important metabolic processes in the body, it has a relatively low profile and is not present in high concentrations throughout the body. Although methionine passes the blood-brain barrier easily, it is not particularly high in the human brain; glutamic acid, glutamine, aspartic acid, alanine, glycine, serine, and taurine well exceed it in concentration. Nor is methionine high in muscle, where its content is low to average compared to other amino acids. A low level of methionine is also found in cerebrospinal fluid.

Methionine performs three major roles in the body—it is a sulfur donor, a methyl donor, and an essential precursor of the important sulfur amino acids cysteine, glutathione, and taurine.

Methionine is the most abundant sulfur-containing amino acid and the principal supplier of sulfur to man and animals. This chemical property enables methionine to initiate translation of the DNA instructions for which of the body's 50,000 proteins are needed and where. Table 5.1 lists some of the important sulfur-containing compounds of which methionine is a component. Among them are the naturally occurring, pain-relieving peptides, enkephalins and endorphins, which contribute to methionine's well-documented antidepressive action. Methionine's high sulfur content helps supply the body with the acidity it needs to stave off chronic disease states that may result when the body's alkaline-to-acid ratio is too high.

As a methyl donor, methionine combines with adenosine triphosphate (ATP), the body's energy molecule, to form active methionine. This compound then contributes a methyl group to the biosynthesis of a number of other important sulfur-containing compounds. Some of these substances are listed in Table 5.1.

One of the more important substances produced as a result of transmethylation (the chemical process of adding a methyl group to a compound) is the antidepressant S-adenosyl-L-methionine (SAMe). Studies have shown SAMe is as effective as the major antidepressants clomipramine (Anafranil) and amitriptyline (Elavil). SAMe can also serve as a methyl donor for a host of methylation reactions similar to methionine. Excessive methylation has been implicated with schizophrenia, psychosis, and disease related to depression. Methyl groups can turn normal brain constituents into hallucinatory substances. In contrast, defi-

TABLE 5.1. COMPOUNDS WITH METHYL GROUPS DERIVED FROM METHIONINE

METHYL GROUP		SULFUR GROUPS
Anserine	Epinephrine	Cysteine
Betaine	Ergosterol	Glutathione
Carnitine	Melatonin	Enkephalins
Choline	Morphine	Endorphins
Cobalamin (vitamin B_{12})	Nicotine	Taurine
Codeine	Pectin	
Creatinine	S-adenosyl-L-methionine (SAMe)	

cient methylation has been implicated in depressive disorders for which SAMe has been used successfully. (For more on SAMe, see "Depression" on page 92.)

From methionine, cysteine, glutathione, and taurine—the body's most powerful antioxidants and detoxifiers—are created. Methionine is also thought to boost levels of all amino acids in the body. Its presence is also vital for the absorption and transportation of the minerals selenium and zinc, and for the formation of choline, a member of the B family of vitamins, that is contained in lecithin and is vital for making the neurotransmitter acetylcholine.

METABOLISM

Methionine, like all the sulfur amino acids, needs adequate amounts of pyridoxine (vitamin B_6), cyanocobalamin (vitamin B_{12}), and folic acid in order to be properly metabolized. Methionine metabolism results in the production of important sulfur-containing nutrients that are necessary to provide adequate and optimal functioning of the cardiovascular, skeletal, and nervous systems such as coenzyme A.

Methionine metabolism is subject to many impairments. Among them is the production of homocysteine. This naturally-occurring, sulfur-containing amino acid, is produced only after ingestion of methionine, which is most commonly in animal proteins. Homocysteine's own metabolic breakdown typical occurs either through remethylation, which regenerates methionine, or trans-sulfuration, which degrades homocysteine into cysteine and then taurine.

Homocysteine is not toxic to the body's systems when present in small amounts. However, when excessive methionine has been consumed and inadequate amounts of pyridoxine, cyanocobalamin, and folic acid are available to convert homocysteine into cysteine or taurine, then homocysteine remains circulating and becomes toxic.

This toxicity is expressed by promoting damage to the epithelial cells that line the circulatory system, encouraging the formation of fibrous plaques that sequester circulating fatty deposits and cellular debris, narrowing the available flow space for blood. This increases the risk for coronary artery disease and arteriosclerosis. We'll talk more about this potentially toxic amino acid in Chapter Six.

Not only are adequate stores of pyridoxine, cyanocobalamin, and folic acid critical for proper methionine metabolism, if depleted, they can throw out of balance the urea cycle amino acids, arginine and ornithine, and lead to the production of polyamines—amino acid compounds that promote the growth of cells, including possibly cancer cells.

REQUIREMENTS

The minimum daily requirement recommended by the National Academy of Sciences for methionine and cysteine is 49 mg/kg for infants, ages four to six months, 22 mg/kg for children, ages one to twelve, and 10 mg/kg for adults. Coauthor Cheraskin and colleagues of the University of Alabama agree with this recommendation although they point out that these may not be the optimal doses.

Minimum requirements for the sulfur-containing amino acids have been reported by investigators to be as high as 1,400 mg per day. The WHO committee established a tentative requirement for all sulfur amino acids (mainly methionine) of 13 mg/kg per day or 910 mg of these amino acids daily for the average 150 lb adult male. Optimal levels of dietary methionine vary greatly from individual to individual. Homocysteine and bacterial flora production can substitute for the requirement for this amino acid in some people.

FOOD SOURCES

In addition to animal foods such as eggs, fish, milk, and meat, sunflower seeds are an excellent good source of methionine (See Table 5.2 on page 89). In contrast, soybeans are very deficient in methionine. According to Fomon and colleagues, methionine is the limiting nutrient in the popular soy-based infant formulas. They found superior results in methionine-supplemented, soy-based formulas. Nonetheless, a human-tinkered formula does not yet equal human breast milk. Another popular baby food, oatmeal, is also deficient in all sulfur amino acids.

An average egg yolk contains 0.165 percent elemental sulfur, which means 165 mg of sulfur per 100 g of yolk. The sulfur amino acids methionine and cysteine account for 91 percent of the sulfur in the yolk, with approximately equal amounts of each. The body needs 850 mg of sulfur each day. The whole egg contains 67 mg of sulfur or 8 percent of the daily need. Sulfur in these amounts is not readily found in any other food.

Although we are just beginning to understand the repercussions of methionine deficiencies in humans, animal studies show that a diet specifically deficient in methionine causes premature atherosclerosis in experimental monkeys. Studies have found that excess methionine with pyridoxine deficiency increased arteriosclerosis and elevated triglycerides.

Rats fed methionine-deficient diets for seven to fourteen days showed a profound increase in the blood concentration of spermidine, yet the total levels of other polyamines and SAMe were not significantly altered in the liver. This polyamine profile (increased spermidine) resembles profiles observed during all repair of regenerative processes. Diets deficient in methionine result in nitrogen retention and cause catabolism or destructive metabolism of protein.

According to Colin, rabbits fed methionine-deficient diets show impaired growth. Sulfur amino acids must make up 6.5 percent of the diet to be adequate for rabbits. Feed efficiency (better use of calories) is achieved by this balanced diet.

TABLE 5.2. METHIONINE LEVELS IN FOOD		
FOOD	AMOUNT	CONTENT (GRAMS)
Avocado	1	0.70
Cheese	1 ounce	0.17
Chicken	1 pound	0.65
Chocolate	1 cup	0.20
Cottage cheese	1 cup	0.20
Duck	1 pound	0.85
Egg	1	0.20
Granola	1 cup	0.20
Luncheon meat	1 pound	1.30
Oatmeal	1 cup	0.20
Pork	1 pound	1.80
Ricotta	1 cup	0.70
Sausage meat	1 pound	0.90
Turkey	1 pound	0.90
Wheat germ	1 cup	0.63
Whole milk	1 cup	0.20
Wild game	1 pound	2.40
Yogurt	1 cup	0.23

FORM AND ABSORPTION

Methionine is available in L- and DL- forms. It is the only amino acid besides phenylalanine that is used in DL- form. Both L-methionine and DL-methionine can be used interchangeably with SAMe. Oral and intravenous supplementation with L- and DL-methionine have proved more effective than SAMe in elevating SAMe levels in the brain. This is because methionine crosses the blood-brain barrier easily with little resistance from other amino acids. In addition, methionine not only improves absorption of tyrosine and phenylalanine, but is also best absorbed by the brain when taken in conjunction with these two aromatic amino acids. Methionine also helps to boost serotonin metabolism in the brain.

D-methionine is utilized by cats but seems to be poorly utilized in humans and monkeys, where it may be excreted essentially unchanged in the urine. Ironically, the DL- form was found to be more effective in lowering histamine, a substance that plays a central role in allergic reactions, than L- or D- forms. Perhaps because of DL salt formation, the DL- form was also more effective than the L-

Methionine Is Key to Healthy Folate Levels

The relationship between methionine and folic acid deficiency has been a subject of controversy for years. When the body is deficient in methionine, the liver will only metabolize histidine to form inoglutamate, an incomplete form of folic acid. From this information, researchers have concluded that methionine is a key factor in regulating the availability of folate—the natural form of folic acid found in food—and is not utilized properly when methionine is lacking. Dark green leafy vegetables and whole-grain products are good sources that are abundantly available.

When methionine levels are low, folate becomes trapped in the liver. This also occurs in cyanocobalamin (vitamin B_{12}) deficiency. Spector and colleagues have further identified the metabolic relationship of methionine, cyanocobalamin, and folate in the brain. Thus, a deficiency in methionine can cause temporary folic acid deficiency because the folic acid can't be used.

It appears that dietary protein restriction of methionine and other amino acids results in alterations in the activity of folate methionine pathway enzymes. Tissues in kidney and spleen are affected first. The liver and brain are spared, however, demonstrating that an organ hierarchy is formed during nutritional deficiencies so that the body's "more important" organs are often saved from damage.

form in reversing central nervous system effects of barbiturates. The DL- isomer form may be more lipid-soluble, according to infrared studies, and may be better absorbed into the brain.

Methionine in the form of selenomethionine is effective at removing parasites from animals.

TOXICITY

Mitchell and Benevenga claim that methionine is the most toxic of the amino acids. Rats on a 5 percent—approximately 50 percent of total dietary protein—methionine supplemented diet show signs of toxicity. However, the human equivalent for an average 150 lb adult male is about 25 g daily. At this large dose, L-methionine produced reduced growth and food consumption and caused hyperactivity, and iron accumulation in the spleen of growing rats. Hematocrit may be lowered. Levels approximately equivalent to 5 g daily in humans may increase iron absorption. Other effects are under investigation.

Anagnostou and colleagues showed that methionine can stimulate erythropoietin, the formation of red blood cells, in rats under certain conditions.

Ekperigin found that 1.5 percent methionine fed to broiler chickens reduced feeding, body weight, hemoglobin, and hematocrit; increased the level of iron in liver and spleen (hemosiderosis); damaged the pancreas, and caused ataxia (loss of ability to coordinate muscle movement).

Similar growth depression occurs when an excess of tyrosine is given. An excess of any amino acid causes an imbalance in protein synthesis, resulting in a homeostatic defense that signals the body to *stop eating*! For example, methionine and threonine are particularly effective in reversing tyrosine toxicity, according to Yamamoto and colleagues, but a beneficial effect has also been achieved with cystine, glycine, tryptophan, and mixtures of branched-chain amino acids. Supplementation of any amino acid can partially correct excess of another, although some are theoretically better for this purpose than others. For example, glycine or serine could reverse methionine toxicity. The level of glycine or serine required is two times the quantity of methionine in cases where methionine is, in low-protein diets, at three to five times its requirement.

High doses of methionine increase urinary calcium excretion, which can be hazardous in osteoporosis, especially for women not taking adequate calcium supplementation.

Doses of 1 to 3 g of methionine have been almost completely without side effects. Idiosyncratic reactions almost completely are reported where methionine is not tolerated; some people may experience intestinal gas on doses as low as 500 mg. DL-methionine doses of 8 to 12 g daily have been shown to affect clotting factors after prolonged therapy. Large doses (20 g) produce hallucinations in some schizophrenic patients.

CLINICAL USES

The group of sulfur amino acids is chemically distinct from other groups of amino acids because they contain a sulfur molecule. The sulfur combines with hydrogen molecules to become a powerful antioxidant that fights free radicals throughout the body. In nearly all conditions, L- and DL-methionine may be used interchangeably with SAMe.

Acrodermatitis Enteropathica

Methionine helps prevent and treat disorders of the hair, skin, and nails. Intravenous methionine and/or intravenous amino acids can temporarily reverse acrodermatitis enteropathica, a rare familial condition that typically begins at the fourth month of life and is thought to be a disorder primarily of zinc metabolism. The most common manifestations are erosions of skin around the mouth, nails, eyelids, anus, genital areas, elbows, knees, and ankles.

Severe paronychia (separation and inflammation of the nail bed) in this condition may lead to loss of nails, alopecia (hair loss), and thrush (a fungal infection of the mouth), which frequently affects the eroded areas. Respiratory infections and diarrhea are common, and malabsorption (particularly of zinc) may occur.

Zinc in combination with methionine is found to be a more useful therapy than zinc alone.

Alzheimer's Disease

Recent studies have shown that methionine is severely decreased in people with Alzheimer's disease and in various forms of depression.

Cancer

Recent studies have shown that methionine and folic acid can prevent cancer because of the benefits of the sulfur amino acid in the diet. It appears that methionine may prevent polyps in the colon from progressing into a cancer state.

Like that of so many nutrients, methionine metabolism differs significantly in people with cancer than in healthy individuals. Cancers seem to require more methionine for transmethylation and synthesis of polyamines, a predisposing factor for cancer growth. Too much methionine may raise levels of some toxic polyamines; therefore, methionine supplementation should be used with caution by cancer patients.

Coronary Vascular Disease

Pyridoxine deficiency is a strong factor in the production of cardiovascular disease. Methionine and pyridoxine are essential for normal homocysteine metabolism and are mild cholesterol-lowering agents. Methionine in high doses without pyridoxine is toxic to blood vessels, because homocysteine may build up in the vessels and cause damage to the lining of blood vessels, weakening and exposing them to the accumulation of plaque. With adequate pyridoxine, this is not a hazard.

Depression

Methionine's antidepressive action is greater than that of any of the other sulfur amino acids. Most studies of depression have been conducted with the modified form of methionine: S-adenosyl methionine or SAMe.

Agnoli and colleagues found that daily intramuscular administration of 45 mg of SAMe had a beneficial effect on depressed mood, suicidal tendencies, intellectual sluggishness, and performance. Improvement occurred in 80 percent of the cases in four to six days. According to Sacchetti and colleagues, circadian rhythms and sex may influence SAMe levels.

Reynolds and colleagues of Kings College, England, reviewed the data in support of methionine's antidepressant properties, and they concluded that methionine as SAMe is as effective as the major antidepressants clomipramine (Anafranil) and amitriptyline (Elavil).

We have used SAMe in low dosages to treat depression. More routinely, we use the familiar DL-methionine form in connection with our Brain Energy Formula containing tyrosine and phenylalanine since methionine improves the absorption of both these amino acids. Tyrosine and phenylalanine help to relieve depression by raising norepinephrine levels.

We have monitored methionine levels in patients at our clinic taking methionine. People taking 1 to 2 g of L-methionine for high blood histamine depression showed levels as high as two to four times normal after one or two months. These elevated levels were without side effects and may be the basis for methionine's therapeutic effects. Even minimal doses of L-methionine (500 mg) usually raise plasma levels to one and a half to three times normal.

Drug Dependence

De Maio and colleagues reported that methionine was useful in reducing withdrawal and depressive symptoms during heroin withdrawal. Coauthor Pfeiffer has suggested that heroin addicts tend to be high-histamine individuals who seek relief from their continued painful state by the use of drugs like heroin. L-methio-

Methionine Controls High Blood Histamine Depression

A sixty-year-old woman with histadelic (high histamine) depression and a history of alcoholism came to our clinic for help. Married with three children, she stated that her skin burned with ordinary sunlight exposure, she had no dream recall, and she was anorexic—her first meal of the day was dinner. She was allergic to animal hair and was taking 200 mg a day of chlorpromazine (Thorazine) with 2 mg of biperiden (Akineton) in the morning and in the evening. She had been given trials of all the tranquilizers. Her symptoms of depression worsened with the onset of menopause at age fifty-one; three years of psychiatric care provided no relief.

Her histamine levels on her first three visits to the clinic were 138, 140, 155; (normal levels are between 40 to 70). Her serum copper levels measured 133, 152, 144 on the first three visits; serum zinc was 81, 144, and 219, reflecting the need for therapy with zinc, manganese, and pyridoxine to correct pyridoxine and zinc deficiency. With this protocol, she experienced dream recall and some relief of her depression. With the addition of 500 mg of L-methionine in the morning and in the evening and 500 mg of calcium in the morning and in the evening, the depression was sufficiently relieved to allow her to stop taking the chlorpromazine. The patient gained employment in a school cafeteria, a job that she still holds. The antidepressant phenytoin sodium (Dilantin) further lowered her high histamine level.

nine's ability to reduce histamine may be the reason for its value in helping heroin addicts. Rats administered 1 mg/kg of intravenous DL-methionine resulted in a 50 percent reversal of the barbiturate pentobarbital (Nembutal)-induced sedation. Taylor found that supplemental methionine decreased the effects of amphetamine on stereotypical behavior in rats.

We have found that methionine in combination with antioxidants, dopamine agents, and tyrosine is the most effective treatment for people attempting to break an addiction to drugs. This protocol is also useful for alcohol addiction.

Parkinson's Disease

Methionine is well-absorbed in the brain where it is converted to SAMe, which can increase adrenalinelike neurotransmitters. Stramentinoli and colleagues supplemented L-methionine and found that of the three neurotransmitters dopamine, norepinephrine, and serotonin, the latter showed the most significant change. Serotonin in telencephalic areas showed a significant increase.

SAMe is one of several body transmethylating substances and is the methyl donor for the conversion of L-dopa to dopamine. Administration of SAMe by Bidard and colleagues produced a change in the urinary ratio of methyldopa to L-dopa. They suggested that SAMe increases the peripheral metabolism of L-dopa. Administration of 100 mg/kg of L-dopa in animals reduced SAMe by 76 percent in the brain and 51 percent in the adrenals, although levels were unchanged in the liver. According to Bidard and colleagues, SAMe's pro-dopamine effect may make methionine an adjunct treatment for Parkinson's disease.

Plasma Levels and Clinical Syndromes

About 15 percent of the people who come to our clinic have low plasma methionine levels. Fifty percent of these people have major depression. In addition, at least two of these patients had kidney disease, two had prolonged illness, two had been institutionalized, one had epilepsy, one had schizophrenia, and one had narcolepsy. One depressed patient's test actually showed no detectable methionine.

Radiation Exposure

Like other sulfur amino acids, methionine has been reported to be beneficial against the toxic effects of radiation and heavy metals. Some essential nutritional elements such as arsenic, chromium, iron, cobalt, molybdenum, and selenium are toxic at high levels or when combined with a methyl group). This is because when methionine is converted to glutathione it becomes a major antioxidant, antiradiation compound.

Schizophrenia

We have successfully used methionine as therapy for schizophrenia. Methionine lowers blood histamine and may also affect histamine metabolism in the brain. Methionine is most successful in those people with schizophrenia who are also depressed (about 20 percent).

Pfeiffer and Iliev demonstrated that either 1.2 g of L-methionine or 1.5 g of DL-methionine lowers blood histamine significantly. Methylation is one pathway by which histamine is degraded and removed from the body. Methionine decreased the intestinal absorption and cell transport of the essential amino acid histidine. One percent methionine in the diet of rats—approximately 10 percent of dietary protein—can result in increased concentration of serum copper. Copper activates the enzyme diamine oxidase, which degrades histamine.

Sluggish Gallbladder

Frezza and colleagues made the remarkable discovery that intrahepatic cholestasis (a sluggish gallbladder) could be reversed in women with 800 mg of SAMe a day. SAMe may also reverse the gallbladder stasis of pregnancy and ameliorate the hazardous effects of estrogen on gallbladder functions.

Urinary Tract Disorders

Methionine appears to protect the urinary tract by regulating the formulation of ammonia and preventing bacteria from adhering to the wall of the bladder. Methionine in doses of 1 to 2 g orally has been reported to be helpful in preventing condyloma acuminata verruccae (vaginal warts) and laryngeal papilloma. Higher doses near 5 g acidify the urine and have been helpful in patients with stubborn urinary tract infections.

METHIONINE LOADING

Loading studies using 5 g of methionine per 150 pounds raise methionine levels to six times normal at two hours, five times normal at four hours, and decrease slowly thereafter. The side effects reported are increased urination and palpitations. These common side effects probably do not occur in individuals undergoing continuous supplementation of 500 to 2,000 mg of methionine. This dose of methionine may lower several other amino acids, for example, leucine, isoleucine, valine, phenylalanine, tyrosine, and tryptophan, during acute loading. High methionine doses lower iron levels slightly, but this, too, does not occur with prolonged nutrition therapy of 500 to 2,000 mg of methionine daily. Methionine supplementation rarely has side effects.

Plasma methionine levels are both useful and accurate in assessing methionine deficiency and response to therapy because they tend to rise quickly with treatment.

SUPPLEMENTATION

Deciding whether to use L- or DL-methionine versus S-adenosyl-L-methionine (SAMe) is dependent upon the condition being treated. Methionine supplements, for example, have proved more effective than SAMe in elevating SAMe levels in brain. In general, however, these forms can be used interchangeably.

Deficiency Symptoms

Signs and symptoms of methionine deficiency include loss of pigmentation in hair, edema, lethargy, liver damage, muscle and fat loss, skin lesions, and slowed growth in children.

Availability

Methionine is available as L-methionine, DL-methionine, or SAMe. It can be found in its free form and DL- form in 500 mg capsules and as SAMe in 25 mg tablets.

Therapeutic Daily Amount

Doses for L- and DL-methionine may range from 1 to 3 g depending upon the condition being treated; the typical therapeutic dose of SAMe is 400 mg taken 3–4 times a day.

Maximum Safe Level

Not established.

Side Effects and Contraindications

When taking methionine, it is critical to take an adequate amount of pyridoxine (vitamin B_6). If not enough pyridoxine is present, some methionine will convert into toxic homocysteine. It can also lead to the production of polyamines, amino acid compounds that promote the growth of cells, including, possibly, cancerous cells.

METHIONINE: A SUMMARY

Claims for methionine in medicine were initiated by Adelle Davis (1970), who suggested that methionine was deficient in toxemia of pregnancy, childhood rheumatic fever, and hair loss. Today, we see a more defined role for methionine as a treatment for some forms of depression, schizophrenia, and Parkinson's disease.

Methionine is one of the essential amino acids needed by humans and higher animals; bacteria can make it from aspartic acid. Some methionine may be absorbed from the bacteria of the gut flora under starvation conditions. The average human needs about 10 mg/kg of methionine and cysteine or as much as 700 mg a day of methionine. This minimal daily requirement is significantly less than the optimal need for methionine.

Methionine-deficient diets in experimental animals result in impaired growth and elevated blood spermidine. Normal methionine metabolism depends on the utilization of folic acid that can be elevated in the serum of methionine-deficient patients. Some foods are rich in methionine. A cup of low-fat cottage cheese can contain up to a gram of methionine. Most cheeses contain 100 to 200 mg per ounce.

Methionine supplements lower blood histamine by increasing the breakdown of histamine. It is also a useful treatment for copper poisoning and for lowering serum copper. Methionine's three major metabolic roles are as methyl donor, sulfur donor, and a precursor to other sulfur amino acids such as cysteine and taurine.

Methionine supplementation is unusual because the DL- form is probably more effective than just the L- form. This is probably due to DL-salt formation. Methionine is well absorbed in the brain where it is converted into SAMe, which can increase adrenalinelike neurotransmitters in the brain. Methionine, the methyl donor, may produce active brain stimulants and degrade blood histamine. Methionine supplementation has been particularly useful in depressing the high-histamine type (histadelia). It has been found to be more effective than MAO inhibitors in depression.

Methionine is a useful adjunct therapy in some cases of Parkinson's disease, because it can stimulate the production of dopa. Methionine may be of value in acrodermatitis enteropathica, a rare disease of zinc deficiency. Methionine, like other sulfur amino acids, protects against the effects of radiation.

Methionine supplementation may help patients with an addiction to heroin, who often are unusually high in histamine and have a low pain threshold. Detoxification and withdrawal from barbiturates or amphetamines may also be assisted by methionine. Methionine may be useful for patients with chronic pain and is thought to lower blood cholesterol.

At present, we use methionine for patients with high blood histamine, depression, high copper, high cholesterol, chronic pain, allergies, and asthma. Measurement of plasma levels is useful for guiding therapy. Doses of 1 to 2 g of methionine can raise plasma methionine levels two to four times above normal.

There are usually small elevations in other amino acids. We have had one case where taurine levels were raised as high as the methionine levels and other cases where taurine was not significantly elevated. Elevated levels of taurine, a methionine metabolite, is a hidden benefit of methionine therapy. These elevations may be the basis of methionine's therapeutic effects.

CHAPTER SIX

Homocysteine: The Predictor of Heart Disease

H omocysteine is an amino acid metabolite that is created naturally in the body from the essential amino acid methionine. This sulfur-containing amino acid occurs only transiently during methionine metabolism before being converted to the amino acid cysteine. The conversion of dietary methionine to homocysteine is controlled by enzyme systems that require pyridoxine (vitamin B_6), cyanocobalamin (vitamin B_{12}), and folic acid. Homocysteine is harmless when present in small amounts; however, when excessive methionine is consumed and inadequate levels of pyridoxine, cyanocobalamin, and folic acid are present in the body to process it, homocysteine builds up and becomes toxic.

This toxicity is expressed by promoting damage to the epithelial cells that line the circulatory system, encouraging the formation of fibrous plaques, which sequester circulating fatty deposits and cellular debris, narrowing the available flow for blood, thereby increasing the risk of numerous cardiovascular diseases, including arteriosclerosis, coronary artery disease, stroke, atherosclerosis, and peripheral vascular disease.

With our understanding of homocysteine, we have finally gone beyond cholesterol, which has proven to be an unreliable predictor of cardiovascular disease, to locate a potent indicator. Many individuals with premature and accelerated forms of cardiovascular disease have elevated levels of homocysteine. The data to support this is so strong that elevated homocysteine, hyperhomocysteinemia, is now considered a major independent risk factor for the development of arteriosclerosis, joining the ranks of hyperlipidemia, hypertension, and smoking.

FUNCTION

Homocysteine is needed to make methionine's most useful metabolites, cysteine and glutathione. As such, it provides a critical chemical link in the transformation of methionine from which cysteine and glutathione, the body's two most powerful natural antioxidants, are eventually derived. An adequate intake of pyridoxine, cyanocobalamin, and folic acid prevent an excess accumulation of this important breakdown product.

Homocysteine is easily measured in the blood, where most of it is oxidized to homocystine, the double-bonded form of homocysteine. Since it was discovered that elevated homocysteine levels increase the risk of heart blockages, heart attacks, and stroke, numerous other disease conditions have been found to exhibit high levels of homocysteine, increasing its importance as a biomarker for health problems.

METABOLISM

Homocysteine metabolism, like the metabolism of all the sulfur amino acids, is dependent upon pyridoxine, cyanocobalamin, and folic acid. It is produced in the body only after eating foods containing methionine. Methionine is most commonly found in animal proteins. Adequate intakes of folic acid, cyanocobalamin, and particularly pyridoxine prevent a toxic buildup of homocysteine. However, numerous surveys of American dietary intake reflect seriously low intake of these nutrients. Unfortunately, many people shun dark green leafy vegetables and whole-grain products that are rich in pyridoxine, cyanocobalamin, and especially folic acid. Supplementation also provides an inexpensive way of getting these nutrients.

The nutrient pyridoxine mediates control of homocysteine metabolism. It may possibly serve as an essential component that acts as the "on-off switch" in the autoregulation of homocysteine synthesis. The addition of excess pyridoxine would, in this hypothesis, permit the homocystine-pyridoxine complex to turn off the defective regulator gene responsible for activating homocystine synthesis.

There is a known stimulatory effect of pyridoxine on other pyridoxine-linked enzymes involved in sulfur amino acid metabolism, specifically the enzyme cystathionine synthase. Extensive research indicates that at least 10 percent of the population suffers—many unknowingly—from an inborn error of homocysteine metabolism called cystathionine betasynthase deficiency or homocystinuria. This liver enzyme converts homocysteine to cystathionine, which is further processed in the liver to cysteine. People with this genetic defect have a 50 to 100-fold elevation in homocysteine blood levels and excrete large amounts of homocysteine in the urine. In addition to causing widespread arterial damage, this enzymatic disorder can affect the eyes (ectopia, myopia), skeletal system (osteoporosis), and the central nervous system (mental retardation).

Chances of homocysteine being present at high levels also increase with a family history of heart disease, using tobacco, being over age fifty, being menopausal, or living a lifestyle that has little to no exercise.

REQUIREMENTS

People and nonruminant mammals (those that don't chew their cud) form homocysteine only from methionine, which is a constituent of all dietary protein. Some researchers have claimed that homocysteine can substitute partially for the daily dietary methionine requirement.

FOOD SOURCES

Homocysteine is a normal breakdown product from the ingestion of methionine-containing foods. Methionine is found in large quantities in all animal protein such as meat and dairy products. (See Table 5.2 on page 89.) Dietary sugar and a diet low in fresh fruits and vegetables help to increase homocysteine levels.

CLINICAL USES

Clinically, the elevation of homocysteine in the blood performs an important function not only as a indicator of heart blockages, heart attacks, and stroke, but also of depression, psychosis, diabetes, kidney failure, neural tube defects, sickle cell disease, cervical dysplasia, HIV, cognitive impairment, and even the progression of some cancers. Low antioxidant levels, copper excess, folic acid deficiency, and inborn errors of methionine metabolism can also be telltale signs of high homocysteine levels.

Cardiovascular Disease

The first indication that homocysteine metabolism may play an important role in arteriosclerosis was discovered by Gibson and colleagues of Queens University of Belfast in 1964. They noticed that a patient with homocystinuria had vascular lesions similar to those found in Marfan's syndrome (a genetic disorder marked by mild mental retardation and tall stature caused by rapid growth in childhood accompanied by long legs, arms, fingers, and toes), with medical degeneration of the aorta and arteries due to thrombosis. There are scientific studies describing coronary and carotid artery occlusion and renal artery sclerosis, as well as livedo reticularis (purple mottling of skin)—a sign of circulatory failure with the homocystinuria of Marfan's syndrome. The increased stickiness of platelets is a frequent cause of death.

Elevated homocysteine accelerates growth of the intimal and medial cells and tissues of arteries, triggering the many processes that lead to loss of elasticity, narrowing, hardening and calcification, and formation of blood clots within arteries.

Homocystine, the double-bonded and most prominent form of homocysteine in the blood, injected intravenously over thirty minutes leads to an increase in the number of circulating endothelial cells (cells that line the arteries). Platelet-

inhibiting drugs or pyridoxine probably can prevent the smooth muscle cell proliferation that is induced by endothelial cell injury.

Homocysteine causes arteriosclerosis in baboons when injected by continuous infusion. Vascular de-endothelialization resulted; platelet consumption increased three times as well.

Homocysteine is similar to the drug penicillamine (N-N dimethyl cysteine);
they both disrupt cross-links (sulfur to sulfur bonds). These compounds are cysteine and glutathione inhibitors.

Skin biopsy from homocystinuric patients shows significantly decreased
cross-links. The collagen of their arteries probably has the same defect. Cross-linking enzyme lysyl oxidase utilizes copper and pyridoxine, and deficiency of either
of these nutrients can produce defective cross-links in the aorta. Copper deficiency is almost nonexistent in the United States because of copper plumbing.

Beyond the treatment of arteriosclerosis by reduction of cholesterol is treatment by reduction of homocysteine. Homocysteine excess is related to pyridoxine deficiency and possibly zinc deficiency, which has a role in the body's ability
to repair cells. Marginal deficiency of pyridoxine and zinc is widespread in this
country.

Marginal deficiency of pyridoxine may result in accumulations of homocysteine even in healthy people. Diets high in meat and dairy products require more
pyridoxine due to the extra intake of amino acids in these foods, and often contain less pyridoxine due to processing.

In addition to heart disease, elevated levels of homocysteine have been implicated in the following conditions.

Psychosis

Homocysteine and glutamic acid are the two most excitatory amino acids in the
human brain. Homocystinuria may be causally related to psychotic symptoms,
since among the several hundred known patients with homocystinemia and
homocystinuria due to cystathionine synthase deficiency, a few have been
reported to be psychotic.

Freeman and colleagues from Johns Hopkins Hospital in Baltimore, Maryland,
reported one possible case of homocysteine "schizophrenia" response (methyl-
tetrahydrofolate deficiency) to folic acid. At our clinic, we have treated thousands
of "schizophrenics" who were clinically responsive to folic acid and pyridoxine.
We have also found some schizophrenics responsive to methionine. Methionine
has pharmacological properties similar to betaine, which has been used successfully in homocystinuria.

Schizophrenia

The homocysteine derivative S-adenosyl L-homocysteine (the energy molecule

ATP plus homocysteine) can inhibit transmethylation reactions. These reactions in excess have been associated with psychosis, hallucinations, and disease related to depression. One possible therapeutic approach for psychotics who show symptoms of over-methylation is to give S-adenosyl L-homocysteine and homocysteine. Schatz and colleagues from the University of Michigan found an effective dose with a level of 200 mg/kg of adenosine plus DL-homocysteine thiolactone. S-adenosyl L-homocysteine (SAH) was markedly elevated and several brain methylation reactions were reduced. SAMe was not affected, but the methyl donor enzymes histamine N-methyltransferase (HMT) and catechol-O-methyl transferase (COMT) were lowered. This suggests that the compound may be useful in high-dopamine, low-histamine schizophrenia. S-adenosyl L-homocysteine also inhibits spermine synthetase, N-methyl tetrahydrofolate, and methyltransferase.

Schatz and colleagues also showed that S-adenosyl L-homocysteine decreases methylation of brain phospholipids N, N-dimethylethanolamine (similar to deanol) and phosphatidylcholine (a component of lecithin). Stritmatter and colleagues from the National Institutes of Mental Health (NIMH) found the B-adrenergic receptors to contain methylated phosphatidylcholine. Some forms of schizophrenia may have increased receptors for catecholamines due to this mechanism. S-adenosyl L-homocysteine is a potent methyltransferase inhibitor and may be useful in some forms of schizophrenia.

DIAGNOSING AND TREATING ELEVATED HOMOCYSTEINE

In our clinic, we measure levels of homocysteine, pyridoxine, folic acid, methionine, and cysteine for every patient with a history of heart disease or diabetes. In general, one out of ten elderly patients we test has high homocysteine levels. Interestingly, we find that patients with elevated homocysteine tend to also have high cholesterol.

Known Methyl Donor Enzymes

- Acetyl serotonin methyltransferase (ASMT)
- Catechol-O-methyltransferase (COMT)
- DNA methyltransferase (DMT)
- Histamine N methyltransferase (HMT)
- Histone methyltransferase (HOMT)
- Phenylethanolamine methyltransferase (PEMT)
- Phosphatidyl ethanolamine methyltransferase (PEMT)
- Protein methyltransferase I-III (PMT)
- S-adenosyl L-methionine (SAMe)
- Tyramine N-methyltransferase (TMT)
- T RNA methyltransferase (RMT)

An adequate intake of folic acid, cyanocobalamin, and particularly pyridoxine can help insure a timely breakdown of homocysteine in the body. We are quickly able to remedy a high homocysteine level through supplementation. Typically we suggest a daily combination of 400 mcg of folic acid and 100 mg of pyridoxine along with a one-time injection (9 mg) or nasal preparation of cyanocobalamin. Increasing dietary fruit and vegetables, which typically have a high pyridoxine and folic acid content, instead of taking supplements may be enough to maintain acceptable levels of pyridoxine and folic acid.

Note: Individuals who supplement with cysteine, N-acetyl-cysteine (NAC), and methionine, without including enough pyridoxine, run the risk of producing excess homocysteine.

HOMOCYSTEINE: A SUMMARY

Homocysteine is a sulfur-containing amino acid involved in methionine metabolism. Homocysteine is not toxic to the body when present in small amounts; however, when excessive methionine has been consumed and inadequate amounts of pyridoxine, cyanocobalamin, and folic acid are available for its deactivation, homocysteine builds up and becomes toxic.

There are several types of inborn errors of homocysteine metabolism. The most prevalent of these is cystathionine synthase deficiency, which is caused by a genetic defect in the liver enzyme cystathionine synthase. This enzyme normally converts homocysteine to cystathionine, which is further processed in the liver to cysteine, and eventually taurine and glutathione.

Extensive research has shown excessive homocysteine accelerates growth of the intimal and medial cells and tissues of arteries, triggering the many processes that lead to loss of elasticity, narrowing, hardening and calcification, and formation of blood clots within arteries. Homocysteine is now considered a major independent risk factor for cardiovascular disease, joining the ranks of hyperlipidemia, hypertension, and smoking.

Homocysteine is easily measured in the blood, where most of it is oxidized to homocystine, the double-bonded form of homocysteine. In clinical use, its elevation in the blood plays an important role not only as a indicator of heart blockages, heart attacks, and stroke, but also of advancing diabetes, kidney failure, neural tube defects, sickle cell disease, cervical dysplasia, HIV, cognitive impairment, and even the progression of some cancers. Low antioxidant levels, copper excess, and folic acid deficiency, and inborn errors of methionine metabolism can also be a telltale sign of high homocysteine levels.

Therapeutically, S-adenosyl L-homocysteine, (the energy molecule ATP and homocysteine) can be a useful therapy in certain forms of psychosis. We have identified a form of psychosis, called pyroluria, which accounts for about 30 percent of psychotic patients. These patients are pyridoxine and zinc dependent.

Chances of homocysteine being present at high levels increase with a family history of heart disease, using tobacco, being over age fifty, being menopausal, or living a lifestyle that has little to no exercise.

Adequate intakes of folic acid, cyanocobalamin, and particularly pyridoxine either through diet sources or supplementation can help insure a timely breakdown of homocysteine in the body.

CHAPTER SEVEN

Cysteine:
The Detoxifier

Cysteine is a nonessential amino acid, yet a biochemical powerhouse. It consists of the basic chemical amino structure—nitrogen, carbon, oxygen, and hydrogen—plus a sulfur-containing thiol group. "Thiol," as in the common antibacterial agent merthiolate, indicates that the compound contains a sulfur and a hydrogen atom bound together. Ever since the ancient Greeks used garlic therapeutically, elemental sulfur has been employed to treat a wide variety of disorders. Cysteine, a higher quality source of sulfur than garlic, turns out to be useful in many of the situations to which sulfur was once applied.

Cysteine is active in many different situations in the body because of the special properties of its thiol grouping at the end of each cystine molecule. Thiol compounds not only help prevent oxidation of sensitive tissues, which can cause aging and cancer, by sacrificing themselves for oxidation first, but they also help the body process and render harmless toxic chemical and carcinogens. It is what makes cysteine, and its well-known star derivatives N-acetyl-cysteine and glutathione, extremely powerful compounds.

FUNCTION

Cysteine's most important functions as a free-radical destroyer, antioxidant, chelator of circulating copper, and general metabolic enhancer, are not performed alone. Cysteine is a highly reactive, versatile, amino acid. Once it enters the body, it is rapidly converted to cystine, the stable form of this sulfur-rich amino acid.

Each cystine molecule is made up of two molecules of cysteine bound together. It derives its stability from an extremely strong bridge called a disulfide bond, or a double bond, that is formed in and between protein chains. Each molecule of cystine consists of two molecules of cysteine joined together. This extra-strength cystine helps proteins maintain their structure as they are carried around the body. It serves as a kind of "solder" at strategic points within structures of crisscrossing chains of molecules and helps determine the form and mechanical properties of many animal and plant proteins. It is the high-cystine content, for example, in the fibrous protein gluten that gives wheat dough its elasticity, and in keratin that makes tortoise shells hard and human hair curly or straight.

From cystine, the body makes N-acetyl cysteine (NAC), one of the most well-documented and effective nutritional agents in medicine today. This slightly modified form of cysteine is thought to be an intermediary in cysteine detoxification mechanisms. That is, as cysteine goes about its business of clearing the cells of toxins, it may be converted temporarily to N-acetyl cysteine. It performs as a detoxifying agent, antidoting more toxins than any other substance in the body—even vitamin C cannot match its antidotal range. It is used in emergency rooms against toxic overdose and commonly for overdoses of acetaminophen (Tylenol). It continues to be one of the best-kept secrets among clinicians who deal with pulmonary, cancer, and cardiac medicine. Like cysteine, N-acetyl cysteine is also thought to increase glutathione production.

Probably cysteine's most exciting and important role in the body, however, takes place in the liver, where it helps the small but ubiquitous protein glutathione detoxify carcinogens and other dangerous pollutants, and in all the rest of the cells of the body, where it serves as the major scavenger of hazardous oxidants. Without its presence, your cells would be destroyed due to the oxidation process and your liver would be destroyed by the level of the toxins within. You would not be able to fight off bacteria, viruses, or cancer.

In contrast to hormones, which are often ten, twenty, or fifty amino acids long, with each amino acid playing only a small role in the hormones' dramatic regulation and enforcement of physiological balances, glutathione is tiny. This amino acid is a tripeptide—a small protein made from just three amino acids: cysteine, glutamic acid, and glycine—yet it serves as the body's toxic waste neutralizer and most abundant natural antioxidant within all cells. Cysteine is the most important of these three contributors because cysteine determines how much glutathione is produced by the body. It is cysteine's thiol group that gives glutathione its power.

In addition to its own potent antioxidant powers, glutathione helps to recycle other antioxidants such as vitamins C and E and lipoic acid. We'll talk more about glutathione later in the chapter.

In addition to the detoxifying function that results from cysteine's conversion to N-acetyl-cysteine and glutathione, cysteine plays an important role in energy metabolism. Like a number of other amino acids, it can be used as fuel if necessary. First it is converted into glucose, which can then either be oxidized for energy or stored as starch. To convert amino acids into simple acids and then sugar, the body must clip off nitrogen from the amino acid and excrete it in the urine as urea. During this same process, cysteine's sulfur is converted to sulfate, a substance that can produce calcium deficiency in people on high-protein diets.

Another important energy system of which cysteine is an active part is fatty acid synthase. Fatty acid synthase is an enzyme that synthesizes fatty acids whenever they are needed by body cells. It uses cysteine's highly reactive thiol group to fasten carbon atoms, two at a time, onto the lengthening chains that make up each fatty acid.

Cysteine's role in the brain is less clear. Unlike the aromatic amino acids (phenylalanine, tyrosine, and tryptophan), which play a paramount role in healthy brain function, cysteine sulphinic acid (a form of cysteine) and glutathione have been identified as neurotransmitters, but their role in the brain is poorly understood. Cysteine deficiencies are sometimes found in psychotic patients, indicating the probable, yet unknown, importance of cysteine in normal mental functioning.

METABOLISM

Cysteine is made by the body only from the essential amino acid methionine. It is a highly unstable molecule and is quickly converted to cystine, a double-bonded form of cysteine. Cysteine, like all the sulfur amino acids, needs adequate amounts of pyridoxine (vitamin B_6), cyanocobalamin (vitamin B_{12}), and folic acid in order for the conversion from one amino acid to another to take place. Cysteine can be converted to N-acetyl-cysteine (NAC), methionine, taurine, thiamine, coenzyme A, and many other organic sulfur molecules needed by the cell.

High doses of pyridoxine are of special value when kidney tumors, thyroid therapy, galactosemia, or pyridoxine deficiency itself can cause the appearance of an error in the conversion of methionine to cysteine, known as cystathioninuria. If this error is not corrected, the result can be mental retardation and decreases in blood platelet and pH (acid/alkaline) levels.

REQUIREMENTS

The National Academy of Sciences has not yet established an RDA for cysteine. However, since methionine, an essential amino acid, and cysteine both raise glutathione levels, they have estimated minimum daily requirements for the two amino acids together.

The minimum daily requirement of methionine plus cysteine for children has been set at 22 mg/kg of body weight, and for adults at 10 mg/kg. Some researchers have suggested that as little as 5 mg/kg of cysteine is necessary for daily use, which is about 350 mg per day. Minimum requirements for total sulfur-containing amino acids (taurine, cysteine, and methionine) have been reported by investigators to be as high as 1,400 mg/day. The WHO committee has established a tentative requirement for all sulfur amino acids (mainly methionine) of

13 mg/kg per day or 910 mg of these amino acids daily for the average 150 lb adult male. Requirements may vary as a result of sex, diet, and age.

FOOD SOURCES

Cysteine is best obtained in the diet from eggs, meat, dairy products, grains, and beans. However, the level of cysteine in foods is difficult to detect just as it is in body fluids. Reliable data on cysteine in foods is not available, but cystine in foods is well known. Foods high in cystine are probably high-cysteine foods. A deficiency in cysteine can result from a strict vegetarian diet low in proteins.

TABLE 7.1. CYSTINE LEVELS IN FOOD		
FOOD	AMOUNT	CONTENT (GRAMS)
Avocado	1	N.A.
Cheese	1 ounce	0.03
Chicken	1 pound	0.40
Chocolate	1 cup	N.A.
Cottage cheese	1 cup	0.30
Duck	1 pound	1.20
Egg	1	0.07
Granola	1 cup	0.30
Luncheon meat	1 pound	0.29
Oatmeal	1 cup	0.20
Pork	1 pound	0.64
Ricotta	1 cup	0.25
Sausage meat	1 pound	0.35
Turkey	1 pound	0.50
Wheat germ	1 cup	0.70
Whole milk	1 cup	0.07
Wild game	1 pound	0.04
Yogurt	1 cup	0.93

FORM AND ABSORPTION

Numerous studies show that cysteine is best absorbed in the modified form of N-acetyl-cysteine. D-cysteine and D-cystine are toxic forms in humans and should not be used.

People who take large amounts of phenylalanine and tryptophan should be alert to the possibility that their cysteine levels will decrease. When cysteine goes down, all antioxidant levels go down, and all aging diseases advance. The concern here with cysteine, as it is with amino acids in general, is balance. Keep in mind that that blood levels of amino acids as well as vitamins, trace minerals, and fatty acids should be routinely measured and monitored by a physician in order to address your individual needs and to optimize your benefits and avoid imbalances.

VITAMIN INTERACTIONS

Cysteine works synergistically in the body with vitamin C and other antioxidants, protecting cell membranes against the dangers of oxidation of lipids and helping to detoxify pesticides, herbicides, plastics, other hydrocarbons, and various drugs. In addition, like vitamin C, cysteine can help kill bacteria and, as part of the glutathione molecule, is an essential element of many parts of the immune system. A further relationship between vitamin C and glutathione is suggested by the discovery that humans, like guinea pigs, cannot manufacture their own vitamin C and produce less glutathione than rats, mice, and hamsters.

TOXICITY

When L-cystine—but not cysteine—builds up in the body, it can be harmful. This occurs in the genetic disorder cystinosis, or Fanconi syndrome. Cystinosis results in kidney dysfunction and occasionally kidney stones. Children with Fanconi syndrome often die by age ten of kidney failure with some organs embedded with thousands of tiny crystals of cystine or suffused with 100-times-normal concentrations of free cystine. While there is no way to reverse the crystallization of cystine, a cysteine derivative called cysteamine (mercaptoethylamine) can quickly rid cells of their excess free cystine; however, its side effects include peptic ulcer, fever, skin rash, lethargy, and a lowered neutrophil count. (A neutrophil is a major constituent of leukocytes, a type of white blood cell important in immune response.)

Because of the damage excess cystine does in children with cystinosis, we are very skeptical of using L-cystine clinically (although some practitioners use it for hair loss and to lower very low density lipoproteins, or VLDL, the "bad" form of cholesterol). Generally, cysteine therapy is used to provide a chemical-reducing or antioxidant environment; using L-cystine, the oxidized form of cysteine, defeats this purpose.

CLINICAL USES

The group of sulfur amino acids is chemically distinct from other groups of amino acids because they contain a sulfur molecule. The sulfur combines with hydrogen molecules to become a powerful antioxidant that fights free radicals throughout the body.

There are dozens of positive reports of L-cysteine's value as an adjunct in treating many types of disease conditions. But because cysteine is a naturally occurring nutrient, and no drug company can patent cysteine itself, there is little incentive to study it directly. Proving that a compound is safe and effective for particular clinical use costs millions of dollars and must be profitable and patentable before industry will undertake the study.

On the other hand, the closely related N-acetyl-cysteine, has been studied extensively. It is a slightly modified form of cysteine, some of which is converted back into cysteine in the body. It is more soluble in water and can be taken as a liquid; therefore many of the studies use N-acetyl-cysteine rather than cysteine. Keep in mind that cysteine is a precursor of glutathione. The conditions described here generally involve deficiencies of cysteine, and therefore of glutathione. Since N-acetyl-cysteine, like natural cysteine, increases glutathione production, either may be used with good results; although N-acetyl-cysteine is considered the better of the two.

Bacterial Infections

Supplemental cysteine or glutathione may prove a useful adjunct like vitamin C in bacterial infection. N-acetyl-cysteine has been found to alleviate the effects of *Clostridium* toxin, an infection that commonly occurs in the colon as a result of the administration of antibiotics. Significant improvement in survival times in experimental animals was noted.

Cancer

N-acetyl-cysteine has been studied extensively in cancer research. N-acetyl-cysteine has been shown to enhance antitumor responses by interleukin 2, a white cell involved in immune response. There have been several interesting studies with laboratory animals showing N-acetyl-cysteine's effectiveness against tumors using dosages equivalent of up to 70 g daily for humans.

N-acetyl-cysteine reduced the toxicity of various highly toxic substances being used in cancer treatment. For example, doxorubicin (Adriamycin)—a commonly used chemotherapy drug—can cause heart damage. N-acetyl-cysteine supplements succeeded in reducing cardiac toxicity in an experiment that dosed dogs daily over an eight-week period with 12 mg/kg—the equivalent of 1 g per day in a 150-lb adult man. In fact, cysteine itself, and several cysteine analogs, including N-acetyl-cysteine, cysteamine (mercaptoethylamine), and D-penicillamine (cysteine with two methyl groupings) all offer protection against doxorubicin toxicity, according to Morgan and colleagues. They report that doxorubicin damages the body when it is metabolized by the liver into the toxic chemicals acrolein and chloroacetic acid. Acrolein is so irritating that it has been used for chemical warfare, and chloroacetic acid is a chlorinated and therefore toxic version of all-too-easily metabolized acetic acid. It can seriously damage the liver.

One study indicated that N-acetyl-cysteine is effective in preventing chemotherapy-induced liver toxicity and heart damage only to the extent that it is converted back into L-cysteine in the body, supporting our own hypothesis that cysteine itself might be as effective as N-acetyl-cysteine.

Glutathione is effective against these toxic breakdown products of doxorubicin, but it is not available in high doses. Cysteine (taken as a pill) or N-acetyl-cysteine (given in liquid form) are the best adjuncts to doxorubicin therapy, and probably in all chemotherapy.

N-acetyl-cysteine helps detoxify another chemotherapeutic agent, namely cyclophosphamide (CPS). Four times as much N-acetyl-cysteine as cyclophosphamide, given a half-hour before the CPS dose, prevented CPS-induced hemorrhagic cystitis—painful inflammation and bleeding of the bladder and urinary tract in humans—and lengthened survival times. A CPS analog used in Europe, ifosfamide (IFX), also damages the urinary tract lining. Eight grams of N-acetyl-cysteine daily provided complete protection against the painful side effects of chemotherapy in a study involving cancers of the pancreas and testicles.

Not only does N-acetyl-cysteine help prevent side effects from chemotherapy, but it can also do the same for radiation treatment. Prepared as an ointment to spread on the skin, N-acetyl-cysteine reduced skin reactions, prevented hair loss, and protected mucous membranes of the eyes. Cystine, and therefore probably N-acetyl-cysteine, also prevents radiation enteritis—inflammation of the mucous tissues lining the small intestine.

Strong exceptions were voiced some years ago about using large doses of N-acetyl-cysteine at 5 to 7 g therapeutic doses for liver cancer. There are very few side effects to N-acetyl-cysteine, even with doses as high as 7 g a day, which we have used at this clinic for severe conditions such as metastatic cancer. (Dosages from 5 to 7 g can be tolerated by most people. Some individuals, however, will develop intestinal gas.) Some research has been done using as much as 20-30 g of N-acetyl-cysteine per day in severe medical conditions. IV solutions should include vitamin C with N-acetyl-cysteine since these substances may work synergistically.

N-acetyl-cysteine has been found to be generally safe in large doses (up to 10 g daily) even during pregnancy. However, it has a nauseating taste and smell and can cause vomiting. Cysteine itself doesn't have this effect.

Dental Cavities

Dental plaque formation may be inhibited by topical applications of silver, tin, and zinc salts to the teeth and gums. Adding cysteine or glutathione to the formula enhanced this effect. It may be its thiol group that enhances the bactericidal properties of the metals. If so, these amino acids may also increase the effectiveness of zinc lozenges in fighting sore throats and colds.

Diabetes

Pangborn of Bionostic Laboratories has studied the urine levels of cysteine in individuals with diabetes and seizure disorders. He believes that cystine metabolism is impaired in both of these illnesses. There are indications that cysteine may help prevent seizures by its conversion to taurine. This suggestion bears further investigation.

People with diabetes have an increased need for cysteine and taurine, a sulfur amino acid, especially during ketosis (abnormal accumulation of ketones) when they excrete increased amounts of sulfur amino acids. Cysteine and methionine, another sulfur amino acid, have been found to be important in the synthesis of lipoic acid from linoleic acid. Lipoic acid can reduce the need for insulin and has been known to be beneficial in diabetes.

A sixty-year-old woman with chronic diabetes had rapidly failing kidneys and appeared to be well on her way to needing dialysis until we gave her 1 g of cysteine in the morning and in the evening. This arrested her kidney failure temporarily.

Damage to the kidneys may also result from taking indomethacin (Indocin) and other nonsteroidal anti-inflammatory drugs, such as phenylbutazone and sulindac (Clinoril). These medications have an unwarranted side effect of depleting glutathione (possibly because glutathione is involved in drug detoxification). Since cysteine is able to raise glutathione levels, it may prevent other side effects as well.

Hair Loss

People who are facing the loss of their hair spend millions of dollars annually on creams, gels, and dietary supplements to restore it. Most of these salves don't work, and the FDA is moving to crack down on those preparations for which exaggerated claims are made.

All the horny layers of the skin, including hair and fingernails (keratin is 12 percent cystine), are high in cystine. There is evidence that the high-sulfur proteins are missing in the hair of people experiencing abnormal hair loss. Dietary supplementation with sulfur-containing amino acids like cystine increases the percentage of high-sulfur proteins in the hair of both experimental animals and humans. Preliminary findings indicate that daily dietary supplementation of cysteine and NAC increases hair-shaft diameter and hair-growth density in certain cases of human baldness and hair loss, and therefore may be useful in treating these conditions.

Heart Disease

Considerable research has found that 2 g of N-acetyl-cysteine administered intra-

Cysteine Stops Abnormal Hair Loss

A twenty-seven-year-old woman came to our clinic complaining of severe hair loss. Tests showed that she was losing several hundred hairs per day as opposed to a normal loss of seventy per day. An amino acid analysis showed low plasma cystine and taurine. We started her on 1 g of L-cysteine in the morning and in the evening. Her hair loss did not improve. When we increased the dose to 5 g daily, the hair loss stopped in one month.

In another case, a thirty-five-year-old woman with excessive hair loss during a depression found that her hair loss stopped after two weeks on 1.5 g of L-cysteine twice daily.

venously increases the efficacy of nitroglycerine medication used by people with angina and coronary artery disease. We recommend N-acetyl-cysteine for most people with cardiac conditions taking such medication as isosorbide mononitrate (ISMO) and isosorbide dinitrate (Isordil). N-acetyl-cysteine prevents these compounds from breaking down, while at the same time promotes their actions in the body. An oral dose of 2 g of N-acetyl-cysteine appears sufficient. N-acetyl-cysteine may also reduce damaging cholesterol proteins in the body.

Heavy Metal Toxicity

Some essential trace minerals are toxic when present in the body in higher amounts than needed. Cysteine supplements have been shown to alleviate toxicity caused by the following trace minerals.

Cobalt and Molybdenum

Both cobalt and molybdenum toxicity have been shown to be alleviated by cysteine supplements. Domingo and colleagues found that cysteine increased the growth rate of rats that had been deliberately stunted by cobalt overdoses and prevented in part a cobalt-induced excess of red blood cells. In pigs, cobalt toxicity was better counteracted by another sulfur-containing amino acid, methionine, which is converted within the body into cysteine and glutathione. We can conclude from these animal experiments that in cases of heavy metal toxicity in humans from mercury, lead, aluminum, copper, and cadmium, cysteine supplementation might be worth a trial.

Arsenic

N-acetyl-cysteine is reported to be a powerful antidote for arsenic poisoning. In one reported case, N-acetyl-cysteine was given intravenously to an individual who had ingested a potentially lethal dose (900 mg) of sodium arsenate. After twenty-four hours, the patient recovered.

Copper

Because cysteine and methionine combine chemically with copper in the body, they can be used to reverse excesses of copper in blood plasma, spleen, liver, and bile. Copper toxicity is an ever-present danger in the United States. Much of our drinking water flows through copper pipes, and copper is commonly added to poultry and pig feed as an antifungal agent and growth promoter. Excess copper in the body can cause psychosis and other mental disturbances, and interestingly, many psychotic patients have elevated serum copper levels. L-cysteine, even better than methionine, can prevent copper buildup.

Note: L-cysteine has yet to be reported as a treatment for Wilson's disease, a genetic disorder characterized by increased intestinal absorption of copper and its accumulation in the brain and other organs. D-penicillamine, a dimethyl cysteine and the copper binder currently accepted as the treatment of choice for Wilson's disease, causes acute toxic reactions in one-third of patients who take it. L-cysteine therapy may be better than D-penicillamine in some cases of Wilson's disease.

Human Immunodeficiency Virus (HIV)

It has been hypothesized that the main human immunodeficiency virus (HIV) mechanism involves depletion of the body's stores of N-acetyl-cysteine. The immune system is exquisitely sensitive to a deficiency of N-acetyl-cysteine. With such a deficiency, the action of CD4 (white cell) count may drop 30 percent.

Research at Stanford suggests that N-acetyl-cysteine could benefit HIV patients. The lingering problem is how to precisely affect blood levels. We think that N-acetyl-cysteine in dosages of 3 to 7 g should be a central component of HIV treatment. HIV is a treatable illness and much can be done therapeutically with nutrition and supplements.

Kidney Stones

N-acetyl-cysteine is an effective treatment for people with kidney stones. It is also useful in treating cystinosis (cystine stones) as is D-penicillamine, a dimethyl cysteine, in doses of 1.5 to 2.0 g a day. (D-penicillamine may inhibit cystine metabolism to some degree, but does not interfere with metabolism of cysteine.)

In our clinic, we have used a combination of magnesium (500 to 1,000 mg), pyridoxine (100 mg), potassium citrate (75 mg), N-acetyl-cysteine (1 g), and fiber (10 g of bran) as a daily program to effectively treat kidney stones. Hundreds of people have been successfully treated with this approach, which is both therapeutic and a preventive against recurrences. Using this protocol, recurrences are extremely rare.

Lung Conditions

There is voluminous research describing the benefits of N-acetyl-cysteine for the treatment of chronic bronchitis, asthma, and emphysema, and for the prevention of lung cancer. In our clinic, we have documented major improvements in dozens of cases of lung disease over the years; it is a fundamental nutrient in our treatment of all lung conditions.

Lung Damage from Smoke

L-cysteine helps protect the vulnerable skin tissue of the alveoli—the tiny sacs that make up the surface of lung tissue—against the damage of cigarette, cigar, or other types of smoke. Hundreds of chemicals in smoke impair the ability of the alveoli's scavenger macrophages to engulf and kill bacteria. Cysteine, or glutathione, improves the bactericidal effectiveness of these cells, and all smokers should take this supplement along with vitamins A and C, selenium, and zinc.

Cigarette, cigar, and other types of smoke also attack the lungs by destroying the cells on the lung's surface. Ingredients in smoke most directly implicated as toxic to lung cells are acrolein, formaldehyde, and acetaldehyde. Oral doses of a food supplement combining L-cysteine and vitamin C gave a high degree of protection against these lethal substances. Adding thiamine to the daily supplement may further increase the effectiveness of the L-cysteine and vitamin C.

N-acetyl-cysteine has been found to be beneficial for breaking up mucous congestion in smoker's cough. Suggested dosages are 500 mg twice a day (or 200 mg three times daily) for all patients with lung disease.

Asthma and Bronchial Conditions

When N-acetyl-cysteine is given in aerosol form, it has the unusual property of helping to liquefy mucus and loosen mucus plugs from the lungs and bronchial tubes. N-acetyl-cysteine in aerosol form is prescribed for chronic bronchitis, asthma, cystic fibrosis, bronchiectasis (chronic dilation of a bronchial tube), emphysema, lung abscess, and chronic obstructive pulmonary disease. N-acetyl-cysteine in tablet form (200 mg in the morning and in the evening), which is converted by the body to cysteine, also has a mucolytic action and can be used to treat chronic bronchitis.

At our clinic, two patients with asthma were able to stop using their asthma medication after taking daily supplements of 500 mg of L-cysteine in the morning and evening. The first patient—a sixty-year-old woman with asthma who had been on an albuterol (Proventil) inhaler and the bronchodilating drug theophylline anhydrous (Theo-Dur) for ten years—was able to discontinue using all drugs with the exception of her inhaler within two months. The second patient, a fourteen-year-old boy also on theophylline anhydrous and an inhaler was able to stop all of his medication once he started supplementing with L-cysteine and vitamin C.

Photosensitivity

A study suggests that N-acetyl-cysteine can reduce photosensitivity in certain patients. We recommend that any individual on medication that may cause photosensitivity take N-acetyl-cysteine. We also suggest beta-carotene for additional antioxidant effect.

Ulcers

It is now known that along with cigarette smoke and stress, the bacteria *Helicobacter pylori* is a factor in causing ulcers. Helicobacter may be ingested from the water supply or may be present in the gastrointestinal tract due to deficient stomach acid. This microorganism has been found to deplete cysteine and glutathione.

Studies suggest that N-acetyl-cysteine improves eradication of helicobacter by the antibiotics omeprazole (Prilosec) and amoxicillin (Amoxil, Augmentin, Polymox, etc.). Other treatments have used bismuth subsalicylate (Pepto-Bismol) and sulfamethoxazole plus trimethoprim (Bactrim). In either scenario, N-acetyl-cysteine was successful.

In our clinic, we use N-acetyl-cysteine along with the antacid Titralac (sugar-free Tums) for ulcers. We are able to wean many ulcer patients off cimetidine (Tagamet) and ranitidine (Zantac) with this approach by using two Titralac pills four times daily, 1 g of N-acetyl-cysteine, magnesium to bowel tolerance, and 30 mg of zinc. If constipation develops, we recommend extra magnesium.

Wound Healing

Because of its importance in protecting skin tissue L-cysteine may be valuable in wound and skin healing. We have used it successfully in treating some cases of psoriasis. Our finding is consistent with previous reports of the antipsoriatic activity of sulfur compounds. L-cysteine is also being investigated for its use in wrinkle prevention.

GLUTATHIONE: CYSTEINE'S MOST IMPORTANT METABOLITE

There are no living organisms on this planet—animal or plant—whose cells do not contain glutathione (GSH). Scientists speculate that glutathione was essential to the very development of life on earth.

One billion years before life appeared on Earth, the environment was gaseous and toxic to any forms of life as it exists now. The atmosphere was made up mostly of hydrogen, carbon monoxide, ammonia, and methane. To protect themselves from the gas, these acid cells had to incorporate antioxidants into their cytoplasm in order to avoid annihilation. Among the first of these antioxidants, as inferred from its present ubiquity, was glutathione.

Glutathione also helped protect against the toxic effects of oxygen produced by the first plants. Apparently very early on, one-celled plants began to use glutathione as an antioxidant to prevent themselves from being destroyed by the oxygen they themselves were freeing. Much later, animal cells incorporated the same compound to help them control oxygen waste products.

Essentially, glutathione still serves these same protective purposes today as the major antioxidant within all cells. It has yet another property that stems from the days when the planet was full of sulfurous and carbon gases; it also helps detoxify various carbon compounds. Now that our polluted environment is gaining chemical characteristics similar to the primordial period, glutathione, through cysteine, is again serving to make existence possible.

Glutathione in the Body

Glutathione is a compound that is synthesized from cysteine and is found in virtually all living cells. It is present in higher concentrations in animals than in plants, and may be more necessary in humans than in other animals. The amount present in the body varies from organ to organ and tissue to tissue. Liver, spleen, kidneys, and pancreas contain the highest concentrations of glutathione; the eye, particularly the lens and cornea, is also rich in glutathione.

The amount of glutathione present in the body decreases with age. Its steady decrease in tissues is a general characteristic of aging, according to Hazelton and Lang. The loss of glutathione by body cells over time has been studied in mice. In addition, the amount present in the tissues of each organ decreases as the mouse ages. For example, in a thirty-one-month-old mouse (the equivalent in age of about a seventy-year-old human), 20 to 35 percent glutathione decreases were found in the heart, liver, and kidneys compared to younger animals.

Another tissue in which high quantities of glutathione have been found is the stomach lining. This has been extensively studied in rats. Gastric levels of glutathione sometimes even exceed liver values; this depends on the time of the day the sample is taken. Gastric glutathione levels are highest in late afternoon and lowest at night. This has to do with glutathione's function of protecting the stomach lining against the highly oxidizing effects of hydrochloric acid, since stomach acid levels are highest in the morning.

Functions

Glutathione has four primary roles in the body. It protects the body against powerful natural and man-made oxidants, and helps the liver to detoxify poisonous chemicals; it is essential to immune function; it promotes the integrity of red blood cells; and lastly, it serves as a neurotransmitter.

Antioxidant

Glutathione, like cysteine, contains the crucial thiol group that makes it an effective antioxidant. Natural and man-made chemicals can do extensive damage in the body by oxidizing fats. This dangerous process is called peroxidation. Lipid peroxidation destroys the body's cell membranes. When hydrogen peroxide is applied to a cut as an antiseptic, it releases so much oxygen that any bacteria present are oxidized and destroyed. Peroxides harm unprotected cells within the body in much the same way. Many industrial chemicals form peroxides as they are metabolized by the liver, including carbon tetrachloride, benzenes, and numerous plastics, dyes, herbicides, and pesticides. Unchecked, such peroxides can virtually render the liver cells into fat.

But glutathione, or cysteine, comes to the rescue in the form of an enzyme complex called glutathione peroxidase, which is designed to reduce peroxides. This glutathione peroxidase antioxidant system, which includes glutathione peroxidase and glutathione reductase, is dependent upon the presence of glutathione. This system scavenges lipid peroxides and prevents other radicals from being produced. Glutathione peroxidase transforms hydrogen peroxide by donating an electron, regaining a free electron, and continually working.

A second enzyme complex in which glutathione plays a role in the liver is the glutathione-S-transferases. Here, glutathione helps detoxify many foreign compounds by chemically transforming them into less harmful products. These are then excreted through the colon via liver bile.

Just how glutathione and glutathione-S-transferases and other liver enzymes work is still under investigation. One clue is found in a study of seven other substances also known to inhibit chemical carcinogenesis. All of these were found to increase glutathione-S-transferase activity in the liver and small intestines of mice.

Whenever the glutathione-producing enzymes are deficient, glutathione becomes a nutrient essential to survival. Hence, it is one of many metabolites that in special situations can become an essential nutrient, or more accurately, cysteine becomes essential. When the body is exposed to toxins, it is crucial to have enough cysteine or glutathione in the diet.

Immune Enhancer

Glutathione is thought to help transport amino acids across membranes. One of these—L-alanine, a threonine amino acid—is essential for the production of the white blood cells called lymphocytes. As previously mentioned, glutathione may be more necessary in humans than in other animals. Human lymphocytes contain more than three times the amount of glutathione in mouse lymphocytes.

Other segments of the immune system that rely on glutathione include phagocytes, which complement a series of proteins in normal blood serum that destroy the membranes of invading bacteria, killing the germs. Glutathione has also been found in high levels in the thymus (of cows, so far), an organ that has important functions in the immune system.

Substances Rendered Less Toxic by GSH

The list of man-made toxins glutathione helps to inactivate is extensive and grows every day as the chemical industry expands its repertoire.

- Allyl compounds, arylamines, arylhydroxylamines, carbamates, and related compounds (phenols)
- Bacterial toxins (*Clostridium difficile*)
- Drugs (steroids/phenolics, quinones, and catechols)
- Dyes and detergents
- Environmental toxins (automobile exhaust, cigarette smoke, and pollution)
- Fungicides
- Heavy metals (lead, mercury, arsenic, and cadmium found in paints, cans, gasoline, dental amalgams, batteries, and plating)
- Herbicides
- Insecticides (organophosphorus compounds)
- Isothiocyanates (methylisocyanate)
- Over-the-counter drugs (substances detoxified by the liver and too numerous to list)
- Pesticides
- Plastics/vinyl chloride
- Solvents and flavorings

In addition to helping the liver clean these chemicals out of the body, glutathione may turn out to be useful in cleaning up the environment itself. Large amounts of glutathione might be dumped into dead lakes and chemical disaster areas. Because the glutathione enzyme systems are the result of such ancient genetic programming, existing in the most primitive plants and animals as well as within the human liver, supplementing the "diet" of whatever is left alive in polluted waters with glutathione may help restore life to dying lakes and streams. Glutathione may be able to reenact the processes that led to the original proliferation of life on Earth.

Glutathione depletion affects the macrophages that function within loose connective tissues and organs, such as the spleen, lungs, and liver. Macrophages have the ability to "swallow" foreign particles, thus protecting the tissues and organs where they are found. When glutathione is low, production by macrophages of the prostaglandin leukotriene C is inhibited. Leukotriene C is essential for cells of the immune system to reach invading organisms. This is another indicator of glutathione's importance in the immune system.

Using inhibitors of glutathione metabolism, researchers have found that glutathione is a precursor, together with arachidonic acid (an essential fatty acid found in unsaturated fats), in the formation of at least one other prostaglandin, E-2, which is involved in inflammation and immune functions.

Oxygen Transporter

Glutathione is involved in the production of red blood cells, although the mechanism is not yet known. Red blood cells contain hemoglobin and are responsible for the transport of oxygen and carbon dioxide throughout the body. A number of studies have documented that when women take birth control pills, their red blood cells respond by producing extra glutathione peroxidase. Since oral contraceptives raise blood lipids, this may be an effort by the body to protect the red blood cell's against the dangers of peroxidation.

One drug that inhibits cysteine metabolism—and thereby glutathione formation—is S-methyl cysteine. S-methyl cysteine has deleterious effects on red blood cells. Tucker and colleagues showed that this inhibitor caused severe anemia and decreased the life span of red blood cells, as measured by increased fragility and a tendency of cell nuclei to fragment. This confirms the role of glutathione in red blood cells.

In animal studies on rats, high red blood cell-glutathione count correlate with increased milk production, as does the uptake of glutathione by mammary gland tissues during lactation. The thyroid is involved following pregnancy in stimulating milk production, and glutathione (or other thiols) may be a cofactor for this activation. More research is needed to determine whether this glutathione trait works similarly in humans. If so, it may prove useful for women with lactation failure.

Neurotransmission

Glutathione, like cysteine, has been identified as a neurotransmitter. The exact role it plays in the brain, however, is still poorly understood. Deficiencies of cysteine, and therefore glutathione, are sometimes found in psychotic patients, indicating the probable, yet unknown, importance of cysteine and glutathione in normal mental functioning.

Metabolism

Glutathione is a tripeptide. It is a small protein made from just three amino acids: cysteine, glutamic acid, and glycine. It requires reduction to its components prior to entering the cellular membrane, and then it is reassembled for use inside the cell. Glutathione is dependent upon pyridoxine, riboflavin, and folic acid for these conversions to occur.

Vitamin E, another important antioxidant, is also involved in glutathione metabolism. Vitamin E deficiency in rats has been shown to reduce the activity of glutathione peroxidase, one of the enzymes that protects cells against oxidation by free radicals and peroxides.

At our clinic, when we give L-cysteine or glutathione supplements to our patients, we nearly always complement them with the mineral selenium to increase the activity of the selenium in glutathione peroxidase. Zinc deficiency also results in reduced GSH in blood plasma. The minerals magnesium, zinc, and vanadium may also enhance glutathione synthesis under specific conditions.

Food Sources

Adequate levels of glutathione in the body depend on adequate availability of cysteine, glycine, and glutamic acid. Of these, only cysteine ever seems to be in short supply. Both glycine and glutamic acid are very abundant in the diet and probably will never be a cause of glutathione deficiency. Cysteine, however, must be made from the essential amino methionine. A small amount of glutathione can also be made directly from methionine. Likewise, when methionine or cysteine is deficient, glutathione levels decrease.

As long as the diet contains enough methionine or cysteine, glutathione levels are likely to be adequate. The exception to this rule is in infants, whose bodies cannot yet manufacture cysteine from methionine, so their cysteine needs are supplied by breast milk. (Cow's milk is an inadequate source of cysteine.)

Foods rich in methionine and cysteine are high in sulfur. Foods containing methionine and cysteine include egg yolks and red peppers. Muscle protein, garlic, onion, and asparagus are also good sulfur sources, along with cabbage, Brussels sprouts, broccoli, cauliflower, mustard, and horseradish. Egg whites and milk protein contain some sulfur, too. (For more foods high in methionine and cystine, see Tables 5.2 and 7.1 on pages 89 and 110, respectively.)

The soil in many areas of the world is deficient in sulfur. Plants absorb sulfur in the form of the sulfate ion and convert it into the many organic sulfur compounds on which animals depend. But the soil in glaciated areas is known to have lost sulfur, selenium, iodide, and zinc. It may not be possible to compensate for those deficiencies with food alone. In such areas, supplementation with methionine or cysteine may be necessary.

Clinical Uses

Most, if not all, clinical uses for glutathione can be achieved by using N-acetyl-cysteine supplements, which raise glutathione levels. Because glutathione is a tripeptide, it is used up quickly once produced, especially in stressful states, such as illness, exercise, fatigue, or the general stress of living. Glutathione's uptake by the body depends upon the delivery systems ability to increase and sustain its blood levels. For this reason, oral N-acetyl-cysteine is the best way to raise glutathione levels. Intravenously, N-acetyl-cysteine or glutathione may be used.

Alcoholism

Glutathione is found in high concentration in liver cells. In addition to preventing fatty liver induced by such chemicals as thionamide and the cleaning compound carbon tetrachloride, glutathione may also help prevent or even reverse alcoholism-induced fatty liver—cirrhosis—as well as hepatitis and liver tumors.

Cancer

It had been believed that in order for glutathione and other antioxidants to inhibit chemical-induced carcinogenesis, they had to be administered either prior to or at the same time as the carcinogen. But Novi reported an astounding finding: Glutathione actually made rat liver tumors regress and even disappear at late stages of tumor growth. Novi produced the tumors by giving the rats the extremely potent natural carcinogen aflatoxin B_1. Within one year, every rat had liver tumors. Four months later—sixteen months after the rats were subjected to aflatoxin—one group of rats were given 100 mg of glutathione intravenously per day. Of the rats given glutathione therapy, 81 percent lived while all the non-treated rats died. The livers of the surviving group were characterized by regression and/or absence of tumor—an extremely impressive finding.

Cataracts

Glutathione is found in particularly high concentrations in the cornea and lens of the eye, where it helps to keep the lens transparent, protecting it against cataracts and loss of visual acuity. Riboflavin (vitamin B_2) deficiency is a factor in cataract formation because the riboflavin-dependent enzyme glutathione reductase is dependent upon adequate stores of this vitamin. Production of glutathione reductase was reduced by 25 percent in the lenses of animals with cataracts due to riboflavin deficiency. Supplemental N-acetyl-cysteine eliminated the effects of riboflavin deficiency, probably by increasing glutathione. Selenium should also be given daily by those at risk of developing cataracts.

People with galactosemia, a genetic disease in which the sugar galactose cannot be properly metabolized and builds up in the body, are particularly prone to form cataracts, and cataracts can be induced in lab animals with massive doses of galactose. When the animals are glutathione-deficient, cataract production is greatly increased.

Animals whose cataracts are induced by X-ray or naphthalene (mothballs) also show decreased glutathione in the lens, starting at the onset of the disease. Glutathione or N-acetyl-cysteine supplements may be valuable in some cases of cataract formation.

Drug Overdose

The standard operating procedure at hospitals is to give N-acetyl-cysteine to patients who have overdosed on the street drug "angel dust" or phencyclidine (PCP). This terribly dangerous hallucinogen can cause psychosislike hallucinations and permanent brain damage. N-acetyl-cysteine prevents these toxic effects and is used in conjunction with lavage, charcoal, and magnesium citrate to protect against liver damage following accidental (or deliberate) ingestion of PCP and other abused drugs.

In the laboratory, doses of PCP high enough to kill 80 percent of the animals subjected to it killed only 20 percent of those treated with N-acetyl-cysteine. N-acetyl-cysteine protects against these toxins by raising glutathione in the liver. The cysteine portion of N-acetyl-cysteine is directly incorporated into glutathione, which then helps detoxify the tissues.

Aspirin or any drug containing salicylates may reduce liver glutathione when taken in large quantities. Glutathione or N-acetyl-cysteine is given in cases of phenacetin and aspirin overdoses. Even in small amounts, these drugs can have toxic side effects. Therefore, at our clinic, we have prescribed L-cysteine in order to raise liver glutathione levels for patients with rheumatoid arthritis who take eight to ten aspirins or other pain medications daily.

Studies continue to document the benefits of N-acetyl-cysteine for liver toxicity, particularly that caused by an overdose of acetaminophen (Tylenol). As much as 10 g of N-acetyl-cysteine can be given over four hours, followed by 5 g of N-acetyl-cysteine every four hours.

Emotional Disorders

Over the last fifty years, there have been occasional reports of low glutathione levels in emotional disorders. Interested in glutathione's role as a neurotransmitter, Altschule reviewed these studies and found low blood glutathione in patients with manic depression and schizophrenic psychosis. He suggested that one mechanism that might explain the effectiveness of electroshock or pineal gland extract administration (therapies used before the introduction of psychotropic drugs) is the fact that they increased blood glutathione levels. At our clinic, we administer N-acetyl-cysteine to all people experiencing classic manic depression or schizophrenic psychosis. N-acetyl-cysteine reduces the side effects of drugs commonly used to treat these conditions, and helps stabilize the brain.

Environmental Pollutants

Glutathione protects both liver and lungs from the effects of automobile exhaust. The liver increases its production of glutathione, but the lungs react differently. Chaudhari and Dutta showed a number of enzyme abnormalities that occur in cells lining the lungs from exposure to exhaust gases, including elevations of angiotensin-converting enzymes, which are involved in raising blood pressure. Since glutathione protects against these lung abnormalities as well as liver toxicity, it might be advisable for those habitually exposed to slow rush-hour traffic or polluted air to take a supplement of 500 mg of L-cysteine every morning and evening. This would produce the necessary raw materials for the extra glutathione such an environment demands. Like cysteine, glutathione can also help protect lungs against cigarette smoke. Smokers usually benefit from at least 500 mg of extra L-cysteine daily.

Heavy Metal Toxicity

Glutathione's most important clinical use is in detoxifying the body of poisons. In addition to the many human-invented chemicals that glutathione renders relatively harmless, it also works against heavy metal overdose. In the case of lead toxicity, the body itself produces extra glutathione to cope with the poisoning. Lead overdose lowers glutathione activity in the liver by 28 percent, but temporarily increases glutathione synthesis. Glutathione is believed to chelate, that is, to bind with and transport, lead, and possibly cadmium from the bloodstream and is therefore useful in treatment.

Glutathione also protects against mercury toxicity. At the age of two to four weeks, the body becomes capable of excreting mercury through the bile. This correlates with the increasing ability of the liver to secrete glutathione. It is no accident that glutathione deficiency, resulting from genetic errors, mimics the acute mercury toxicity effects of Minamata disease—a condition that can cause hair loss, heart ailments, and psychosis. Without adequate glutathione, mercury from the environment cannot be detoxified and eliminated from the body.

Arsenic poisoning is another heavy metal toxicity glutathione can alleviate. Experimental animals poisoned by arsenic-contaminated milk were treated for forty days with 100 mg/kg of glutathione. Within ten days, their blood arsenic levels were back to normal. Anemia and leukopenia also improved, and fever (due to arsenic) abated within twenty days. Overpigmentation of the skin diminished, and other clinical symptoms of arsenic poisoning improved. Glutathione is an adjunct to the drug dimercaprol (a thiol sulfur drug), the usual treatment of arsenic poisoning, and may even replace it.

Oxygen Toxicity

In keeping with its function as an antioxidant, glutathione is used as an adjunct to hyperbaric oxygen treatment, in which oxygen is administered under pressure. This therapy is used with stroke victims, where there is some risk of damage to lungs and other delicate tissues, depending on a number of factors such as age, nutrition, and endocrine status. In mice administered glutathione and then subjected to high doses of oxygen under pressure (at one, or one-and-a-half atmospheres considered close to normal pressure) only slight oxygen toxicity occurred, which glutathione could not alleviate. But at six atmospheres of pressure, where oxygen can do extensive damage, glutathione provided excellent protection.

Parkinson's Disease

Antioxidants like glutathione and N-acetyl-cysteine have shown tremendous potential in protecting the diseased part of the brain in individuals with Parkinson's disease. Although still anecdotal, the best results have been achieved with intravenous rather than oral doses of glutathione and N-acetyl-cysteine.

Radiation Prevention

Glutathione and several sulfhydryl compounds (substances that contain sulfur and hydrogen) protect cells from the lethal effects of ionizing radiation. It is suggested that these substance act as a reducing agent, detoxifying by donating hydrogen atoms to organic "free radicals," thereby turning them into water. Studies conducted by Kuna and colleagues indicate that glutathione is of little value following radiation injury such as from a nuclear accident. Rather glutathione's primary use is preventive. In most types of laboratory animals, a 400 mg/kg dose of glutathione reduced the number of deaths, increased the number of white blood cells present, and lowered weight loss and sensitivity to trauma in animals subjected to 2 MEV of X-rays. Some form of glutathione supplementation should be considered prior to radiation therapy for cancer. Sulfur amino acids like cysteine may be the most powerful natural antiradiation compounds.

Stroke Injury

Glutathione has been shown to improve the prognosis of stroke victims. Fritz and colleagues have noted that patients who lose glutathione from the brain in the cerebrospinal fluid following a stroke have a poorer prognosis than those who do not. It may be that one day glutathione, like cysteine, will be added to the standard sugared-salt IV solution in hospital emergency units.

Ulcers

There is solid evidence that glutathione protects the stomach lining against stomach acid. A variety of stress situations that lead to ulcers in experimental animals, including cold, restraint, starvation, or the administration of ulcer-causing chemicals, decrease gastric glutathione levels, according to Boyd and colleagues. This finding implies that glutathione or cysteine may be useful in preventing ulcers caused by medications such as aspirin, phenylbutazone, and other similar nonsteroidal anti-inflammatory agents. It has already been shown that these drugs decrease glutathione levels in rats and that gastric lesions can be prevented by injecting the rats' abdomens with glutathione or cysteine before administering phenylbutazone or piroxicam (aspirinlike derivatives).

Ironically, one chemical analog of cysteine (that is, a chemical very similar to cysteine in structure) actually stimulates ulcer formation. Cysteamine, unlike cysteine, causes histamine to be released, which in turn increases gastric secretion. Lysolecithin, a form of lecithin, protects against cysteamine-induced ulcers.

CYSTEINE AND CYSTINE LOADING

L-cysteine and L-cystine are poorly absorbed forms of cysteine. Six grams of cystine did not elevate blood cystine levels. Yet, this oxidized form of cysteine can break down protein and lead to an increase in hydroxylysines (toxic forms of lysine). Oral cystine had no significant effect on a variety of other biologic parameters. A significant body of research has confirmed that cysteine is best absorbed in the form of N-acetyl-cysteine.

SUPPLEMENTATION

The most effective way to boost glutathione levels is with N-acetyl-cysteine supplements. Supplemental glutathione is expensive, and the effectiveness of oral formulas is questionable. Glutathione, a tripeptide, is used up quickly once produced, especially in stressful states, such as illness, exercise, fatigue, or the general stress of living. To raise glutathione levels, it is better to supply the body with the raw materials to make this compound. Although L-cysteine supplements may also be used with good results, N-acetyl-cysteine is particularly effective for this purpose. N-acetyl-cysteine also appears to be a core antioxidant that needs to be taken daily in conjunction with vitamins C and E, selenium, beta-carotene, and lipoic acid to ensure optimal health and protection. It is especially important for people exposed to high levels of pollutants, smokers, the aging, and those with liver disorders.

Deficiency Symptoms

There are no known signs of cysteine deficiency.

Availability

L-cysteine (free form): 500 mg capsules; N-acetyl-carnitine: 600 mg capsules. Intravenously, either N-acetyl-cysteine or glutathione may be used.

Therapeutic Daily Amount

For most people, 2 g of N-acetyl-cysteine daily for health maintenance is sufficient. The dosage range for L-cysteine is 500 mg two times per day; dosages for N-acetyl-cysteine may vary widely from 2 g to 20 to 30 g daily depending upon the condition being treated.

Maximum Safe Level

Not established. Cysteine and N-acetyl-cysteine appear to be a very safe supplement even in high doses.

Side Effects and Contraindications

In severe conditions, as much as 7 g of N-acetyl-cysteine can be utilized without significant side effects. If L-cysteine is used, we suggest a limit of 500 mg of cysteine twice per day except under medical supervision. Starting with a larger amount can lead to indigestion. Cysteine supplements should be taken with large doses of vitamin C to prevent cysteine from being converted to cystine, which may form kidney stones. Doses greater than 7 g can be harmful. People with cystinuria, an inherited disorder marked by excretion of large amounts of cystine and other amino acids in the urine, are at increased risk of forming cystine gallstones. Excessive intake of cysteine can also result in liver damage or even in some forms of schizophrenia.

CYSTEINE: A SUMMARY

Cysteine is important in energy metabolism. As cystine, it is a structural component of many tissues and hormones. But what makes L-cysteine and all its chemical variants—N-acetylcysteine, D-penicillamine (dimethylcysteine), gamma glutamyl cystine, and cysteamine—so active pharmacologically is that cysteine is a precursor of the ubiquitous tripeptide glutathione.

Glutathione has many roles; in none does it act alone. It is a coenzyme in various enzymatic reactions. The most important of these are redox reactions, in which the thiol grouping on the cysteine portion of cell membranes protects against peroxidation and conjugation reactions, in which glutathione (especially in the liver) binds with toxic chemicals in order to detoxify them. Glutathione is also important in the formation of red and white blood cells and throughout the immune system.

Through these basic functions, glutathione is important. Everyone is likely to be exposed to many of the pollutants that glutathione detoxifies, including lead, mercury, radiation, pesticides, herbicides, fungicides, plastics, nitrates, cigarette smoke, birth control pills, and some pharmaceutical drugs. At the same time, cysteine, by its rapid conversion to glutathione, protects against these toxins.

Glutathione's clinical uses include the prevention of oxygen toxicity in hyperbaric oxygen therapy, treatment of lead and other heavy metal poisoning, lowering of the toxicity of chemotherapy and radiation in cancer treatments, and reversal of cataracts. In one study, oral glutathione was able to reverse advanced liver cancer in rats. Other potential uses may include increasing the recovery chances of stroke victims, preventing liver cirrhosis, and alleviating arthritis, psychosis, and allergies.

Cysteine itself, in addition to the detoxifying function that results from its ability to increase glutathione levels, has clinical uses ranging from baldness to psoriasis to preventing smoker's cough. N-acetyl-cysteine is available in liquid or aerosol form and is great for mucus-burdened bronchial passages. In some cases, oral cysteine therapy has proved excellent for the treatment of asthma, enabling patients to stop using theophylline and other medications.

Cysteine also enhances the effect of topically applied silver, tin, and zinc salts in preventing dental cavities. In the future, cysteine may play a role in the treatment of cobalt toxicity, diabetes, psychosis, cancer, and seizures.

Cysteine levels fall with advancing age, and supplements should be taken to boost blood levels. Cysteine is best absorbed in the form of N-acetyl-cysteine and at present is the preferred form for raising gluthione levels orally. For most people at our clinic, 2 g a day is sufficient for health maintenance, though dosages as high as 7 g a day can be used without significant side effects for treating severe conditions. Measurement of plasma sulfur amino acids provides a guide to therapy and is essential for scientific treatment.

CHAPTER EIGHT

Taurine:
The Seizure Fighter

Taurine is a lesser-known essential amino acid. For many years, it was considered a nonessential amino acid because it is not incorporated into the structural building blocks of protein. Yet taurine is critical in preterm and newborn human infants and in many species, where it is essential for normal growth and development.

Recent research indicates that this amino acid enhances the immune system and plays a major role in the brain and other electrically excitable tissues within the central nervous system, heart, retina, and muscle. Although the body can manufacture taurine from cysteine, it is not known whether the body can manufacture enough taurine to satisfy these needs.

FUNCTION

Taurine has many diverse biological functions where it is found in every cell and in great quantity throughout the body. It has been identified in the kidney; liver; pituitary, thymus, and adrenal glands; nasal membranes; and salivary glands, as well as the mucous membranes lining the digestive tract. Taurine is most concentrated, however, in the central nervous system, heart, white blood cells, muscle, and retina, where its most important function is to facilitate the passage of the minerals sodium, potassium, and possibly calcium and magnesium ions, into and out of cells and to electrically stabilize the cell membranes.

Brain and Central Nervous System

Taurine is the most plentiful free amino acid in the developing brain and the second most plentiful, after glutamic acid (a glutamate amino acid), in the adult brain. Within the brain, taurine is concentrated in the olfactory bulb, which is concerned with taste and smell; in the hippocampus, which is the memory center; and in the pineal gland, a tiny area involved in the body's responses to light and dark. In addition, taurine protects and stabilizes the brain's fragile membranes and acts as a neurotransmitter.

It appears to be closely related in its structure and metabolism to other amino acid neurotransmitters such as gamma-aminobutyric acid (GABA) and glycine. Taurine, like GABA, is inhibitory, that is, it suppresses the release of excitatory neurotransmitters like norepinephrine and acetylcholine. Its concentration in the hippocampus is thought to play a role in memory by increasing histamine and acetylcholine, neurotransmitters believed to be involved in remembering. Within the brain, taurine is also involved in calcium metabolism, which plays a major part in the release of neurotransmitters.

The Heart

Taurine is the most important and abundant free amino acid in the heart, surpassing the combined quantity of all other amino acids. It modulates the activity of important enzymes in heart muscle and contributes to the muscle's contractility. Taurine also plays a role in the metabolism of calcium in the heart and may affect the entry of calcium into the heart muscle cells where it is essential in the generation and transmission of nerve impulses.

The Eyes

Taurine is the most abundant amino acid in the retina of every species studied. Cats make less taurine than humans and can become blind on diets deficient in taurine, cysteine, or methionine. This blindness is due to degeneration of the light-sensitive cells in the eye and can be reversed if caught early enough and the animal's diet is supplemented with taurine.

Although there have not yet been reports of taurine-deficiency blindness in humans, Voaden and his colleagues found that people suffering from retinitis pigmentosa, a disorder characterized by the progressive degeneration of the retina, show abnormal blood levels of taurine. Taurine levels within the eye have also been shown to be decreased in this disease. Taurine has also been found to protect the eye and body from various toxins.

METABOLISM

Taurine is formed primarily from cysteine. Pyridoxine (vitamin B_6) is the most critical nutrient to support the manufacture of taurine in the body. As the most abundant urinary sulfur metabolite after sulfate, a modified form of sulfur, some taurine may be made directly from sulfate, thus bypassing the need for cysteine.

REQUIREMENTS

The National Academy of Sciences has not yet established an RDA specifically for taurine. Minimum requirements for the entire group of sulfur-containing amino acids (taurine, cysteine, and methionine) for infants is 49 mg/kg of body weight. Taurine is an essential for newborns where it is needed to assist in normal growth and development. As the infant grows, they begin to manufacture their own taurine. By age ten, the estimated requirement for the sulfur-containing amino acids is 22 mg/kg.

Adults normally make their own taurine, but it is not known whether the body can manufacture enough to satisfy its own needs. For adults, the estimated minimum requirements for the sulfur-containing group of amino acids is 13 mg/kg per day or 910 mg of these amino acids daily for the average 150 lb adult male. Some reports estimate the tentative requirement to be as high as 1,400 mg/day.

According to Gaull and colleagues, because human beings never developed a high level of cysteine sulfinic acid decarboxylase, an enzyme necessary for the formation of taurine from cysteine, it is likely that all people are somewhat dependent upon dietary taurine. For reasons not yet understood, men have higher levels of the enzymes needed for taurine synthesis than women. In animals, dietary taurine deficiency has a greater effect on females than on males.

Also, human needs for taurine increase under certain high-stress conditions or disease states such as hypertension, seizure disorders, and many forms of heart disease, to make up for either an accompanying impairment of taurine metabolism or for increased requirements by the body. In these cases, taurine plays an important pharmacological as well as nutritional role. Domestic pets (the meat-eating carnivores) also need taurine in their diets. Cats and, to a lesser extent, dogs make none of their own taurine and so depend completely on dietary sources. Herbivores such as horses get no taurine in their diets and so must make all that they need. Humans, monkeys, and other omnivores that eat both meat and vegetables are somewhere in between.

Unfortunately for pets, taurine is largely absent from processed pet food. Dogs and cats may suffer from taurine deficiencies that can lead to degeneration of the retina of the eye and ultimately to blindness. It is a good idea to feed pets raw meat or fish as a regular part of their diet. Organ meats such as kidneys, brains, heart, and liver are inexpensive sources of taurine, which they will greedily eat.

FOOD SOURCES

Organ meats, particularly brains, are excellent food sources of taurine; however, these parts of an animal can be toxic to eat, so we do not recommend them. Taurine, in general, is not found in significant concentrations in food; therefore, in the various disease states in which taurine is depleted or its manufacture by the body is inadequate, food sources alone will probably not supply sufficient taurine, and supplements are necessary.

The Advantages of Taurine for Nursing Mothers

Newborns have very little, if any, capacity to synthesize taurine, and are dependent upon their mothers to provide optimum nutrition. A very important early function of breast milk is to provide taurine to aid normal brain development.

Babies fed formula or cow's milk derive none of the immunological benefits of breast milk, nor do they receive nutrients in the correct amounts or ratios. Low–birth-weight infants fed synthetic formulas were found to have a progressive decrease in taurine concentrations in their blood and urine. Formula-fed infants readily become taurine deficient.

In the mother, taurine increases levels of the hormone prolactin, which triggers the production and release of milk. Therefore, taurine or N-acetyl-cysteine, which is readily converted to taurine, can be a useful supplement for nursing mothers. In a study of three groups of mouse pups on high-, normal-, and low-protein diets, taurine added to the mother's drinking water increased the pups' survival rate by increasing the supply of milk. Failure to thrive may be the first sign of taurine deficiency in an infant, shown by studies in experimental animals. As an infant grows and begins to manufacture its own taurine and obtains taurine from food, the taurine content of the mother's milk drops.

Newborns fed formula often develop higher levels of bilirubin, a red bile pigment that causes the yellow color (jaundice) of some babies at birth. This yellowing is due probably to the stress of birth, and to the fact that neither the liver nor the gallbladder is functioning to capacity. The primary danger of high bilirubin levels at birth is their potential for causing brain damage. When infants are breastfed or sufficient taurine is added to infant formula, jaundice is rare.

Recommendations have been made that baby food, especially infant formula, should be supplemented with taurine since it is also important for the developing nervous system.

FORM AND ABSORPTION

Taurine is a well-absorbed amino acid. Like all nutrients, taurine's absorption is enhanced or decreased by the action of other nutrients. The amino acids alanine and glutamic acid, as well as pantothenic acid, inhibit taurine's action while vitamins A and pyridoxine and the minerals zinc and manganese help build taurine and increase its effects. If monosodium glutamate (MSG)—the sodium salt of the amino acid glutamic acid—is given, as is sometimes done with alcoholics, it tends to reduce taurine. MSG itself can also reduce taurine levels.

CLINICAL USES

The group of sulfur amino acids is chemically distinct from other groups of amino acids because they contain a sulfur molecule. The sulfur combines with hydrogen molecules to become a powerful antioxidant that fights free radicals throughout the body. In its converted form, taurine helps build levels of glutathione, and therefore can help protect against oxidation states and conditions associated with aging. Taurine is particularly effective against hypochlorite, a free radical that contributes to many autoimmune diseases and infections.

Alcohol Withdrawal and Toxicity

Ikeda effectively used 3 g of taurine daily for seven days in the treatment and prevention of alcohol withdrawal symptoms. Taurine, like glutathione and N-acetylcysteine, has been shown to reduce the toxicity of alcohol damage to the liver. *Note:* Taurine may worsen the depressant effects of alcohol. Tachiki and colleagues of Indiana University Medical Center found significantly decreased levels of taurine in depressed patients. Hereditary mental depression has been found in some taurine-deficient patients.

Cardiovascular Conditions

Taurine content in the heart is increased during chronic stress as part of the body's adaptive response. Following ischemia (low oxygen in the heart) or necrosis (heart attack), taurine levels drop sometimes to as low as one-third of normal.

Taurine is now widely used in Japan to treat various types of heart disease. The Japanese are treating acute ischemia of the heart successfully with up to 5 g of taurine a day for three weeks. Although this treatment could produce the unpleasant side effect of ulcers in the digestive tract, none have been reported. In addition, taurine's anti-atherosclerotic effect in the brain has been found to prevent ischemic changes and damage.

Arrhythmia

It is known that both taurine and magnesium are depleted in arrhythmia, or abnormal heartbeats, and may be useful in treating some types of it. Sebring and Huxtable found that intravenous administration of taurine prevented arrhythmias caused by the digitalis commonly used to treat heart failure.

Taurine was also found to inhibit the drop in potassium levels inside heart cells, which can cause electrical instability and thus arrhythmias. It acts in this way to treat poisoning from oleander, an herbal diuretic, and from ouabain, a substance used by African tribesmen in the preparation of poison arrows, which was formerly used in the treatment of heart failure.

Findings have been mixed with regard to taurine's role in other types of arrhythmias. It has been found to prevent supraventricular beats and arrhythmias due to epinephrine (adrenaline), intravenous potassium, and heart stimulants such as digitalis.

According to a Japanese study, taurine can also promote the pumping action of the heart. Taurine alone may be better than low-dose coenzyme Q_{10} (CoQ_{10}) for congestive heart disease. At our clinic, we recommend up to several grams of taurine daily, plus 30 mg of CoQ_{10}.

Cardiomyopathy

Taurine supplements given to experimental animals prevented development of induced cardiomyopathy. Cardiomyopathy is a serious chronic heart condition in which the heart's ability to provide sufficient blood flow to the body is reduced. Taurine is also thought to help lower blood pressure slightly and prevent deterioration in cardiomyopathy patients.

Congestive Heart Failure

A study by Azuma and his colleagues has had a major impact on the treatment of heart disease in Japan. His group ran a double-blind study using taurine to treat congestive heart failure. They found that 4 g of oral taurine a day for four weeks brought improvement to nineteen out of twenty-four patients. The only side effect of the treatment was a tendency to produce loose stools. Taurine content naturally increases in failing hearts, which is thought to be the body's attempt at metabolic correction.

Large doses of taurine, in the range of 2 g per day, appear to help in congestive heart failure by acting as a diuretic and causing sodium and water to be excreted. Taurine also acts as a heart stimulant like digitalis, yet may be safer than the conventional treatments, which do not nourish the heart muscle.

Mitral Valve Prolapse

Some patients with mitral valve prolapse (MVP), a condition in which the mitral valve, which controls blood flow from the left atrium to the heart's main pumping chamber, protrudes too far, have been found to have depressed levels of heart muscle taurine. This inborn error underscores taurine's importance in the heart and suggests that there may be some cases of the common diagnosis MVP that respond to taurine therapy.

Cholesterol Reduction

High cholesterol levels often accompany cardiovascular disease. According to studies by Yamori and his colleagues, dietary taurine stimulates the formation of taurocholate, a substance that increases cholesterol excretion in the bile. Taurine-dependent rats that were fed less sulfur amino acids and more cholesterol showed a rise in blood cholesterol. Adding cystine or taurine to the diet normalized the rats' cholesterol levels.

Taurine also improves fat metabolism in the liver and seems to accelerate the regression of atherosclerotic plaques inside arteries. It should be taken with lecithin and olive oil, which also lower cholesterol, to prevent an increase in stomach acid, a side effect of taurine.

Diabetes

Experimental studies using taurine in insulin-dependent diabetes show the amino acid counteracts oxidative stress and enhances nerve growth factor, slowing the progression of diabetic neuropathy (nerve damage). In insulin-dependent diabetes, taurine is thought to improve utilization of glucose and potentiate the action of insulin. *Note:* Because insulin can have a hypoglycemic effect, taurine should be given with caution to patients with blood sugar problems.

Epilepsy

Since taurine is found primarily in areas of high electrical activity such as the brain, it is not surprising that it exhibits a potent and long-lasting anticonvulsant action that shows great promise in the treatment of seizure disorders such as epilepsy, head or brain trauma, and various forms of encephalopathy.

Taurine's most important function is to stabilize nerve cell membranes, which continuously receive and transmit electrical impulses as the result of the movement of sodium, potassium, calcium, and other ions back and forth across the cell membrane. If the cell membrane is electrically unstable, the nerve cell may fire too rapidly and erratically, which may be the cause of some forms of epilepsy. By making the nerve cell membranes more electrically stable, taurine helps to prevent this erratic firing.

It has also been proposed that epilepsy is caused by abnormal amounts of glutamic acid (a glutamate amino acid) in the brain. According to this theory, taurine works by normalizing the level of glutamic acid. Findings in mice indicate that lack of protein or taurine during the first two weeks of life permanently affects the level of some amino acids, among them glutamic acid, in the brain. This increased level of glutamic acid may make an organism more seizure-prone during certain stressful situations such as high fever, excessive stimulation, trauma, dietary changes, or any of these circumstances in combination with genetic factors and brain damage.

Bonhaus and Huxtable have shown that the uptake of taurine by a special strain of seizure-susceptible rats is only half that of normal control rats. Taurine increases the rate of action of glutamate decarboxylase, an enzyme that breaks down glutamic acid. If epilepsy is caused by an excess of glutamic acid in the brain, taurine's anticonvulsant action must be due to its ability to lower brain glutamic acid levels.

In the brain (as well as in the light-sensitive cells of the retina), taurine is closely associated with or bound to zinc and manganese. These minerals, together with pyridoxine, which is necessary for the synthesis of taurine and all other neurotransmitters, may also be helpful in epilepsy. Since stress can deplete the body of zinc and pyridoxine, it may also lead to lower taurine levels. This is consistent with the fact that certain types of seizure disorder are worsened by stress.

Most studies find that taurine is diminished in the brains of people with epilepsy and that it is an anticonvulsant in most models of experimental epilepsy. Overall evidence suggests that brain taurine deficiencies can be corrected by oral taurine therapy, although other data suggest that taurine has one of the lowest penetrations into the brain of amino acids when given orally. Transport of taurine also can be impaired in people with epilepsy. Bergamini and colleagues may have been the first to use taurine in epilepsy, giving as much as 10 to 15 g intravenously—equivalent to 3.5 to 7 g daily in a 150-lb adult male, with good results, in otherwise untreatable cases.

Recent research shows that taurine has the ability like the amino acid gamma-aminolbutyric acid (GABA) to stabilize cell brain membranes. It is possible that used in high doses it can work as a mild antianxiety agent similar to lithium.

Eye Disorders

Taurine is thought to play a major role in preserving retina health. Taurine deficiency in experimental animals produces degeneration of light-sensitive cells. The lens of the eye acts as an optical filter for the retina and is exposed to high levels of free radicals from ultraviolet radiation, air pollution, cigarette and cigar smoke, and other environmental toxins. It is thought that oxidation might contribute to cataracts by damaging proteins within the lens. Taurine in combination with zinc has been shown to inhibit the development of cataracts. Low levels of taurine are found in the hereditary disorder retinitis pigmentosa.

Taurine Helps Free Patient of Seizures

At our clinic, we have given taurine successfully to many patients with seizure disorders. A sixty-six-year-old man with a history of seizures came to us for help. He had been put on phenytoin (Dilantin), but it had failed to control his seizures. We maintained his dose of phenytoin yet supplemented it with optimal doses of taurine (4 g), manganese (100 mg), and zinc (60 mg). Six months later, he was still free of seizures and his dose of phenytoin had been reduced.

Gallbladder Function

Taurine, glycine, and methionine are the three amino acids most essential to healthy gallbladder function. Taurine is needed for the formation of taurocholic acid, one of the two primary bile acids necessary for the breakdown of fats in the small intestine. Bile formation and excretion may be increased by taurine supplements.

Because of the male's greater ability to make taurine, women may need a higher amount of dietary taurine than do men. Insufficient taurine intake may be one reason women have a higher incidence of gallbladder disease than men. Women with gallbladder disease may benefit from up to 1,000 mg of supplemental taurine per day.

Hypertension

The Japanese's understanding of taurine's role in heart disease naturally led them to explore its role in hypertension. Taurine may act as antagonist to the blood pressure–increasing effect of angiotensin, a circulating protein that is activated by renin, a hormone secreted by the kidneys in response to a drop in blood pressure.

Kohashi and his colleagues have shown that urinary taurine is decreased in essential hypertension (hypertension of unknown origin). This would suggest that overall taurine levels were low and that the body was holding on to its remaining taurine. It is presently unknown whether low taurine levels occur in hypertension because it has been depleted or because the body can't produce enough or obtain enough from the diet.

When both blood and urine taurine levels decrease, renin is activated, angiotensin is formed, and blood pressure rises. Taurine can suppress renin and thus act to break the renin-angiotensin feedback loop, which is believed to be one mechanism of hypertension. In contrast, when rats are given taurine by injection, they show a sharp drop in blood pressure followed by a gradual return to normal. Taurine injected directly into the brain of cats produces a rapid lowering of blood pressure. In hypertensive patients, taurine was found to act as a protector of the central nervous system.

Yamori and colleagues did studies using a strain of rats that are genetically programmed to develop hypertension. He found that these rats had a much lower incidence of stroke if their diet was supplemented with methionine, taurine, and lysine; their stroke rate fell from 90 percent to 20 percent on this diet. Since stroke is often a complication of hypertension in humans, it would be wise for hypertensive individuals to take supplements of these amino acids and to eat a diet high in fish protein, which contains high levels of the sulfur-containing amino acids taurine and its precursor methionine.

Taurine has also been found to reduce the incidence of pulmonary hypertension in individuals who use weight-loss drugs.

Immunostimulation

Taurine is found in high concentration in white blood cells. White blood cells function in fighting infection and in wound repair. Taurine enhances the immune system by stimulating the release of macrophages and increasing the activity of neutrophils, both white blood cells. Taurine has been used to treat the toxicity associated with pneumonia.

Plasma Levels and Clinical Syndromes

At our clinic, we have treated many patients with low plasma taurine. The lowest levels observed were found in a young psychotically depressed female, an eleven-year-old boy with histiocytosis, and a person with chronic schizophrenia. An assorted group of patients showed borderline low levels, among them three hypertensive patients, four depressed patients, and one patient each with obesity, kidney failure, high triglycerides, gout, mental retardation, and infertility. Taurine was particularly helpful in the treatment of the hypertensive patients.

Mildly elevated taurine levels can occur in patients taking other amino acids. Elevations of 25 to 200 percent above normal occur with taurine therapy. Five hundred milligrams of taurine usually raises taurine levels 25 to 50 percent above normal; 1 g generally raises levels from 50 to 100 percent above normal. With prolonged therapy, levels may continue to rise, increasing to three times normal values of taurine in plasma without ill effects. Indeed, taurine levels may be a way of monitoring therapeutic response.

Morphine Withdrawal

Yamamoto and colleagues found that the amino acid neurotransmitters taurine, gamma-aminobutyric acid (GABA), and glycine antagonized the painkilling effect of morphine. Conteras and Tamayo have suggested that taurine may lessen the discomfort of morphine withdrawal. Taurine may also increase the effect of the opiate antagonist naloxone, which is given to drug addicts to block the pleasant effects of opiates such as heroin and morphine. For best effect, taurine should be given thirty minutes prior to administration of naloxone.

Ulcers

Early studies found that taurine and glycine enhanced the ulcerogenic effect of aspirin and other salicylic acid derivatives such as magnesium salicylate. However, a more recent study by Kimura and colleagues showed that taurine protects the stomach and liver from aspirin-induced irritation under some circumstances.

TAURINE LOADING

Taurine is a well-absorbed amino acid with few side effects. We loaded healthy subjects with 5 g of taurine. At two hours, taurine levels increased to more than twenty times normal. At four hours, taurine levels fell to ten times normal. Given acutely, this amino acid had no significant effects on blood pressure; pulse; levels of copper, zinc, iron, manganese, and polyamines; or general chemistry screen variables. Only patients with a tendency to increased stomach acidity have difficulty. Five hundred milligrams of taurine daily will elevate plasma taurine to one and one-half times normal, which may be therapeutic in some diseases.

SUPPLEMENTATION

Taurine is a well-absorbed amino acid with a low rate of side effects, making supplementation easy for individuals to tolerate.

Deficiency Symptoms

Signs and symptoms of taurine deficiency include epilepsy, anxiety, hyperactivity, and impaired brain function.

Availability

Free-form L-taurine is available in 500 mg capsules.

Therapeutic Daily Amount

We continue to lack the data necessary to establish known dosage ranges for taurine. Double-blind controlled studies are not yet available. However, those who are seeking natural remedies for blood pressure, diabetes, arteriosclerosis, atherosclerosis, neuropathy, and anxiety can easily use 1 to 5 g daily without significant documented risk. Higher doses up to 15 to 20 g have been used intravenously.

Maximum Safe Level

Not established.

Side Effects and Contraindications

Taurine may elevate stomach acid and increase risk of ulcers, but only in individuals with a tendency toward increased stomach acid. Taking taurine with food, milk, or milk of magnesia will alleviate this problem. Taurine should never be taken with aspirin. Although rare, taurine in excess may cause depression.

TAURINE: A SUMMARY

Taurine is a sulfur amino acid like cysteine and methionine. It is a lesser-known amino acid because it is not incorporated into the structural building blocks of protein. Yet taurine is an essential amino acid in preterm and newborn human infants and many other species. Adults can synthesize their own taurine, yet are probably dependent in part on dietary taurine. Taurine is abundant in the brain, heart, breasts, gallbladder, and kidneys and has important roles in health and disease in these organs.

Taurine has many diverse biological functions, serving as a neurotransmitter in the brain, a stabilizer of cell membranes, and a facilitator in the transport of minerals such as sodium, potassium, calcium, and magnesium. Taurine is highly concentrated in meat and fish, which are good sources of dietary taurine. Taurine can be synthesized by the body from cysteine when pyridoxine is present. Deficiency of taurine occurs in premature infants and neonates fed formula milk, and in various disease states.

An inborn error of taurine metabolism has been associated with mitral valve prolapse, a disorder involving a defect in one of the heart's valves. People with this condition have elevated urinary taurine levels and depressed levels of myocardial (heart muscle) taurine. Some individuals with mitral valve prolapse may respond to taurine therapy.

After GABA, taurine is the second most important inhibitory neurotransmitter in the brain. Its inhibitory effect is one source of taurine's anticonvulsant and antianxiety properties. It also lowers glutamic acid in the brain, and preliminary clinical trials suggest taurine may be useful in some forms of epilepsy. Taurine in the brain is usually associated with zinc or manganese. The amino acids alanine and glutamic acid, as well as pantothenic acid, inhibit taurine metabolism while vitamins A and pyridoxine and the minerals zinc and manganese help build taurine. Cysteine and pyridoxine are the nutrients most directly involved in taurine synthesis. Taurine levels have been found to decrease significantly in many depressed patients.

Low levels of taurine are found in retinitis pigmentosa. Taurine deficiency in experimental animals produces degeneration of light-sensitive cells. Therapeutic applications of taurine to eye disease are likely to be forthcoming.

Taurine has many important metabolic roles. Supplements can stimulate prolactin and insulin release. The parathyroid gland makes a peptide hormone called glutataurine (glutamic acid-taurine), which further demonstrates taurine's role in endocrinology. Taurine increases bilirubin and cholesterol excretion in bile, critical to normal gallbladder function. It seems to inhibit the effect of morphine and potentiate the effects of opiate antagonists.

Low plasma taurine levels have been found in a variety of conditions, including depression, hypertension, hypothyroidism, gout, infertility, obesity, and kidney failure.

Megataurine therapy has been proven to be useful in those with post myocardial infarction, congestive heart failure, elevated cholesterol, and supraventricular arrhythmias. Dying heart muscle quickly becomes depleted of taurine. Taurine may prove to be useful in patients with epilepsy, gallstones, mitral valve prolapse, hypertension, hyperbilirubinemia, retinitis pigmentosa, photosensitivity, and diabetes. Effective supplemental doses range from 1 mg to 5 g orally. Therapy can be guided by plasma amino acid determination. Taurine is usually well absorbed, and taurine levels can increase to five times normal during therapy without ill effects.

SECTION FOUR

Urea
Amino Acids

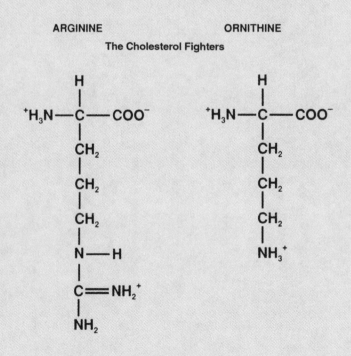

ARGININE **ORNITHINE**

The Cholesterol Fighters

CHAPTER NINE

Arginine and Its Metabolites: The Cholesterol Fighters

A rginine is a nonessential amino acid that the body can synthesize in the liver at a sufficient rate for health maintenance. Yet during periods of growth, stress, infection, or trauma, the body's ability to produce enough arginine to meet these demands may not be rapid enough. At these times, arginine is deemed essential.

Arginine is important for the transport and elimination of the end products of protein metabolism, or nitrogen-containing compounds. Unlike fats and carbohydrates, proteins produce waste material when metabolized. What substances cannot be recycled to build other amino acids and proteins, the body must excrete primarily in the urine before they build up and become toxic. This final biochemical pathway for the breakdown of protein is called the urea cycle.

Major interest in arginine has focused on its role as a precursor to the neurotransmitter nitric acid (NO). With merely one atom apiece of nitrogen and oxygen, nitric oxide is the smallest, lightest molecule and is the first known gas to act as a biological messenger in humans and other mammals. It helps to regulate the dilation and constriction of small blood vessels and plays a crucial role in the treatment of peripheral vascular and cardiovascular conditions throughout the entire body.

FUNCTION

Arginine's primary function in the urea cycle is to maintain a proper nitrogen balance by acting as a vehicle for the transport, storage, and excretion of excess nitrogen. Urea, the main nitrogen-containing constituent in urine, is the final product of protein metabolism.

After nitrogen, the second most abundant waste material is ammonia. Ammonia is produced in the body during deamination (the metabolic process whereby the nitrogen portion of an amino acid is removed), from intestinal tract bacteria, and primarily—although indirectly—from the metabolism of glutamic acid, aspartic acid, and the purines, adenine and guanosine, basic constituents of DNA. A certain amount of ammonia aids the body in keeping a healthy acid/alkaline balance. But because ammonia readily transverses the blood-brain barrier, where high levels of it in the brain can cause irreparable neural and cell damage, it is neutralized and turned into urea almost as soon as it is produced.

Five major enzymes participate in the urea cycle. Arginine stimulates the activity of the first enzyme, carbamyl phosphate (CP) synthetase, which starts the cycle. The liver, which contains all the enzymes involved in the urea cycle in proper proportions, is by far the most important organ for the start of urea cycle reactions. The kidney also contains all the urea cycle enzymes, but only a small amount of arginine is made in the kidney. With the exception of the liver and kidney, deficiencies of one or more urea cycle enzymes have been found in most other tissues and cells tested throughout the body.

The activity of the urea cycle depends on the intake of dietary protein. When rats are fed an arginine-deficient diet, the specific activities of the enzymes involved in arginine's biosynthesis are increased twofold to the level found in urea products. Hence, about half of the body's need for arginine is connected with its action in the urea cycle. Arginine also activates the enzyme acetyl glutamate synthetase, which aids in the synthesis of the glutamate and other stimulatory amino acids.

Arginine is not alone in its role in the urea cycle, which is actually a series of reactions. Early in the cycle, the urea amino acid ornithine, and glutamate and aspartate (derivatives from the family of glutamate amino acids) stimulate the formation of urea; later in the cycle, the urea amino acid citrulline helps keep the body free of toxins by excreting excessive ammonia.

Ornithine and citrulline are primarily found in the liver. Arginine produces ornithine during the urea cycle. Ornithine, in turn, makes glutamic acid, proline, and when combined with ammonia and carbon dioxide, it produces citrulline. Ornithine can regenerate arginine thus perpetuating the urea cycle. Citrulline, if attached to aspartic acid, can create arginosuccinic acid that is further metabolized into arginine. Although ornithine and citrulline are similar to arginine in their biological activity—and therapeutically at times may be used interchangeably—they are not incorporated into body proteins. In fact, citrulline is one of the few amino acids that is not a part of any major proteins or enzyme systems.

Even though ornithine and citrulline and glutamate and aspartate are key to successful nitrogen metabolism in the urea cycle, none has been effective in lowering blood and tissue amounts in several clinical situations because of its key role in this cycle.

Deficiencies or imbalances of essential amino acids will result in increased urea production and excretion. Thus, any amino acid deficiency increases the demands upon the available supplies of arginine. It is thought that a deficiency of arginine increases urea formation. Increased urea synthesis, resulting from increased amino acid deamination is limited by the internal and external (dietary) supplies of arginine. Thus, arginine has a key role in the regulation of protein metabolism throughout the body, and is an indispensable amino acid for optimum growth.

Arginine also serves as a vehicle for transport, storage, and excretion of nitrogen within muscle. Guanidophosphate, phosphoarginine, and creatine are a few of the high-energy compounds used in muscle that are derived from arginine. With excess nitrogen, arginine boosts the production of nitric oxide in the endothelial cells that line the band of muscle that encircles blood vessels. Nitric oxide helps relax blood vessels and keep arteries flexible, making it potentially useful as an alternative agent in the treatment of peripheral vascular and cardiovascular conditions such as high blood pressure, angina, congestive heart failure, diminished cerebral circulation, erectile dysfunction, and high cholesterol.

Arginine is important in the synthesis of polyamines and guanidinoacetic acid (substances that act as markers of cell growth). It helps to increase sperm and collagen production and prompts the release the insulin, glucose, and glucagons (hormones that help maintain normal concentrations of glucose in the blood) from the endocrine gland, and enhances the utilization of glucose. Arginine also stimulates the pituitary gland to release growth hormone.

Arginine is found in highest concentrations in the skin and connective tissues and affects virtually every system in the body.

METABOLISM

Arginine is manufactured in the liver during the urea cycle from its metabolites

Arginine Reserves for Ailing Livers

Because the liver is the primary site of protein metabolism, when conditions such as liver injury, hepatic cirrhosis, and fatty liver degeneration occur, the liver loses a great deal of its capacity to metabolize urea. This results in excessive and toxic levels of ammonia, which can lead to serious health problems, including encephalopathy (brain disease) or hepatic coma. When arginine deficiency develops, supplemental arginine therapy works only some of the time. Supplemental arginine can be toxic because of the way the liver handles nitrogen from amino acids. The success of arginine therapy depends on having some natural arginine reserve within the liver. If there is a liver reserve, arginine can help restore the liver. If there is no reserve, supplemental arginine will only speed the already guaranteed decline.

ornithine and citrulline. When arginine is hydrolyzed by the enzyme arginase, it creates ornithine; ornithine, in turn, is the precursor of citrulline and arginine. Both ornithine and citrulline can regenerate arginine after it has been used up in the urea cycle. Arginine is the primary end product of ornithine and supplemental arginine is immediately converted back to ornithine.

The amino acid lysine antagonizes the breakdown of arginine by inhibiting arginine enzyme activity necessary for proper metabolism.

Inherited urea-cycle disorders most frequently associated with the inability to properly metabolize arginine are arginase deficiency (arginemia), argininosuccinate lyase deficiency (argininosuccinic aciduria), and argininosuccinate synthetase deficiency (citrullinemia). All three arginine enzyme disorders are characterized by insufficient ornithine and excess ammonia.

REQUIREMENTS

There is no RDA for arginine. This amino acid is essential for birds and conditionally essential to humans and most mammals. Arginine-deprived cats become seriously ill within twenty-four hours due to rapid decrease in arginine concentration in blood and tissues. Cats cannot make either arginine or ornithine, but ornithine could essentially replace arginine as a dietary supplement in these animals. Rats fed a 14 percent protein diet without arginine showed significantly reduced growth. Pau and Milner of the American Institute of Nutrition found that rats on arginine-deficient diets showed delayed maturation and delayed puberty.

Arginine can be produced in the human body; however, it is considered to be essential in newborn infants and during early childhood development when production may not occur quickly enough to keep up with the requirements. The amount of arginine made by ornithine and citrulline in the urea cycle is deemed sufficient enough to meet adult needs.

Although the body typically makes sufficient quantities of arginine to maintain health, we know that arginine deficiency can occur under many conditions. In the presence of excessive ammonia, excessive lysine, rapid growth, pregnancy, trauma, or protein deficiency and malnutrition, arginine deficiency may occur.

FOOD SOURCES

A high content of arginine is found in fish, poultry, meat, oats, peanuts, soybeans, walnuts, dairy products, carob or chocolate, brown rice, wheat and wheat germ, raisins, and sunflower seeds. It is higher in oats, wheat, and rice than other amino acids, and it is very difficult to find significant amounts of arginine in vegetables, fruits, and oils.

When the diet is low in arginine, it may eventually lead to a deficiency in orotic acid (OA), which is marked by excess excretion of orotic acid in the urine; a condition known as orotic aciduria. Orotic acid is an intermediate compound

TABLE 9.1. ARGININE LEVELS IN FOOD		
FOOD	AMOUNT	CONTENT (GRAMS)
Avocado	1	0.70
Cheese	1 ounce	0.17
Chicken	1 pound	0.65
Chocolate	1 cup	0.30
Cottage cheese	1 cup	1.40
Duck	1 pound	2.20
Egg	1	0.40
Granola	1 cup	0.90
Luncheon meat	1 pound	3.20
Oatmeal	1 cup	0.60
Pork	1 pound	5.24
Ricotta	1 cup	1.60
Sausage meat	1 pound	1.70

in the synthesis of pyrimidines, one of the essential nonprotein nitrogenous constituents of deoxyribonucleic acid (DNA). Hassan and Milner showed that arginine deficiency leads to deficiencies of various nucleotides and nucleic acids. Diets that are high in the amino acid lysine, relative to arginine, can cause high orotic acid excretion in the urine. Therefore, it is important to maintain an adequate intake of arginine.

FORM AND ABSORPTION

Arginine is one of the more poorly absorbed amino acids. Its effectiveness is dependent upon the adequate availability of ornithine, or by high doses of 4 to 5 g or more of supplemental L-arginine. The uptake of L-arginine in supplement form is inhibited by L-lysine just as it is when in the form of dietary protein.

Research is currently being conducted on the D-form of arginine for inhibiting the effect of pain relievers and antibacterial agents.

TOXICITY

Strong arginine supplements of 5 g or more may produce diarrhea. Life-threatening kidney failure can be induced by arginine in people with severe liver disease and moderate renal insufficiency. These contraindications occurred after extremely high doses of 40 to 60 g were administered in experimental trials. Oral doses of L-arginine greater than 40 g are likely to be dangerous.

Arginine, ornithine, and citrulline have very similar adverse effects in most cases. An excess of ornithine, citrulline, or arginine succinic acid can produce ataxia, Hartnup's disease (characterized by disturbances of gait and coordination), and elevated tryptophan levels. Amino acids are natural substances, and like everything in nature, they have the power to heal and occasionally to harm.

Note: When used in the proper dose, arginine supplementation based on low blood levels of arginine may be beneficial for individuals suffering from kidney failure.

CLINICAL USES

Urea amino acids are unique in that they have nitrogen urea attached to them. They can exchange and eliminate waste products and control nitric oxide in the blood. Almost all recommendations given for therapeutic uses of arginine likely apply to ornithine. It is thought that ornithine may enter the mitochondria—rod-shaped structures within cells that manufacture and trap ATP (energy)—more readily than arginine. It is possible that L-ornithine may be a better arginine supplement than arginine itself.

Arginine Vasopressin

Arginine is a component of vasopressin, a natural hormone made by the pituitary with antidiuretic and blood–pressure-elevating effects. One peptide form of vasopressin contains arginine—as one of nine amino acids—and is called arginine vasopressin (AVP). Although arginine may indirectly contribute to these effects, because AVP contains such a small amount of arginine, it is doubtful that this hormone can be induced by arginine supplements alone.

Bacterial Infection

An aggressive and deadly disease-causing bacterium known as pseudomonas that often attacks chronically ill individuals can be very dependent upon arginine in the diet. Low-arginine diets may be helpful in controlling this infection.

Cancer

Arginine has been found to inhibit tumor growth. Weisburger reported that rats given a particular carcinogen, acetamide, responded favorably to arginine supplementation. Takeda found that diets supplemented with arginine significantly inhibited the growth and development of mammary tumors in rats. Additional evidence suggests that arginine may have beneficial effects in treating tumors other than those that are chemically induced.

Milner and Stepanovich of the University of Illinois have closely studied the effects of arginine on cancer. Their research suggests that arginine in some manner inhibits cellular replication of Ehrlich ascites tumor cells found in certain types of cancers. A diet of 5 percent arginine freed mice of tumor cells. A 3 percent diet of arginine was also found to be effective. Neither the 3 percent nor the 5 percent diet inhibited growth in normal mice.

There appears to be a positive correlation between increased activity in the ornithine decarboxylase, an enzyme that helps to break down ornithine and increased tumor growth. Arginine supplementation decreases the activity of ornithine decarboxylase, and thus retards tumor development and reduces polyamine synthesis from ornithine. (Polyamines, as you may remember, are substances that mark cell growth.) Extra arginine probably does not increase polyamines, according to plant studies by Schuber and Lambert. Although the pathway in humans is poorly defined, it is thought that ornithine probably raises polyamines while arginine decreases them.

Arginine deficiency is associated with severe alteration in pyrimidine biosynthesis. Therefore, supplemental arginine may reduce pyrimidine biosynthesis, causing a shortage of nucleic acids for tumor cell growth. Reduced pyrimidines, in turn, lead to a reduction in polyamine biosynthesis. Polyamines are usually high in both blood and urine of cancer patients.

Drugs that are gathered from normal arginine metabolism, such as L-canavanine, can cause low cell counts in blood and produce a lupus-like skin irritation (erythematosus). These analogs have antitumor activity.

Barbul and colleagues working at Albert Einstein College of Medicine showed that dietary arginine inhibits the size, incidence, and regression of tumors in mice with a sarcoma virus. These effects may again be due to arginine's blocking of polyamine, specifically spermine (a type of polyamine) synthesis. We have found that an arginine loading with 6 g can reduce blood spermine by 25 percent, while spermidine (a type of polyamine) remained unchanged. High blood spermines are also characteristic of various cancers.

Diets of 1 percent arginine in mice protect against thymus involution (shrinking of the thymus) of normal aging and injury in rats. The thymus is a small organ located behind the breastbone that produces hormones important for immune response. This effect may be a result of the stimulation of growth hormone.

A diet of 5 percent arginine significantly inhibits tumors induced by the chemical 7,12 dimethylbenzanthracene and transplanted Walker 256 sarcoma. Arginine and glutamine prevent the carcinogenic effect of acetamide in rats. On the other hand, arsenic is a toxic metal that provokes cancer formation by inhibiting arginine and zinc metabolism, according to a study by Nielson.

Arginine can stimulate T lymphocytes, a type of white blood cell that is a crucial component of the immune system, by increasing their numbers and response to mitogens, or unwanted, harmful substances.

Ornithine and arginine inhibit tumor growth in laboratory animals. In mice inoculated with tumor cells, vitamins in combination with L-arginine increased survival times and decreased the incidence of tumor by 30 percent. The effect of L-arginine supplements has promising possibilities in preventing cancer and aging. Further studies are necessary to establish effective anticancer dose ranges, which most likely will be in the 5 to 20 g range.

Cholesterol Regulation

Arginine is even more effective than methionine, taurine, or glycine in lowering blood cholesterol in experimental animals. Diets enriched with 18 percent arginine produced varied reductions in cholesterol. Arginine inhibits fat absorption. The higher the arginine-to-lysine ratio, the lower the cholesterol level. Meats contain more lysine than do vegetable proteins. Lysine inhibits arginine enzyme activity and the breakdown of arginine.

High-lysine diets cause more arginine to be incorporated into atherogenic, arginine-rich apoproteins, for example, apoE, a protein that transports fat and cholesterol in the bloodstream. The lysine-arginine ratio may be important in the regulation of plasma cholesterol. Addition of lysine to soy protein causes an increase in the lysine-arginine ratio, which results in greater severity of atherosclerosis in experimental animals. Vahouny and colleagues of George Washington University School of Medicine have shown that the addition of soy to diets decreases lipid absorption.

Citrulline is high in cholesterol-lowering foods such as onions, scallions, and garlic. These foods may lower cholesterol because citrulline is converted to arginine.

Circulation

There have been dozens of studies showing that arginine as a precursor of nitric oxide improves circulation throughout the body. Nitric oxide is produced by arginine in the endothelial cells that line the band of muscle that encircles blood vessels. It dilates these vessels by signaling neighboring smooth muscle cells to relax. Nitric oxide is thought to enhance circulation and performance in the arteries, immune system, liver, pancreas, uterus, penis, peripheral nerves, lungs, and brain.

Fat Reduction and Increase in Lean Muscle Mass

Arginine helps to reduce body fat and increase lean muscle mass. Because arginine forms the building blocks of creatine, a protein that is needed for making energy in the muscles and for muscle growth, many in the body-building world feel arginine supplementation helps to reduce body fat and increase lean and muscle mass. That view was based on original intravenous studies years ago with 30 g of L-arginine that showed a growth hormone connection (see "Growth Hormone Stimulation" on the following page).

Growth Hormone Stimulation

When 30 g of L-arginine is administered intravenously, a prompt increase in levels of blood glucose, insulin, glucagons, and growth hormone is observed. The elderly respond with a significantly greater elevation of glucose and growth hormone.

Weldon and colleagues showed that 125 to 500 mg of L-dopa and 0.5 g/kg of L-arginine (equivalent to 30 to 40 g in an average adult male) if given intravenously, help to release growth hormone in children of short stature by two different mechanisms. These two substances also help to identify more than 40 percent of growth hormone–deficient children.

Growth hormone stimulates the growth of bone and cartilage systems and favors the retention of amino acids incorporated into proteins and the release of fatty acids from adipose tissue. Growth hormone increases catecholamines and serotonin derivatives in the brains of experimental animals. Growth hormone release via arginine may be beneficial in treating fractures and wounds.

Arginine deficiency produces symptoms of muscle weakness similar to muscular dystrophy. This may be a growth hormone or glucagon deficiency effect. Arginine deficiency often results in insufficient estrogen in developing rats.

Arginine stimulation of growth hormone release may be effective only by the intravenous route of administration. Claims that growth hormone release can occur with low doses of arginine may be unwarranted. We did not find any elevation of growth hormone following oral loading of 6 g of L-arginine in normal controls. Maximum growth hormone release with arginine occurs at four to six times normal arginine levels. (This means that arginine releases growth hormone at about a 30 g dose.) Other amino acids, such as glycine, may be more effective releasers of growth hormone. Arginine may also increase serum gastrin release— a factor in ulcers—and this is a consideration in regard to oral dosing. The hormone somatostatin, taken intravenously, can add to the growth hormone response of arginine.

Many people now choose to inject growth hormone directly instead of stimulating the production of growth hormone naturally. Although growth hormone is available by prescription only, it has proven to be far superior to arginine's ability to stimulate its release.

Hypertension

Arginine has been noted to help reverse high blood pressure. There are numerous anecdotal reports from people who feel arginine helps to lower their blood pressure. Several studies suggest that this effect may be caused by an increase of nitric oxide by arginine. People with high blood pressure may produce insufficient nitric oxide in the blood vessel walls, or may destroy nitric oxide too rapidly.

Lack of adequate relaxation may lead to chronically narrowed arteries, causing hypertension.

Kidney Disease

Arginine aids in kidney disorders and trauma. Arginine deficiency may cause alkalosis and increased urinary ammonia. Arginine supplements were found to decrease orotic acid excretion significantly following partial removal of the liver and with three other types of liver damage and regeneration. Arginine supplementation will promptly decrease urinary citrate concentration during kidney disease.

Male Infertility

Several studies have been reported in the treatment of male infertility with arginine supplementation. Schacter and colleagues found a 100 percent increase in the sperm counts of forty-two male animals shortly after arginine was given. Sperm motility also increased. When treatment was withheld, a decline in sperm counts was noted. After reinstitution of arginine treatment, an immediate improvement again occurred. Arginine deficiency may cause metabolic disorders in tissues where mitosis (cell division) frequently takes place, such as the testes. Arginine therapy not only enhances production of sperm, but also serves to rebuild those substances necessary for normal sperm motility.

Pryor and colleagues from England, however, found arginine supplements did not improve sperm count density and motility. The patients' studies may not have had a long enough trial (three months) at too low a dose (4 g daily). Yet, L-arginine, unlike D-arginine, and lysine, stimulates human sperm motility in test tubes. Further study in man rather than animals is needed. L-ornithine and L-aspartate may also be as effective as L-arginine. Test tube studies suggest these amino acids have positive effects on sperm activity.

Pau and Milner, working at the University of Illinois, found that arginine deficiency appeared to have a specific effect on the development of reproductive functions because with deficiency, puberty was delayed. Only mildly deficient diets resulted in reduced ovarian weight and the rate of first ovulation.

Plasma Levels in Clinical Syndromes

We have found low plasma arginine levels in thirteen patients, four of whom had been chronically institutionalized and the majority of whom were women. Four of the patients were depressed; five other patients presented with one of the following: psychosis, thought disorder, phenylketonuria, severe allergies, and asthma. In general, these patients were of reduced weight and had chronic disease. It is worth noting that in general, patients with lower arginine levels also have lower ornithine levels.

We have not found elevated arginine levels in any of our patients. The highest levels were in patients supplemented with amino acids. Chronic mega amino acid therapy may concomitantly elevate several plasma amino acids. It is important to remember that higher plasma amino acids are found in youth more often than in adulthood; the decline as the body ages is probably a natural, healthy one.

Urea, a byproduct of the urea cycle, is controlled to some extent by arginine. Urea in plasma often follows a distribution similar to that of arginine in plasma. Plasma urea levels are significantly lower in women. Individuals with elevated levels of urea usually have some type of chronic disease like arthritis, myeloma, heart failure, or hypertension.

Wound Healing

In one animal study, 4.3 g a day of L-arginine was given to rats three to four days prior to surgery, and three to ten days postoperatively. Incisions healed more quickly and greater collagen synthesis resulted. Collagen is the main supportive protein of skin, tendons, bone, cartilage, and connective tissues. Arginine, by its conversion to ornithine and proline, leads to proline's conversion to collagen. (Proline supplementation reduces the dietary requirement for arginine.) Results are mixed when comparing the benefits of arginine versus glutamic acid in collagen conversion. Arginine-deficient animals rapidly lose collagen according to Barbul and colleagues. Skin incisions are also weaker in these rats.

Enzymes that break down collagen, known as collagenases, are dependent on zinc for activity. Large loading doses of 6 g of L-arginine can significantly lower whole blood zinc levels by as much as 25 percent.

Lee and Fisher from Rutgers University, New Jersey, found that arginine (2 percent) increased posttrauma growth in rats. The basis for arginine's role in controlling cancer and healing wounds may be related to the thymus, the organ that produces hormones important for immune response. Three to five grams of L-arginine daily may be thymotropic, or thymus stimulating. Diets that consist of 1 percent arginine protect mice and rats against thymus involution (shrinking of the thymus) caused by normal aging or injury. This protection may be a result of the stimulation of growth hormone. Ornithine is also thymotropic, while citrulline responses may not be.

TWO IMPORTANT METABOLITES

Citrulline

Citrulline is one of the few amino acids that is not a part of any major proteins or enzyme systems. It is made when carbon dioxide, ammonia, and orthinine are combined in the liver. If attached to the amino acid aspartic acid, citrulline creates arginosuccinic acid, which is further metabolized into arginine. Its mechanisms of action include participating in the urea cycle to keep the body free of toxins and to excrete excessive ammonia.

It appears to play the part of a diuretic, tonic, and an immune-system enhancer. Studies have also noted that citrulline appears to play a part in rheumatoid arthritis and its associated inflammation, regulation of blood pressure, and cardio-protectiveness, as well as perhaps having a positive impact on learning abilities.

A rare genetic defect that prevents proper conversion of citrulline to arginine has been identified in a few individuals. This results in an elevation of the level of citrulline in the blood and a decrease in the circulating level of arginine. This condition is associated with ammonia buildup in the body and symptoms such as irritability and mental confusion. Zinc and pyridoxine are needed for proper conversion of citrulline to arginine.

Dietary sources of citrulline are melons, watermelons, cantaloupe, and cucumber, but not the citrus fruits as we might expect from the name. Citrulline supplementation can be helpful in chronic fatigue patients. Further studies to determine specific treatment guidelines for this amino acid continue.

Ornithine

Ornithine is the most important constituent of the urea cycle. Due to its ability to enhance liver functions, it is often used in hepatic crisis states. Ornithine is also the precursor of citrulline, proline, and glutamic acid. When hydrolyzed by the enzyme arginase, arginine creates ornithine.

Ornithine has been associated with an increase in polyamines. Ornithine decarboxylase is a rate-limiting enzyme in the synthesis of polyamines. Because its activity is associated with tissue growth and differentiation, ornithine decarboxylase can be used as a marker of cancer activity. Stimulation of B-adrenergic receptors accounts for increase in the activity of the enzyme. Hence, B-agonists can raise polyamine levels while B-blockers may artificially lower them.

Decarboxylation of ornithine is the most important step in polyamine synthesis. Thus, ornithine supplements may raise polyamine levels.

Salt-Free Salt

First came aspartame, the amino acid sweetener. Now, researchers have created ornithyltaurine, the amino acid combination that tastes salty without any sodium. Recently developed in Japan, this new nutritive salt may eventually provide significant amounts of ornithine to people's diets. For this and other reasons, we studied ornithine loading.

A number of pharmaceutical agents have been developed to inhibit the enzyme ornithine decarboxylase in an attempt to block cancer growth. Initial research into this aspect of ornithine metabolism bears watching.

Ornithine has been claimed to improve the immune system, stimulate growth hormone release, and suppress tumor activity. It is found in the largest concentration in the skin, explaining its ability to assist with wound healing and repairing damaged tissues.

Several studies with bodybuilders have been conducted on the benefits of ornithine. Some studies have found that a combination of ornithine and arginine may promote muscle-building activity, as well as increases in lean muscle mass and strength.

Clinical studies have found different uses for ornithine. For example, a study done in 1994 with acutely ill patients noted that supplementation with ornithine improved the patients' appetites, allowed weight gain, and improved their over-all quality of life. In 1998, a study showed that ornithine alpha-ketoglutarate sup-plementation improved wound healing and decreased hospital stays in people with severe burns.

A rare cross-linked recessive disorder marked by the blockage in conversion of ornithine and carbamyl phosphate (CP) to citrulline is called ornithine trans-carbamylase deficiency. Most commonly, it is identified by excessive levels of ammonia, elevated orotic acid with normal levels of citrulline, argininosuccinic acid, and arginine.

Low ornithine levels have also been found in patients with growth defects. The lowest significant plasma ornithine levels we have seen have been in two patients with delayed maturation and one patient with low sperm count. We are presently treating these patients with ornithine. Ornithine has been suggested to produce increased motility in human sperm during test tube studies.

Ornithine levels are low in most patients with overall low amino acids, i.e., institutionalized patients, those with kidney disease, those with inborn genetic errors such as phenylketonuria, patients in depression and women with chronic illness (women generally have lower plasma amino acids). Among patients at our clinic who were found to have low ornithine, three patients had hypertension. The significance of this unusual finding is unclear.

Of our patients with higher ornithine levels, eight were depressed, two had problems of leg edema, and one was hypothyroid. The significance of these find-ings is also unclear.

Ornithine is produced naturally by the body, but can also be found in meat, fish, dairy products, and eggs. The normal diet provides about 5 g of ornithine per day.

Studies suggest that ornithine can only be of benefit by assuring production and metabolism are not blocked, thus resulting in decreased hair production or decreased cancer cell growth. Ornithine is sold as a topical hair-growth inhibitor.

Almost all recommendations given for therapeutic uses of arginine likely apply to ornithine. It is thought that ornithine may enter the mitochondria more readily than arginine. It is possible that L-ornithine may be a better arginine supplement than arginine itself.

ARGININE LOADING

Arginine loading shows that arginine is one of the more poorly absorbed amino acids. Six grams administered to a 180-lb man increased plasma levels only slightly more than 100 percent at two and four hours. It is possible the arginine was more rapidly utilized. Ornithine levels rose concomitantly. Of all the amino acid conversions thus far studied, the arginine-ornithine conversion is the most rapid. Other conversions, such as lysine to carnitine, take six hours to become significant.

Arginine loading affects other amino acids as well. It is thought to raise the sulfur amino acids and decrease tryptophan and glycine. Other biological parameters, such as growth hormone, most chem-screen items, trace metals, and polyamines showed little or no change.

SUPPLEMENTATION

Almost all recommendations given for therapeutic uses of L-arginine likely apply to L-ornithine. It is thought that L-ornithine may enter the mitochondria more readily than arginine.

Deficiency Symptoms

Signs and symptoms of arginine deficiency include rash, hair loss and breakage, poor wound healing, muscle weakness, constipation, decreased sperm count, a fatty liver, hepatic cirrhosis, and hepatic coma.

Availability

Free-form L-arginine and L-ornithine are available in 500-mg capsules. These amino acids may also be found in a combination formula in a ratio of 500 mg of L-arginine to 250 mg of L-ornithine. L-arginine and L-lysine should not be taken together, as lysine is a direct antagonist of arginine.

Therapeutic Daily Amount

The typical dose of L-arginine or L-ornithine is 3 g twice daily. This is dependent upon the condition being treated. Large doses of 5 g or more of L-arginine may be necessary to achieve desired effects. Monitoring of plasma arginine levels may be necessary to guide therapy.

Maximum Safe Level

Not established.

Side Effects and Contraindications

L-arginine and L-ornithine should always be supplemented with great care in patients who have diagnoses or distinct characteristics of schizophrenia due to the possibility of exacerbating the psychiatric symptoms. Side effects of nausea, vomiting, and insomnia have been noted when taking more than 10 g of L-ornithine a day.

ARGININE: A SUMMARY

Arginine is a basic amino acid involved primarily in urea or ammonia buildup and excretion, as well as DNA, polyamine, and creatine synthesis. Arginine is an essential nutrient in cats, rats, and other mammals. In humans, arginine is essential only under certain conditions. Conditional deficiency of arginine occurs in the presence of excess ammonia, excess lysine, amino acid imbalances, rapid growth, pregnancy, trauma, protein deficiency, or enzyme deficiency. As much as 20 g of L-arginine can be used to treat several inborn errors of urea cycle enzymes. Arginine deficiency is associated with rash, hair loss and breakage, poor wound healing, constipation, fatty liver, hepatic cirrhosis, and hepatic coma.

Arginine supplementation is marked by many endocrine effects. In high doses of 20 to 35 g given intravenously, arginine releases growth hormone, glucagons, and insulin. Doses as low as 1 g have been claimed to increase growth hormone quite significantly, although our studies have been unable to document this claim. Large doses of arginine given to rats increase collagen deposition, promote wound healing, and positive nitrogen balance. Even larger levels in the diets of rats, 1 percent or more, protect the rats against thymus involution and provide anticancer effects. We have found that large doses of arginine can lower polyamines, which are elevated in various cancers. Arginine, like ornithine and aspartic acid, has a positive effect on viability of sperm and may have a role in the treatment of male infertility.

Metabolic arginine deficiency can be measured in blood or cerebrospinal fluid, or by orotic acid excretion in urine. Several of our cancer patients have shown decreased arginine in blood and have been treated with amino acid supplements. We have characterized patients with low plasma arginine as being primarily women of small structure who have reduced protein mass with a history of chronic disease or prolonged hospitalization. Many of these patients have multiple amino acid deficiencies and respond to multiple amino acid formulas. Arginine excess occurs in several inborn errors of metabolism and may be useful in treating cancer.

Doses greater than 40 g daily of arginine can result in dangerous kidney failure in patients with liver or kidney disease.

Arginine, like methionine, taurine, and glycine, lowers cholesterol. We have found arginine loading doses of 6 g to reduce cholesterol by as much as 10 percent. The cholesterol-lowering effect is enhanced by diets high in arginine and low in lysine, probably cereals such as whole grains and oats as opposed to meat protein.

Arginine supplements may be of value in many disease conditions. As part of the body's health-maintenance system, this amino acid is just beginning to be understood.

SECTION FIVE

Glutamate Amino Acids

GLUTAMIC ACID, GAMMA-AMINOBUTYRIC ACID, AND GLUTAMINE
The Brain's Three Musketeers

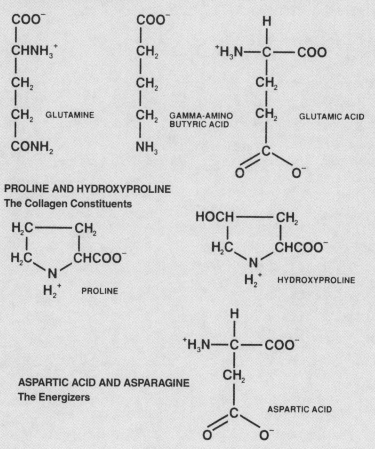

PROLINE AND HYDROXYPROLINE
The Collagen Constituents

ASPARTIC ACID AND ASPARAGINE
The Energizers

CHAPTER TEN

Glutamic Acid, Gamma-Aminobutyric Acid, and Glutamine
The Brain's Three Musketeers

Glutamic acid (GA), gamma-aminobutyric acid (GABA) and glutamine (GAM) are three closely related, nonessential amino acids that are intricately involved in sustaining proper brain function and mental activity. They work as a powerful trio to ensure smooth running of brain reactions and nerve signals throughout the central nervous system with each dependent upon the other for their role in the brain's message-delivery system. Glutamic acid can be converted into either glutamine or GABA and—vice versa—can be formed from both GABA and glutamine.

Glutamic acid is an excitatory neurotransmitter that acts as a brain stimulant by increasing the firing of neurons; GABA is an inhibitory neurotransmitter that creates a calming effect by decreasing neuron activity and nerve cells from overfiring; and glutamine, which can readily pass the blood-brain barrier, is a primary source of brain fuel and a mediator of both glutamic acid and GABA activity. Because of their metabolic teamwork, we call them "the three musketeers."

FUNCTION

Among the three musketeers, glutamate, the salt form of glutamic acid, is the most prolific neurotransmitter; it exists everywhere in the body and is present in almost all nerve cells. Glutamic acid is a major excitatory neurotransmitter that is found in the cranial nerves and in the nerves of the hippocampus—the memory center of the brain. It is also involved in all brain cells and in photoreceptor transmission in the retina, an extension of the brain. Of all the amino acids in the brain, glutamic acid has the highest concentration with the exception of aspartic acid, another glutamate amino acid.

Glutamic acid performs critical roles in disorders of the brain such as schizophrenia, Parkinson's disease, and epilepsy, and it helps to correct childhood

165

behavioral disorders. It is useful in treating hypertension, chorea, dyskinesia, and alcoholism, and in the metabolism of sugars and fats.

Optimal functioning of the brain requires that excitation is balanced with inhibition. GABA was identified some fifty years ago as the most prevalent inhibitory neurotransmitter in the central nervous system. Many neurologic, psychiatric, and impulse disorders and addictive behaviors that have agitation and manic behaviors or high levels of anxiety associated with them such as Parkinson's disease, epilepsy or any seizure disorder, alcohol or drug addictions, sleep disorders, chronic pain syndromes, or even chronic stress and illness are conditions affected by GABA receptors. GABA blocks stress and anxiety-related messages from reaching the motor centers of the brain by occupying their receptor sites.

GABA works in the body in much the same way as diazepam (Valium) and chlordiazepoxide (Librium) and other tranquilizers and barbiturates, but without the undesired side effects and the potential for addiction. New pharmacologic agents have been formulated that create similar effects by activating GABA neurons and receptors in the brain. In recent years, research on GABA's role in controlling seizures and mood swings has intensified and resulted in new, important compounds that augment GABA uptake in the brain.

Two of the best examples of the blending of medical technology and nutritional science are gabapentin (Neurontin) and tiagabine (Gabitril), which are almost identical to the chemical structure of GABA. They represent one of the largest breakthroughs in medicine to assist individuals to remain calm without having to resort to using a narcotic. GABA is found in particularly high concentrations in the hypothalamus, a region of the brain that regulates the hormonal functions of the pituitary, an endocrine gland, where it appears to exert an effect on the pituitary's release of prolactin. GABA has also been found to be important in glands controlled by the sympathetic nervous system, such as the pancreas, duodenum, and thymus.

Although not as clear-cut in its functions as glutamic acid and GABA, the neurotransmitter glutamine is known to be a major fuel source for the brain and for various cells of the immune system. It is the most abundant amino acid in muscles and blood. The concentration of glutamine in the blood is three to four times greater than all other amino acids, and glutamine is ten to fifteen times more concentrated in cerebrospinal fluid than in the blood.

In muscle, glutamine is readily available when needed to make skeletal muscle proteins. Because glutamine helps maintain and build muscle, it helps protect against muscle wasting that can occur in diseases such as cancer and AIDS, or as a result of stress or trauma to the muscles, and it is a critical component in wound repair.

Glutamine is unique in that each of its molecules contains two nitrogen atoms instead of one like all other amino acids. This construction particular to glutamine enables it to serve as an important vehicle for nitrogen transport from one place to another. In cells, it performs a major role in DNA synthesis by contributing nitrogen atoms in the manufacture of purines and pyrimidines (major components of DNA). Glutamine also donates one of its nitrogen atoms to form niacin (vitamin B_3) and participates in the metabolism of arginine. It helps clear ammonia from the tissues, especially the brain, and assists in maintaining the proper acid/alkaline balance in the body.

Glutamine can be converted to glutamic acid and can boost levels of GABA in the brain, depending upon which is needed at the moment to maintain balance in the central nervous system. The combined concentration of this trio makes the three musketeers the most abundant amino acid group in the brain. Their motto is "one for all and all for one."

METABOLISM

Although glutamic acid and its family of neurotransmitters are made primarily from glutamine and GABA, it can be synthesized from many different sources. Glutamic acid can also be formed from aspartic acid, ornithine, arginine, proline, and alpha-ketoglutarate (a carbohydrate involved in glutathione metabolism from which glutamic acid may form).

It was once thought that the degree of glutamic acid's potency depended on its source; however, it is now known that all these substances make a significant metabolic contribution. Arginine, in particular, makes a significant contribution in the brain to the formation of nitric oxide, whereas glutamine, aspartic acid, and alpha-ketoglutarate play a major role in the formation of the stimulatory amino acids. Metabolism of GABA results in the derivatives gamma-hydroxybutyrate (GHB), a natural sleep-inducing compound in the brain, and gamma-butyroplactone; both are found in small amounts in the brain where they function as inhibitory neurotransmitters.

As in the normal metabolism of all amino acids, pyridoxine (vitamin B_6) is the most important physiological compound that regulates the manufacture of glutamic acid, GABA, and glutamine in the body and brain, where the metabolism of these three musketeers is widespread and active.

REQUIREMENTS

There is no RDA for glutamic acid. Its levels are easily affected by disease states, but in general, this amino acid is widely available in the body. It can be synthesized in the body from many different sources and glutamic acid is one of the more abundant amino acids found in food.

FOOD SOURCES

Glutamic acid is plentiful in foods, whereas glutamine and GABA are absent. Glutamic acid makes up 43 percent of wheat gluten, 23 percent of casein, and 12 percent of gelatin proteins. Meat, poultry, fish, eggs, and dairy products are all rich sources of in glutamic acid.

FORM AND ABSORPTION

Dietary and supplemental sources of glutamic acid, GABA, and glutamine are most potent in their L- form. Of the three, glutamine and GABA are better absorbed than glutamic acid. Their effectiveness appears to be based on individual biochemistry as some individuals benefit more from GABA (in the form of gabapentin) and some from glutamine.

Aspartic acid is an excitatory neurotransmitter that is competitively trans-

TABLE 10.1. GLUTAMIC ACID LEVELS IN FOOD		
FOOD	AMOUNT	CONTENT (GRAMS)
Avocado	1	0.40
Bacon	1 pound	6.00
Cheese	1 ounce	1.51
Chicken	1 pound	0.65
Chocolate	1 cup	1.70
Cottage cheese	1 cup	6.70
Duck	1 pound	4.50
Egg	1	0.80
Granola	1 cup	2.60
Ham	1 pound	13.00
Luncheon meat	1 pound	10.00
Oatmeal	1 cup	1.40
Peach	1	0.14
Pork	1 pound	5.24
Ricotta	1 cup	6.00
Rolled oats	1 cup	2.00
Sausage meat	1 pound	1.70
Turkey	1 pound	6.00
Wheat germ	1 cup	5.60
Whole milk	1 cup	0.30
Wild game	1 pound	12.0
Yogurt	1 cup	2.30

ported with glutamic acid and can hinder its absorption. The inhibitory neuro-transmitters taurine and glycine are competitively transported with GABA and can block its absorption. Lysine, through its metabolite pipecolic acid, however, seems to amplify GABA action in the brain.

NUTRIENT INTERACTIONS

The enzyme glutamine synthetase is a manganese-containing enzyme, so manganese is obviously important in the synthesis of glutamine and in the overall proper metabolism of glutamic acid. Many patients seen at our clinic are low in manganese because of poor dietary habits and poor food quality.

An analysis of the relationship of vitamin C and the three musketeers found that GABA stimulates the release of vitamin C from rat striatal tissue and appears to promote its utilization and metabolism.

TOXICITY

Certain acidic amino acids—glutamic acid, aspartic acid, cysteic and cysteine sulfinic acid, and homocysteinic acid—are excitatory neurotransmitters and can be damaging to the brain. Extremely large doses of glutamic acid can produce brain damage in experimental animals. Animals given 2.5 to 5 percent of glutamate (a salt form of glutamic acid) or aspartate (a salt form of aspartic acid) in drinking water would voluntarily drink enough to result in hypothalamic injury. Studies reviewed by coauthor Pfeiffer while at the University of Chicago initially suggested that 2 g/kg of glutamic acid, or 140 g for the average male adult, could produce symptoms of toxicity, primarily nausea and vomiting. The level in blood that results in clinically documented toxicity is twenty times normal.

However, other studies found that much lower levels of glutamic acid could cause acute loss of brain neurons, particularly in young animals because they lack a well-developed blood-brain barrier. Monosodium glutamate (MSG) becomes toxic at .75 g/kg or about 55 g a day and glutamic acid at 1 g/kg or 70 g a day, producing severe necrosis (tissue death) of hypothalamic neurons of the brain. In contrast, cysteine at 3 g/kg reduced hypothalamic neurons in experimental animals; this would be the equivalent of 200 g per day of this amino acid in a human diet.

Remarkably, even at this high dose of 3 g/kg, glycine, serine, alanine, DL-methionine, leucine, phenylalanine, proline, and arginine given to experimental animals did not produce any observable neurological side effects. At high doses between 70 to 280 g of glutamic acid, severe retinal lesions and degeneration occurs. It is worth noting that while chickens will tolerate a 15 percent diet of L-glutamate, a 5 percent diet of D-glutamate results in a 40 percent depression of growth in chickens in just two weeks. The D-form amino acids are usually more

Monosodium Glutamate (MSG): "Chinese Restaurant Syndrome"

For at least 1,000 years, the Chinese have added an extract of seaweed to enhance the flavor of food. In the early twentieth century, the agent that was responsible for the flavor-enhancing effects was chemically analyzed from the seaweed extracts and found to be monosodium glutamate (MSG), a salt form of glutamic acid. Today, MSG is a meat tenderizer and food additive used throughout the world in processed and restaurant foods. Its usage is estimated to be as much as 30,000 tons per year worldwide.

About 30 percent of diners who ingest Chinese food regularly suffer from Chinese restaurant syndrome (CRS). Ingestion of large amounts of MSG may be followed by headaches, nausea, weakness, thirst, flushing in the face, burning, abdominal pain, cramps, dizziness, vomiting, chills, depression, and dryness of the mouth. Excessive sweating, a sense of fullness after eating relatively little food, sleepiness, tingling sensation of the gums, and weakness have also been reported. The most frequent side effects are blurred vision, dizziness, and headaches. MSG also increases heart rate. The cause of these effects may be due to a transient increase in acetylcholinelike substances.

The sodium salt of glutamic acid is significantly more toxic than glutamic acid alone. Minimal toxicity has been observed with doses as low as 2 or 3 g when administered to average adult males on an empty stomach. MSG in high doses can cause damage to all brain structures in infants and animals, particularly the hypo-

---

toxic than the L- forms. In experimental animals, the equivalent of as little as 3 g of glutamic acid per 150 pounds can lower seizure threshold.

CLINICAL USES

The glutamate group of amino acids primarily serves to modify GABA and its dominating inhibitory effects upon the central nervous system. They control the excitatory and relaxation pathways of the brain by turning on and off the GABA and glutamate pathways. There are therapeutic uses for glutamic acid and glutamine, but GABA has the most therapeutic potential of the three musketeers.

Aging and Mental Performance

Aging greatly alters the metabolism of the brain. With aging, the enzyme glutamic acid decarboxylase, which forms GABA from glutamic acid, decreases markedly. Manganese supplements can correct the problem of reduced GABA synthesis in aging brains.

thalamus and all structures that are adjacent to the ventricular cerebrospinal fluid chambers. Large doses of 4 g of MSG per kg—a dose equivalent to 280 g per day—when given to an average adult male, produces increased body weight and decreased pituitary, thyroid, and testis size. Stunted growth and various reproductive dysfunctions may also occur with chronic MSG intake.

The body's water retention after eating soy sauce, which is more than 50 percent MSG, can be so extreme as to inhibit normal urination for twenty-four hours. Large doses of common salt will produce the same effect. Two years of prolonged studies of feeding 4 percent MSG to rats resulted in increased urine volume, sodium excretion, and significant kidney damage. In another study, feeding of 10 percent MSG to rats increased the excretion of sodium in urine, but there were no adverse effects on body weight gain, general behavior, eyes, blood, or hematological or blood chemistry. The kidneys did not show any permanent damage.

Studies using MSG in amounts similar to normal human exposures, such as 0.1 percent or 0.4 percent in the diet of rats for twelve weeks, had no adverse effects on motor activity, food consumption, weight, blood, fertility, or survival. In fact, it is possible that MSG at low doses has no permanent side effects and no sign of toxicity.

Typically, when MSG is used as a flavor enhancer, it is added only at a rate of 0.2 to 0.8 percent in foods and is relatively nontoxic. Those susceptible to CRS, however, should ask for MSG-free food when ordering Chinese food and should avoid any use of soy sauce with its high level of MSG. As a possible antidote to reduce symptoms caused by MSG, we recommend 1g of GABA with inositol.

Measured intelligence quotient (IQ) also decreases with aging. Both GABA and glutamic acid in megadoses have been reported to raise IQ in the elderly, and these nutrients, along with glutamine, have been found effective in treating various forms of age-related decreased mental performance.

Twelve grams of glutamic acid per day were given orally to a group of individuals. Although the subjects complained of gastric distress, the glutamic acid brought about improved intellectual performance, alertness, and attentiveness. Several studies have been done since with experimental rats at low dosages of glutamic acid that were equivalent to a human dose of about 6 g. The rats' abilities to learn mazes and other tasks improved. Doses as high as 20 g given intravenously produced some nausea and vomiting in human subjects. It appears that doses up to 10 g per day given to humans are probably safe. Whether or not these have lasting intellectual benefits has not been followed up adequately. Most likely there exists a therapeutic window for glutamic acid therapy in patients with decreased IQ. In a study using a GABA-like compound at 1 to 3 g in mentally retarded patients, 63 out of 106 patients showed a significant increase in IQ.

An inhibitor of the synthesis of glutamine called methionine sulfoximine, a byproduct of methionine, has been known for a long time to produce convulsions and Alzheimer's disease or senile dementia–like changes in the brain of animals. This further reinforces the essential role of the three musketeers in cognitive performance.

Alcoholism

Glutamic acid and glutamine therapy may reduce cravings for alcohol. In one impressive study, alcoholics were given 2 g of L-glutamine three times a day, or 6 g daily, for one month. The second month, they received 12 g, and in the third and fourth months, the dose was increased to 15 g daily. Compared to a placebo, 75 percent of the alcoholics reported to have a definite improvement or control over their alcoholism.

In follow-up studies, vitamins containing large amounts of MSG (approximately 7 or 8 g a day) were used. These alcoholics experienced a 70 percent improvement. However, in later studies, patients using 10 g of MSG showed no improvement.

Some nutritionists continue to use L-glutamine and report good results in the treatment of alcoholism. Obviously, further research is necessary. For those who are chronically resistant alcoholics, trials of 6 to 15 g of L-glutamine would be justified. The theoretical basis for glutamine's action may relate to glucose metabolism; glutamine can provide adequate energy for the brain in the absence of glucose.

No clear role for GABA in alcoholism has been identified. Stress seems to increase GABA in the brain, while alcohol or diazepam and other benzodiazepine drugs seem to deplete GABA. Thiamine-deficient encephalopathy due to alcoholism also depletes GABA, glutamic acid, and aspartic acid in the brain. Because it raises GABA, chlordiazepoxide is now known to be useful in curbing alcohol cravings.

Alzheimer's Disease

Increased levels of glutamic acid have been found in patients with Alzheimer's disease. The significance of this finding is unclear, but these levels are doubtless related to the seizures that frequently occur following loss of memory.

Anxiety

Levels of GABA, like glutathione, go down with chronic illnesses and can result in chronic anxiety symptoms. Everyone becomes anxious and burned out when they suffer from continuous levels of stress and/or illness, secondary to the GABA deficiency that occurs. The level of stress that can precipitate this physiological change can be anything from day-to-day activities or chronic back pain to high levels of physical or mental traumas.

Antianxiety medications work by stimulating GABA receptors. Because of its inhibitory effects on the central nervous system, GABA can help to decrease message transmissions in neurons. This helps prevent nerve cells from firing too fast, which can overload the system, and allows for a calming effect to predominate.

A forty-year-old woman with severe anxiety came to our clinic. She was taking both diazepam and lorazepam (Ativan) daily. We started her on 200 mg of GABA four times a day. Soon she was able to stop taking the diazepam and could reduce the dosage of lorazepam. The only side effect she experienced was fatigue, which was most likely brought on by the inositol in the GABA preparation.

We had inconsistent results with supplemental forms of GABA. Nevertheless, over the years, many anxiety patients who have been willing to take 2, 3, and 4 g a day, in multiple doses, claim that GABA works well for them. They use GABA the way other people use the antianxiety drug alprazolam (Xanax); they claim that it helps them to sleep and relax. Still others have used lower dosages and claim benefit. It is possible that some of these patients have an individually enhanced sensitivity; for some, there may be a placebo effect. We believe a modified version of GABA such as gabapentin or tiagabine is more effective, not only for treating anxiety, but also for use in impulse disorders, addictive behavior, and many other psychological conditions.

GABA can be nauseating, but this side effect is infrequent with gabapentin and tiagabine. We have also been able to replace the anticonvulsant clonazepam (Klonopin, Rivotril) with GABA. We believe that GABA as an antianxiety agent is worth a try in some severely anxious people dependent on benzodiazepines.

Appetite Suppression

Several studies have analyzed the role of GABA in dietary habits. It was found that GABA can reduce appetite and in experimental animals to inhibit insulin hyperphagia (an excessive intake of food beyond that needed for basic energy requirements due to an abnormality in regulation of pituitaty hormones) or increased eating. Other studies are in progress on the role of GABA in diet.

Benign Prostatic Hypertrophy

Glutamic acid may play a role in the functioning of the prostate. Fluid produced by the prostate contains significant amounts of glutamic acid. This finding has led some scientists to speculate that glutamic acid may be correlated to a decrease in benign prostatic hypertrophy (enlargement of the prostate with no signs of cancer).

Cancer

Glutamine provides cells with fuel for growth. Unfortunately, a substantial body of evidence indicates that glutamine serves as respiratory fuel for tumor cells. The enzymes glutaminase, which breaks down glutamine, and asparaginase, which breaks down the amino acid asparagine, have been used as components in an effective drug for cancer. The drug, known as asparaginase (Elspar), is particularly useful in treating acute leukemia and lymphocytic malignant cells because these cells depend on glutaminase whereas normal cells do not, and exemplifies the rare situation of an enzyme being absorbed by the stomach. Asparaginase is particularly useful in treating acute leukemia and lymphocytic malignant cells because these cells depend on glutaminase whereas normal cells do not. This action may also explain why a vegan diet can be useful in cancer treatment (glutamic acid and glutamine occur mainly in animal protein).

The primary side effects from the glutaminase destruction of glutamine include renal or liver injury, infertility, pancreatitis, hyperthermia, depression, clotting factors, abdominal cramps, headache, weight loss, irritability, anorexia, nausea, vomiting, fever, chills, elevation of blood ammonia, and rare occurrence of a severe Parkinson-like syndrome with tremor and a progressive decrease in muscular tone. Interestingly, its side effects have not been found to include psychotic or other major psychiatric abnormalities.

GABA and its analogs have been found to exhibit some anticancer properties against experimental sarcomas, particularly when combined with chemotherapeutic agents.

Depression

GABA metabolism may be abnormal in depressed patients. Many depressions have an anxiety or stress-related component associated with them. GABA can help prevent anxiety-related messages from reaching the motor centers of the brain by occupying their receptor sites. GABA and drugs that potentiate GABA's effects such monoamine oxidase (MAO) inhibitors, valproate (Depakote), and phenytoin (Dilantin), have been extremely useful antidepressants. Many schizophrenic episodes are induced from the stress of drug and alcohol abuse and benefit from GABA therapy.

Diabetes and Hypoglycemia

Administration of 2 to 4 g of GABA to fifty people with diabetes resulted in significant decrease in blood sugar in approximately half the individuals. It is thought that GABA increases insulin's effect and, hence, is hypoglycemic. Although GABA may be useful in treating people with diabetes, it may need to be avoided by those with hypoglycemia.

Encephalopathy

Glutamine is greatly increased in the brain and the cerebrospinal fluid of patients with hepatic encephalopathy—a form of liver damage in alcoholics. This condition is marked by a decline in brain function manifested as speech difficulties, altered sleep, tremors, and other symptoms due to the accumulation of toxins in the brain caused by abnormal functioning of the liver. Abnormal levels of glutamate are also found in the brain and cerebrospinal fluid. The breakdown of glutamate is the major involvement of the amino acid system in kidney and liver ammonia metabolism.

During dialysis encephalopathy, GABA is decreased or normal in cerebrospinal fluid but decreased significantly in the brain. Glutamic acid and glutamine should be used with caution in these patients, but GABA may be an important therapy for them.

Hypertension

GABA has been shown to help regulate cardiovascular mechanisms related to hypertension. Agents that stimulate GABA receptors and drugs that modify GABA in the brain clearly have important roles in blood pressure regulation. When glutamate is injected into certain regions of the brain, particularly the hippocampus, it produces a decrease in heart rate and a drop in blood pressure. It is doubtful that glutamic acid is hypotensive when given orally, but 3 g of GABA given orally have proved to be an effective treatment in lowering elevated blood pressure. Many analogs of GABA, substances that enhance its activity, also lower blood pressure. The blood pressure drug verapamil (Calan), a calcium channel blocker, may function through a mechanism similar to that of GABA.

Involuntary Muscular Movement Syndromes

It has been observed that decreased levels of GABA are usually present in either the cerebrospinal fluid or the brain in people with one of a group of syndromes characterized by involuntary muscle movement. Occasionally, GABA levels may be normal or increased depending upon the condition as Table 10.2 illustrates.

Glutamic acid is also decreased in the brain of people with Friedreich's ataxia, an inherited, progressive, nervous system disorder marked by loss of balance and coordination. Individuals with spinal conditions and movement disorders show abnormal results from glutamine loading tests and abnormal metabolism of glutamic acid. Spastic animals show increased needs for GABA and glutamic acid. Drugs that act as GABA antagonists are frequently prescribed as muscle relaxants.

Plasma Levels in Clinical Syndromes

Glutamic acid. Five of our patients have had low glutamic acid levels and suffered

TABLE 10.2. GABA IN SYNDROMES INVOLVING MUSCLE MOVEMENT		
SYNDROME	GABA FOUND IN CEREBROSPINAL FLUID	GABA FOUND IN BRAIN
Action tremors	decreased	
Friedreich's ataxia		decreased
Huntington's chorea	normal	decreased
Multiple sclerosis	decreased	
Parkinson's disease	normal	increased
Tardive dyskinesia	decreased	decreased

from one of the following: depression, thought disorder, hair loss, phenylke-tonuria (PKU), and psychosis.

Most of our patients with elevated glutamic acid levels have been male. The one female found to have high glutamic acid levels was an institutionalized mentally retarded girl with severe hypothermia. The other patients had elevated levels of many amino acids. These patients were taking amino acid supplements, which concomitantly may raise the levels of other amino acids, including glutamic acid.

Glutamine. We have not been able to measure glutamine effectively in our patients because of its rapid decay. However, the diversity of syndromes associated with abnormal levels of this family of amino acids demonstrates the importance of measuring them.

GABA. About 10 percent of patients at our clinic have had detectable GABA levels. Of these patients, six were depressed, one was psychotic, one suffered from migraine headaches, one had Alzheimer's disease, and one exhibited no symptoms.

Schizophrenia

Some people with schizophrenia have elevated glutamic acid levels. While glutamine levels have been found to be normal in the brains of schizophrenics, occasionally GABA levels have been found to be decreased in both brain and cerebrospinal fluids. Research has also shown that GABA mechanisms are involved in catatonia, a condition in which a person lacks the will to talk or move and sits or stands motionless. Thus, some people with schizophrenia may benefit from mega GABA therapy. GABA may also release the hormone prolactin, which has been found elevated after antipsychotic drug use.

Seizure Disorders

Study of the three musketeers is particularly relevant to seizure disorders. As we discussed earlier in this chapter, glutamic acid in the form of MSG is a high-potency glutamate that can produce a seizurelike syndrome and convulsions in some infants because the blood-brain barrier at that age is not well developed. MSG in high doses also can produce convulsions in experimental animals. It is thought that MSG is the cause of the seizure-inducing action of glutamic acid. GABA and glutamic acid depletion occur in seizures that are induced by an excess of ammonia in the brain. In contrast, glutamic acid is increased in the brains of some people with epilepsy.

While the data are contradictory concerning glutamic acid levels and seizures, GABA is almost always deficient in clinical and experimental seizure disorders. All GABA-like drugs, given orally, are effective in cases of status eplipeticus, a form of epilepsy characterized by long-lasting seizures that can be life-threatening. Some studies suggest that oral dosages of GABA do not enter into the brain significantly. Yet, just 100 mg of GABA given orally to mice has prevented some experimental seizure disorders. Anticonvulsant drugs like valproic acid (Depakene) increase GABA, particularly in cerebrospinal fluid.

Antagonists of the excitatory neurotransmitters glutamic acid and aspartic acid, particularly methylaspartate, have an anticonvulsant action, which antagonizes these two amino acids. Glutamic acid has been found to be depleted in the cerebrospinal fluid of some seizure patients and elevated in others. Glutamine levels have also been found to be elevated in some seizure patients.

Taurine, an anticonvulsant amino acid, is effective in epilepsy because it increases the breakdown of glutamate to GABA. Many attempts have been made to develop a drug that can mimic GABA action, thereby proving useful in the prevention and treatment of epilepsy. It is well recognized that the drugs used in the treatment of status epilepticus, such as the benzodiazepines clonazepam, oxazepam (Serax), and alprazolam (Xanax), mimic GABA. These drugs, which raise GABA levels in the brain and thereby decrease neuron activity, have been used successfully for treating all types of seizure-, manic-, or anxiety-like states. Diazepam has also been successful as a standard therapy in status epilepticus, and probably works in a similar way to GABA. In our clinic, we find the use of 300 mg of gabapentin twice daily to be extremely beneficial for rapidly building up significant levels of GABA to achieve a calming effect for the control of seizures and mood swings.

Several strategies have been used to decrease glutamic acid and to increase the synthesis of GABA, taurine, and purines (inhibitory neurotransmitters with anticonvulsant properties). GABA or taurine supplements may increase GABA content and affect the brain. However, at the time of this printing, it is not completely clear how to increase GABA with amino acid supplements while decreasing glutamate.

Manaco and colleagues have found as many as ten amino acids to be low in the spinal fluid of epileptic patients. However, overwhelming evidence indicates that most epileptics have decreased levels of taurine, GABA, and glycine with increased levels of aspartic acid and glutamic acid. Because GABA is a major inhibitory neurotransmitter, failure in its synthesis or loss of its action promotes excitatory neurotransmitters. This situation occurs when the enzyme glutamate decarboxylase, which makes GABA from glutamic acid, is reduced. Glutamate decarboxylase is a pyridoxine-dependent enzyme, and it is not surprising that drugs that inhibit pyridoxine are potent seizure-producing agents. Extra pyridoxine and manganese can be used to elevate GABA in the brain. One major study on GABA and pyridoxine found 50 percent of the 699 epileptics given these two supplements showed improvement.

Stroke

Glutamine is greatly increased in both the brain and the cerebrospinal fluid of stroke victims. Considerable research has been devoted to blocking the damaging actions of glutamic and aspartic acids following stroke; their neurotoxic effect exacerbates damage to brain cells. New drugs such as memantine (Ebixa) and are being developed that stop the toxic cascade of glutamic and aspartic acids. The target of these pharmaceutics is the N-methyl-D-aspartate receptor and the excitory amino acid transporters (EAATs), which modulate levels of these amino acids in the brain. (See Chapter 12 on aspartic acid for more information.)

Until effective blockers are available, we can attempt to use antioxidants to slow the neurotoxic activity of these amino acids following stroke. In our clinic, we also use L-cysteine, N-acetyl-cysteine, and GABA in the form of gabapentin, as well as our Brain Energy Formula (see "Energy in a Capsule" on page 43) which contains tyrosine, phenylalanine, and methionine.

This multinutrient approach works well to help prevent damage from the action of glutamic and aspartic acids in Parkinson's patients. Five out of eleven cases of patients with symptoms such as difficulties in speech and defects in memory caused by stroke, showed improvement when 2 to 3 g of GABA was given daily for one to two months. An increase in the activity of the GABA-synthesizing enzyme gamma amino decarboxylase (GAD) is probably the best marker of brain ischemia or injury.

Other Potential Uses

The World Health Organization (WHO) has suggested that glutamine be added to certain sugar solutions to aid in the treatment of diarrhea, cholera, and other infectious conditions. It appears that glutamine may augment rehydration solutions, particularly oral solutions, used for these conditions.

Glutamine and sugar are also considered part of the ideal solution for treating total parenteral nutrition and patients with low blood sugar. It has been suggested that glycine also be added. However, it does not appear that supplementation with either glutamine or glycine offers much benefit for healthy individuals. Both glutamine and glycine are abundant in the body and almost as common as glucose.

Gout. High plasma glutamic acid concentrations have been reported in primary gout. Studies of plasma glutamic acid is a useful measurement in a variety of diseases. Elevated plasma GABA may be an indicator of central nervous system stress.

Migraine. Brenner and colleagues reviewed GABA in plasma and reported elevated levels in migraine headaches, cerebrovascular disease, and other brain diseases.

Additional uses currently under investigation for glutamic acid include its role in muscular dystrophy, cancer, and detoxification after exposure to hydrocarbons, chlorine, air pollution, radiation, and peroxides. Research on glutamine involves ulcer protection and ability to increase the growth of mucosal epithelial cells. All of these uses at this time are speculative.

GABA LOADING

In studying the effects of amino acids in large doses, we were continually impressed by their lack of toxicity. I (Pfeiffer) found by testing myself that I had no trouble tolerating 20 to 30 g a day of most amino acids. The largest single dose of GABA that had been given to a human subject we could find described in medical literature was 3 g. Overly confident, I (Pfeiffer) took 10 g of GABA on an empty stomach. Ten minutes after taking the GABA, I started to wheeze, my breath rate increased, and I felt anxious and nauseated for the next two hours. This dose of 10 mg of GABA also caused a constant flush sensation, like that of niacin (vitamin B_3), although my skin was not red. I had a tingling sensation in my hands and throughout my entire body. This effect occurred even at the lesser dose of 3 g of GABA and is likely to be neurologic, unlike the effect of niacin, which is primarily vascular. This unusual tingling and flushing, nausea, and shortness of breath, has been confirmed by several volunteers taking oral doses of 1 to 3 g of GABA.

SUPPLEMENTATION

There are therapeutic uses for glutamic acid and glutamine, but GABA has the most therapeutic potential of the three musketeers. As glutamic acid is abundant in common foods, and glutamine is the most abundant amino acid in blood, supplementation is not necessary unless directed by a physician.

Deficiency Signs

Deficiencies of glutamic acid, GABA, and glutamine are rare. Glutamic acid and GABA can become depleted with chronic illnesses. Low levels of glutamic acid may manifest as low energy, of GABA as anxiety, and of glutamine as fluctuating energy levels.

Availability

Supplemental glutamic acid is available as free-form L-glutamic acid in 500-mg tablets; supplemental glutamine is available as free-form L-glutamine in 500-mg to 1,000-mg capsules and tablets; and supplemental GABA with inositol and niacinamide is available in 200- to 500-mg capsules.

Therapeutic Use

The normal range of supplemental GABA is .5 g to 3 g. This is dependent upon the condition being treated. Doses greater than 3 g may cause nausea. In times of crisis involving anxiety and stress, 10 g of inositol or L-glutamine or gabapentin administered intravenously is one of the most powerful ways of delivering a high loading dose of GABA.

Maximum Safe Level

Not established.

Side Effects and Contraindications

Glutamic acid (glutamate): People who are hypersensitive to monosodium glu-tamate (MSG), such as those who suffer from Chinese restaurant syndrome, should *not* take supplemental glutamic acid, as it can exacerbate their symptoms.

Glutamine: People who are hypersensitive to monosodium glutamate (MSG), such as those who suffer from Chinese restaurant syndrome, should take supple-mental glutamine with caution, as the body converts glutamine into glutamate. Glutamine should not be taken by persons with cirrhosis of the liver, kidney prob-lems, Reye's syndrome, or any other disorder that can result in an accumulation of ammonia in the blood.

GABA: Side effects can include a tingling sensation in the face and hands and a slight shortness of breath shortly after taking the supplement. This effect lasts only a few minutes.

GLUTAMIC ACID, GABA, AND GLUTAMINE: A SUMMARY

Glutamic acid is a nonessential amino acid that can normally be synthesized in the body from many substances, such as alpha-ketoglutarate and the amino acids ornithine, arginine, proline, and glutamine. Glutamic acid is used by the body to make proteins, peptides (glutathione), amino acids (proline, histidine, glutamine, and gamma-aminobutyric acid or GABA), and DNA.

Glutamic acid, GABA, and glutamine function as neurotransmitters in the brain. Glutamic acid has excitatory effects and GABA has inhibitory effects upon the central nervous system. Glutamine serves primarily as a brain fuel. Pyridoxine (vitamin B_6) and manganese increase the amount of GABA made from glutamic acid. Aspartic acid is an excitatory neurotransmitter that is competitively transported with glutamic acid, whereas taurine and glycine are inhibitory neurotransmitters that are competitively transported with GABA.

Glutamic acid and glutamine are extremely abundant amino acids in the body. Glutamic acid is the second most concentrated amino acid in the brain; glutamine is not far behind. Glutamine is the most abundant amino acid in the blood. Glutamic acid is one of the most abundant amino acids found in food; about 7 g are contained in a cup of cottage cheese and as much as 13 g in a pound of pork.

Initial studies with glutamic acid using 10 to 12 g in mentally retarded individuals were found to raise IQ. One to 3 g doses of GABA orally also have been used effectively to raise the IQ of mentally retarded individuals.

Initial studies in alcoholics using a daily dose of 10 to 15 g of L-glutamine were effective in controlling this addiction. These results have not been carefully reproduced, but suggest therapeutic promise.

As a major fuel for the brain, glutamine also unfortunately fuels lymphocytic cancer cells. An enzyme that destroys glutamine is useful in acute leukemia and other cancers. Some effects of the excessive breakdown of glutamine are infertility, depression, abdominal cramps, headache, weight loss, anorexia, increased blood ammonia, and, rarely, a Parkinson's-like syndrome. Other deficiencies of the glutamate family of neurotransmitters relate to the metabolism of glutathione.

Glutamic acid given as MSG can produce a seizurelike disorder in infants. In contrast, various drugs that inhibit glutamic acid, aspartic acid, and their metabolites are effective anticonvulsants. In many studies of experimental and human epilepsy, GABA is found to be deficient in the cerebrospinal fluid and brain. Benzodiazepines such as diazepam (Valium) are useful in status epilepticus because they act on GABA receptors. GABA increases in the brain after administration of many seizure medications. Hence, GABA is clearly an antiepileptic nutrient, while the data is mixed regarding glutamic acid. Inhibitors of glutamine metabolism can also produce convulsions.

Muscle spasticity and involuntary movement syndromes, for example, Parkinson's disease, Friedreich's ataxia, tardive dyskinesia, and Huntington's chorea are all marked by low GABA levels when amino acid levels are studied. Trials of 2 to 3 g of GABA given orally have been effective in various epileptic and spasticity syndromes.

Agents that elevate GABA also are useful in lowering hypertension. Three grams orally have been effective in blood pressure control. GABA is decreased and glutamic acid is increased in various encephalopathies. GABA can reduce appetite and is decreased in people with hypoglycemia. GABA reduces blood sugar in diabetic individuals. Chronic brain syndromes can also be marked by deficiency of GABA, as well as by a deficiency of glutamic acid and glutamine. GABA has many promising uses in therapy.

There may be therapeutic uses of glutamic acid and glutamine, but GABA has the most therapeutic potential of the three musketeers. GABA levels are difficult to detect in plasma and urine, while glutamine and glutamic acid are easily measured. GABA therapy should be considered when glutamic acid is elevated and glutamine is deficient. Cerebrospinal fluid levels of GABA may be useful in diagnosing very serious diseases.

With further study, it is likely that GABA, glutamic acid, and glutamine will prove to have an even greater therapeutic potential in the near future.

CHAPTER ELEVEN

Proline and Hydroxyproline: The Collagen Constituents

Nearly all proteins contain proline. It is a nonessential amino acid and the third most abundant amino acid in the body, exceeded in concentration only by glutamine and alanine. Approximately half of the body's total proline content is contained in collagen, which makes up 30 percent of all protein in the body. Collagen is essential for healthy skin, connective tissues, and bone. It serves as the major reservoir for proline, and its breakdown product hydroxyproline.

Proline is present in human amniotic fluid at an unchanging concentration throughout pregnancy. It is low during the growth period of children—and may not be present in sufficient quantities to support the body's nutritional requirement. Hence, proline, like many other "nonessential amino acids," is a conditionally essential amino acid. Proline levels become slightly higher in adults.

FUNCTION

Proline is critical for the production of collagen and reducing the loss of collagen through the aging process. It also helps in the healing of wounds and cartilage; maintaining the integrity of joints, tendons, ligaments; and maintaining and strengthening heart muscle. Proline's function in brain metabolism is presently unknown. It is the only amino acid that is readily soluble in alcohol.

Hydroxyproline is a breakdown, or waste, product of proline. In higher than normal levels in the body, it is a signal that collagen and bone are breaking down.

METABOLISM

Proline synthesis starts with the breakdown of glutamic acid and ornithine. Metabolism of glutamic acid is first required to stimulate and ready the brain for proline production in the liver while ornithine is responsible for preparing cells for growth. Hence, the building of bone and muscle, or proline synthesis, begins with the metabolism of these two other amino acids. Enzymes using niacin, pyridoxine (vitamin B$_6$), and vitamin C are required for these conversions to occur. Studies have shown that collagen is not properly formed or maintained if vitamin C is lacking, so proline is most effective when adequate vitamin C is supplied at the same time. A deficiency of vitamin C may be an indication of elevated levels of hydroxyproline.

REQUIREMENTS

There is no RDA for proline. Proline is a nonessential amino acid that can be synthesized from other amino acids within the body. Proline's immediate precursor, glutamine, is the most abundant amino acid in the bloodstream and is also abundant in food; therefore, the raw material for making proline is readily available. Low proline levels are found almost exclusively in women and in poorly nourished individuals.

FOOD SOURCES

Proline is concentrated in high-protein foods such as meat, cottage cheese, and wheat germ. There is more proline in dairy protein than in meat, whereas for most amino acids, the reverse is true. Hydroxyproline is found in large concentration, usually about 15 percent or more, in gelatin.

FORM AND ABSORPTION

Proline is a well-absorbed amino acid and occurs only in the L- form. D-proline does not occur naturally in human metabolism.

NUTRIENT INTERACTIONS

In some mammals, proline has been shown to reduce the dietary requirement for the lipid-lowering amino acid arginine. Arginine, as you may remember, can be synthesized from ornithine, and ornithine, in turn, is synthesized from proline.

In elderly people, vitamin C deficiency results in the loss of proline in the urine. This comes from the breakdown of collagen and is an early sign and precursor of degenerative disease.

Fed in high concentrations to experimental animals, hydroxyproline reduces the animals' growth rate. Growth depression is particularly great in pyridoxine-deficient animals, because this vitamin is so important to normal hydroxyproline metabolism.

TOXICITY

High doses of D-proline injected intraventricularly into the brain of two- and five-day-old chickens induced convulsions and death. The mortality rate was not sig-

TABLE 11.1. PROLINE LEVELS IN FOOD		
FOOD	AMOUNT	CONTENT (GRAMS)
Avocado	1	0.16
Cheese	1 ounce	0.71
Chicken	1 pound	1.20
Chocolate	1 cup	0.77
Cottage cheese	1 cup	3.59
Duck	1 pound	1.97
Egg	1	2.41
Granola	1 cup	0.65
Luncheon meat	1 pound	3.39
Oatmeal	1 cup	0.55
Ricotta	1 cup	2.62
Sausage meat	1 pound	1.36
Turkey	1 pound	1.60
Wheat germ	1 cup	1.75
Whole milk	1 cup	0.78
Wild game	1 pound	3.50
Yogurt	1 cup	0.93

nificantly different between L- and D-proline when extremely high doses were placed directly into the brain. At present, there is no therapeutic use for either the L- or D- form of proline.

CLINICAL USES

Presently, there are few therapeutic roles established for proline. It is primarily used as a diagnostic tool.

Alcoholism

Proline levels are frequently elevated in the blood of alcoholic patients with liver cirrhosis like many other amino acids that are abnormally high when the liver is cirrhotic. Proline is also elevated in liver cells after chronic exposure to alcohol or ethanol and its toxic metabolites.

One distinctive feature of liver damage in alcoholic patients, compared to other chronic liver diseases, is the presence of hyperprolinemia (excess proline in the blood). In alcoholic cirrhotics, blood lactate is also significantly increased when compared to normal, nonalcoholic cirrhotic patients. Proline synthesis also seems to be increased in alcoholic liver disease, an indication that the body is unable to metabolize proline into muscle and bone.

Blood lactic acid and serum proline values may possibly be used as markers in liver fibrogenesis (a condition common to liver disease involving the accumulation of connective tissue) and alcoholic liver disease.

Cancer

Proline has attracted some interest with regard to cancer because certain carcinogenic nitrogen substances, for example, N-nitrosoproline, are carcinogenic. Smokers given a 500-mg supplement of proline an hour after taking 325 mg of nitrate have increased synthesis of this carcinogen. The ingestion of proline and nitrate, a common preservative used in meats and to cure or pickle foods, in smokers produces significantly greater amounts of N-nitrosoproline than in nonsmokers; smokers produce two and a half times as much N-nitrosoproline as nonsmokers. Evidence indicates that dietary nitrate can convert this harmless amino acid into a carcinogen.

Interestingly, the cancer drug thioproline is a derivative of proline that may block proline metabolism. In doses of 400 mg/kg, thioproline causes acute neurological toxicity, convulsions, and death. Yet lower doses can restore some normal characteristics to cancer cells and have been reported to have clinical efficacy against head and neck cancers, with fewer toxic side effects. Thioproline did not inhibit the development of cancer in several experimental cell models, however. At this time, proline therapy should be used judiciously in cancer patients.

Cognitive Learning

Substance P is a neurotransmitter in the brain of which proline is a component. Several other proline neuropeptides have been identified, suggesting that proline peptides and proline itself have neurological functions that promote learning.

By directly injecting proline into the brains of experimental animals, Versaux-Botteri and Legros-Nguyen found an increase in the growth of dendritic spines. These spines of brain cells are thought to be a form of brain growth that contributes to learning.

Penetration of the blood-brain barrier by proline and acetylproline was found to be low as compared to high penetration rates for the proline derivatives prolinethylester and N-acetylprolinethylester. Intravenous injection of prolinethylester was found to be effective in elevating the level of free proline in the brain. The dose injected was 250 mg of prolinethylester per kg of body weight in experimental animals, equivalent to 15 g in the average male adult. Modification of proline to N-ethylester increases its penetration into the brain tenfold. This amazing effect needs to be investigated, but at this point, any application in human beings is only conjectural.

Collagen Synthesis

If an abnormality is noted in the synthesis of collagen, the breakdown of tissue, ligaments, and tendons; easy bruising; and even internal bleeding may occur. In such cases, there is most often an elevation in the concentration of hydroxyproline in the urine; this may also represent a vitamin C deficiency.

Osteoporosis

Osteoporosis is a progressive disease in which the bones gradually become less dense, making the individual extremely susceptible to bone fractures and breaks. If a person is maintained on an adequate osteoporosis treatment, bone healing or renegeration will occur. Hydoxyproline is a byproduct of proline and an indicator of bone and collagen deterioration. A derivative of hydroxyproline known as telopeptides are breakdown parts of bone that can be measured in the urine. Monitoring their levels can be used as a continuous check to assess whether osteoporosis treatments such as growth hormone, calcitonin (sold under the brand names Calcimar, Cibacalcin, and Miacalcin), alendronate (Fosamax), or some of the new intravenous prescription drug therapies such as Ariveda are working to control osteoporosis and improve bone healing.

Plasma Levels in Clinical Syndromes

Proline. Three of our patients with low proline levels had been institutionalized for long periods of time in mental hospitals; inferior protein nutrition is characteristic of patients in psychiatric hospitals. Among the patients with low proline levels, one had anorexia and was emaciated; another patient had a problem in protein metabolism, resulting in hair loss; another was manic depressive; several were depressed; one was psychotic; one had phenylketonuria (PKU); and one had a learning disorder.

Two of our patients with learning disabilities had high proline levels in blood; another had Raynaud's disease, a circulatory condition characterized by constriction of blood vessels in the extremities. The significance of these 10 to 25 percent elevations is unclear. We did have one patient with severe allergies whose proline levels were four times normal. This thirty-five-year-old female with multiple allergies of unknown origin had showed normal proline levels following nutrient therapy high in vitamin C and experienced significant but not complete improvement in her allergies.

Hydroxyproline. Hydroxyproline was found to be low in plasma of eight patients at our clinic. Five patients were depressed, one was psychotic, and two were healthy. The clinical significance of these values is unclear. Elevated levels of hydroxyproline, three times normal, was found in a psychotically depressed fifty-year-old man. Among his treatments were high doses of vitamin C; he showed a gradual return to normal function over two months with normalization of his plasma hydroxyproline level.

Of four patients with mild 25 to 100 percent elevations in hydroxyproline, two were depressed, one was impotent, and the other had petit-mal seizures, a type of seizure most common in children characterized by a blank stare. All were given extra vitamin C. Their subsequent improvement in function is difficult to correlate to this unusual finding.

Wound Healing

The efficacy of proline to stimulate wound healing the way that glycine and arginine do has been studied with mixed results. It is postulated that because proline is highly concentrated in collagen and is involved in collagen synthesis, which is essential to wound healing, it may have some value in certain types of wounds resistant to healing. Its presence may help wounds heal by the deposition of more collagen in the affected area. Indeed, accumulation of collagen in certain tissues, particularly the liver, directly parallels proline concentration.

Wrinkle Prevention

Proline improves skin texture by assisting in the synthesis of collagen and reducing the loss of collagen through the aging process. Proline is used in a variety of cosmetic products designed to decrease the visual effects of wrinkles and aging. These products usually contain vitamin C to assure maximum uptake of proline.

PROLINE AND HYDROXYPROLINE LOADING

Five grams of proline loaded in a volunteer was well absorbed, increasing in plasma to eight times normal at two hours and falling to four times normal at four hours. Aluminum levels almost doubled at two hours; however, the significance of this increase is unclear. Other amino acids were not significantly changed by loading, but creatinine levels were significantly increased by proline supplementation. The significance of this finding is also unclear.

Hydroxyproline loading of approximately 1 to 2 g raised hydroxyproline levels to ten to twenty times normal. Other biological parameters were not significantly affected, except for a slight decrease in iron and uric acid levels. The significance of these findings requires further investigation.

Hydroxyproline loading had no effect on polyamine, histamine, copper, and zinc levels, chem screen, and biologic parameters. Iron was lowered when 5 g was given. Heart rate also dropped significantly, and one patient's pulse fell from seventy-eight to fifty-four hours after the initial dose. In contrast, similar doses of proline may actually raise iron, polyamine, and histamine levels. Proline loading, however, has no effect on blood pressure or pulse.

SUPPLEMENTATION

Knowledge of proline supplementation is limited. Until there is definitive proof that proline has a therapeutic role in the prevention or restoration of bone, collagen, or muscle, its use as a supplement is unwarranted. Supplementation may be advisable in tissue-damage states, joint abnormalities, and in cases of decreased tenacity of skin secondary to the natural aging process, but only under the supervision of a healthcare practitioner.

Deficiency Symptoms

An abnormal breakdown of tissue, ligaments, and tendons and a loss of collagen; easy bruising; and even internal bleeding may indicate a deficiency in proline or vitamin C.

Availability

Supplemental free-form L-proline is not readily available but can be obtained in in 250 to 500 mg tablets. Most proline, however, is not found in supplement form.

Therapeutic Daily Amount

Not established.

Maximum Safe Level

Not established.

Side Effects and Contraindications

None known.

PROLINE AND HYDROXYPROLINE: A SUMMARY

Proline is a nonessential amino acid that is highly concentrated throughout the body, except in cerebrospinal fluid. Collagen is an important protein and the major reservoir for this amino acid. Proline can be synthesized in the body from either ornithine or glutamic acid; it can be broken down into ornithine and thereby reduce the body's requirements for ornithine and arginine.

Excess proline due to genetic errors can lead to convulsions, elevated blood calcium, and osteoporosis. Dietary restriction is a useful treatment, probably because the body depends on dietary proline to meet some of its proline needs. Therefore, proline deficiency probably can occur under some conditions. At least one patient with Parkinson's disease with low blood levels of proline has been identified at our clinic.

Elevated proline levels can occur in alcoholics with cirrhosis of the liver and probably in those with depression and seizure disorders. We have observed elevated hydroxyproline levels in cases of psychotic depression. These patients also may require extra vitamin C.

Proline is modified in smokers and becomes a carcinogen. Drugs that inhibit proline metabolism have anticancer properties. Diets low in proline may be useful in some forms of cancer treatment.

Proline also may be of value in wound healing since it is part of the collagen process. Proline peptides are involved in important neurological proteins that may promote learning, although this is only conjecture at this point.

Knowledge of proline supplementation is limited. Proline is concentrated in high-protein foods like meat, cottage cheese, and wheat germ. There is more proline in dairy protein than in meat protein, whereas for most other amino acids, the reverse is true.

CHAPTER TWELVE

Aspartic Acid and Asparagine: The Energizers

Aspartic acid and asparagine are two structurally similar, nonessential, amino acids that are influential in the metabolic pathways responsible for generating energy and for the transportation of energy throughout the body.

Aspartic acid, most well known for its role in the production of the synthetic sweetener NutraSweet, is manufactured in the liver from glutamate and in small amounts from bacteria. Asparagine is synthesized from aspartic acid and adenosine triphosphate (ATP), a high-energy compound that triggers many of the body's activities, along the same pathway as glutamic acid to glutamine. Both asparagine and glutamine release this energy, which is used by the brain and nervous system, when they are converted back to aspartic acid and glutamic acid respectively.

FUNCTION

Aspartic acid is highly concentrated throughout the body and brain. As an energy amino acid, it helps trigger two of the body's most important metabolic pathways: the Krebs and urea cycles.

In the Krebs cycle, where carbohydrates are broken down for energy, aspartic acid helps activate the process by transporting energy into the mitochondria. Mitochondria, also known as the "powerhouse of the cell," are microscopic bodies found in the cells of almost all living organisms that contain enzymes responsible for the conversion of food to usable energy.

Aspartic acid helps stimulate the urea cycle, where waste products from protein metabolism are detoxified and formed into urea, by helping to form carbamyl phosphate (CP), the key enzyme that starts the urea cycle. It also helps in the removal of excess ammonia and nitrogen.

Aspartic acid contributes its energy to the building of pyrimidines, important constituents of DNA and RNA, the carriers of genetic information, and enhances the production of immunoglobulins and antibodies (immune system proteins). It helps move the minerals magnesium and potassium across the intestinal lining into the blood and cells, and when combined to form the mineral salts magnesium aspartate and potassium aspartate, respectively, it can improve energy production in muscles.

Aspartic acid, like glutamic acid, functions as a major excitory neurotransmitter in the brain, where it is particularly concentrated in the hippocampus and hypothalamus. A highly active form of aspartic acid known as N-acetylaspartic acid is considered the brain's most highly concentrated amino acid neurotransmitter. Godfrey and colleagues, however, suggest that aspartic acid has a larger role in brain energy metabolism than as a neurotransmitter.

At small doses, aspartic acid, again like glutamic acid, excites nerve cells to higher levels of activity. At higher doses, these amino acids can overstimulate these cells, causing cell damage or death. This is thought to happen in stroke, when aspartic acid triggers a cascade of neurotransmitters activity that can result in further damage. Researchers are currently investigating ways of short-circuiting aspartic acid's neurotransmitter action.

Asparagine, like glutamine, is needed to maintain balance between too much or too little stimulation in the central nervous system. When asparagine's extra amino group is removed during its conversion back into aspartic acid, it releases energy that the brain and central nervous system can use for metabolism.

METABOLISM

Aspartic acid is synthesized in the liver from glutamate and is dependent upon the cofactor pyridoxine (vitamin B_6) for this conversion. Asparagine is synthesized primarily from aspartic acid and ATP, but also can be manufactured from glutamic acid. Its manufacture from aspartic acid appears also to require the mineral magnesium.

REQUIREMENTS

Because aspartic acid is a nonessential amino acid that can be made from adequate stores of glutamate, no RDA is listed for this amino acid. Depleted levels of aspartic acid may occur temporarily within certain tissues during stress states or under trauma, but because the body is able to make its own aspartic acid to replace any depletion, deficiency states do not occur often.

FOOD SOURCES

Like most amino acids, aspartic acid is highly concentrated in protein foods. Plant protein, especially that found in sprouting seeds, contains an abundance of aspartic acid.

TABLE 12.1. ASPARTIC ACID LEVELS IN FOOD

FOOD	AMOUNT	CONTENT (GRAMS)
Avocado	1	0.6
Cheese	1 ounce	0.4
Chicken	1 pound	2.2
Chocolate	1 cup	0.6
Cottage cheese	1 cup	2.1
Duck	1 pound	3.2
Egg	1	0.6
Granola	1 cup	1.0
Luncheon meat	1 pound	4.7
Oatmeal	1 cup	1.0
Pork	1 pound	6.4
Ricotta	1 cup	2.5
Sausage meat	1 pound	2.5
Turkey	1 pound	3.3
Wheat germ	1 cup	3.0
Whole milk	1 cup	0.6
Wild game	1 pound	7.4
Yogurt	1 cup	0.6

FORM AND ABSORPTION

Aspartic acid and asparagines occur in L- and D- form. Dietary proteins are made from the L- form of aspartic acid and asparagine. Aspartic acid and glutamic acid compete for absorption in the cerebrum, cortex, and spinal cord. Competition for absorption by similar functioning amino acids is one of the body's methods of metabolic regulation.

The uptake of aspartic acid and glutamic acid is decreased in people who have conditions in which the brain has been damaged. Like other excitory neurotransmitters, aspartic acid is frequently decreased in unipolar depression. Trials are underway to study the effects of aspartic acid therapy in some depressed patients.

TOXICITY

Research on aspartic acid toxicity shows that it is quite similar in toxicity to monosodium glutamate (MSG). High doses of aspartic acid given to experimental animals will produce similar destruction in the central nervous system, partic-

Aspartame Claims

There are increasing claims that aspartic acid, which is commonly used with phenylalanine in the artificial sweetener NutraSweet, is unfortunately associated with the excitory brain pathways. These excitory pathways can contribute to increased pain, irritation, mood swings, and even psychosis. They can precipitate damage throughout the body, including the lungs and the brain as in Alzheimer's disease.

NutraSweet is a unique sugar trick. Because it is a dipeptide and breaks down quickly, it gives the sensation of a very intense sugar that is hundreds of times sweeter than glucose, yet is low in calories.

In our own study, initial loading of aspartame, which contains aspartic acid and phenylalanine, in dosages of 34 mg/kg (approximately 2 g of aspartic acid for an average 150-lb adult), was not sufficient to significantly elevate aspartate, asparagine, or glutamine levels in plasma. Therefore, we see that dosages of 2 g of aspartic acid—an amount far higher than that found in NutraSweet—is safe in normal doses to all except phenylketonurics.

ularly in the hypothalamus, resulting in obesity, stunted body length, and reproductive dysfunction. Aspartic acid treatment can decrease locomotor and exploratory behavior in animals. It can also reduce fertility (aspartic acid enzymes have been noted to be abnormal in conditions characterized by abnormal sperm), decrease pituitary, thyroid, ovary, or testis size, and cause disassociation of retinal activity and injured retina. D-aspartic acid is even more toxic than L-aspartic acid, as evidenced by growth depression of experimental animals.

The dosages of aspartic acid used in these studies were approximately 2 to 4 g/kg in animals, equivalent to 140 to 280 g equivalent in the average 150-lb adult male. These values are far above any physiological or therapeutic use at this time. Indeed, oral doses as high as 25 to 100 g of aspartic acid probably are not toxic in humans.

CLINICAL USE

Few studies have been conducted solely using aspartic acid. Most research has involved the use of aspartate, the salt form of aspartic acid. However, since aspartic acid is relatively nontoxic, studies are now in progress that will elucidate aspartic acid's pharmacologic and therapeutic roles.

Cancer

Cells require the amino acids asparagine to fuel their growth. Some malignant cells, particularly leukemia cells and lymphocytic malignant cells, have an enzymatic defect. Such malignant cells must acquire the asparagine needed to fuel their growth from fluid such as blood, whereas normal cells can make their own. The drug asparaginase (Elspar) is formed from L-asparaginase—the enzyme that deaminates asparagine to aspartic acid—and is used for treating acute lymphoblastic leukemia. It works by depriving the tumor cells of the asparagines for protein synthesis; normal cells, on the other hand, can survive its rapid depletion and synthesize the amount needed without cell death. When combined with other chemotherapeutic drugs, asparaginase has been effective in the induction of remission. This therapy is not as prevalent as it has been in the past.

Chronic Fatigue Syndrome

Because aspartic acid functions as an energy amino, it is thought that chronic fatigue syndrome may be associated with low levels of aspartic acid. Chronic fatigue syndrome (CFS) is a condition with a complex array of symptoms that often resemble those of the flu and other viral infections, but which is always marked by persistent, debilitating fatigue. There have been some human trials using magnesium aspartate and potassium aspartate to treat chronic fatigue syndrome, but as of yet the findings are inconclusive.

Epilepsy and Stroke

N-methyl-D-aspartic acid, a high-energy form of aspartic acid, has been used to produce experimental seizures in animals. Antagonists of this compound, particularly 2-amino-7-phosphoheptanoic acid, act as anticonvulsants and can block these experimentally induced seizures.

Both status epilepticus (a form of epilepsy characterized by long-lasting seizures) and stroke can produce similar patterns of brain damage characterized by elevated neurotransmitter activity of N-methyl-D-aspartate. Antagonists of this neurotransmitter such as the stimulant receptor blocker memantine (Ebixa) are useful in the treatment of experimentally induced strokes.

Honda and colleagues found elevated levels of asparagine following seizures. Elevated asparagine levels have also been found in a few cases of schizophrenia.

Magnesium is a natural calming agent and a natural inhibitor of N-methyl-D-aspartic acid in certain experimental models. Magnesium therapy may be used to treat elevated levels of aspartic acid and its metabolites in blood, as well as stroke and epilepsy. Zinc injected into experimental animals also becomes an inhibitor of aspartic acid neurotransmission. People with epilepsy who have had elevated levels of plasma aspartic acid may need to avoid artificial sweeteners containing aspartame.

Exercise Endurance

Recent studies on asparagine shows that this amino acid can help individuals maintain muscle mass, and possibly increase stamina and endurance. Further research needs to be done to validate this finding.

Immunostimulation

Studies in mice by Pipalova and Pospisil found that as little as 25 mg of aspartic acid can increase the weight of the thymus gland, which makes cells and hormones instrumental in immune response. Great interest was generated when it was discovered that aspartate in the form of potassium aspartate and magnesium aspartate could stimulate proliferation and differentiation of the cells of the thymus, bone marrow, and spleen tissue in mice. Mice that were exposed to a single whole body x-ray after pretreatment with potassium and magnesium aspartate exhibited a conspicuous regeneration of the red blood cell–producing organs. Furthermore, treatment with potassium aspartate and magnesium aspartate increased post-irradiation survival, suggesting that potassium and magnesium aspartate may be useful for protection against radiation damage.

Plasma Levels in Clinical Syndromes

Aspartic acid. In our first amino acid studies, 15 percent of the patients showed elevated aspartic acid in blood plasma. They were marked by a variety of diseases such as epilepsy, depression, schizophrenia, impotence, narcolepsy, allergy, cardiomyopathy, and delayed growth. Approximately 25 percent of the patients who had elevated aspartic acid levels were depressed.

In patients with elevated aspartic acid, several amino acids may be abnormal such as high branched-chain amino acids and low ornithine. The correlation of amino acid abnormalities with aspartic acid levels requires continued research. Under certain conditions of hepatic failure, aspartic acid may be elevated.

Asparagine. We have had twenty-one patients at the clinic with low asparagine levels. Eight patients were depressed, three were mentally retarded and institutionalized, two had high blood pressure, another two had high triglycerides, one was healthy normal, while the remaining five patients had one of the following: kidney disease, migraine, narcolepsy, cancer, thyroid disease.

Asparagine levels were found elevated in three depressed patients, two psychotic patients, and one girl with delayed maturation. The elevations in these patients have led us to consider therapy with the enzyme asparagine, but we have not done so at present.

Other Claims

Other conditions for which potassium aspartate and magnesium aspartate have been reported to be useful are certain myocardial disorders, shock states, muscle fatigue, and cell electrolyte disorders. These two compounds are thought to be well absorbed. The kidney eliminates more potassium and magnesium when they are taken as aspartate than when they are taken as chloride salt, an indication that aspartic acid apparently increases the absorption of magnesium, potassium, and possibly other important minerals from the intestine.

ASPARTIC ACID LOADING

We have explored the effects of large doses of aspartic acid in individuals who were fasting. Five grams of aspartic acid raises plasma aspartic acid levels from nondetectable to the normal-to-high range. At four hours, aspartic acid was again undetectable. Since aspartic acid is very soluble and rapidly metabolized, it should be tested at different intervals to accurately evaluate its effects. No change in the levels of aspartic acid metabolite asparagine was observed with loading studies using 5 g of aspartic acid. This dose is obviously too small to produce any toxic effects. Aspartic acid loading also did not change levels of trace metals, polyamines, or any of the other biological parameters tested.

SUPPLEMENTATION

Studies are now in progress to elucidate aspartic acid's pharmacological and therapeutic roles. However, to date no proven therapeutic purpose for L-aspartic acid or L-asparagine supplements are known. We have considered but not yet tried aspartic acid or asparagine therapy because rarely do low aspartic acid or asparagine occur as isolated abnormalities. Supplements made solely of L-aspartic acid, however, are not readily available.

Deficiency Symptoms

Signs and symptoms of low levels of aspartic acid include fatigue, mental sluggishness, and decreased stamina and endurance.

Availability

Supplemental free-form L-aspartic acid is not readily available but can be obtained in 250 to 500 mg tablets. Aspartic acid may be taken in the form of potassium aspartate and magnesium aspartate. However, while the salt form of aspartic acid improves the absorption of magnesium and potassium, these supplements supply negligible amounts of aspartic acid.

Therapeutic Use

Not established.

Minimum Safe Level

Not established.

Side Effects and Contraindications

None known.

ASPARTIC ACID AND ASPARAGINE: A SUMMARY

Aspartic acid is a nonessential amino acid that is made from glutamic acid by enzymes using pyridoxine (vitamin B_6). The amino acid has important roles in the Krebs and urea cycles and DNA metabolism. Aspartic acid is a major excitatory neurotransmitter, which is sometimes found to be increased in epileptic and stroke patients. It is decreased in depressed patients and in patients with brain atrophy.

Asparagine is a nonessential amino acid that is manufactured from aspartic acid, and if necessary from glutamic acid in the liver. It combines with ammonia and creates aspartic acid; this is a reversible chemical reaction. It has glycogenic properties and plays a role in the synthesis of glycoproteins. A low level of asparagine may be reflective of the need for additional magnesium to assist in the conversion from aspartic acid. Low levels of aspartic acid may result in nitrogen-containing toxic metabolites.

Some malignant cancer cells such as leukemia and lymphoma cells have a metabolic enzymatic defect that prevents them from making asparagine in order to grow. The drug asparaginase (Elspar) is formed from L-asparaginase—the enzyme that deaminates asparagine to aspartic acid—and when combined with other chemotherapeutic drugs is effective in inducing remission in people with acute lymphocytic leukemia.

Aspartic acid supplements are being evaluated. Five grams can raise blood levels. Magnesium and zinc may be natural inhibitors of some of the actions of aspartic acid.

Aspartic acid, with the amino acid phenylalanine, is a part of the natural sweetener, aspartame. This sweetener is an advance in artificial sweeteners, and is probably safe in normal doses to all except phenylketonurics.

Aspartic acid may be a significant immunostimulant of the thymus and can protect against some of the damaging effects of radiation. Many claims have been made for the special value of administering aspartic acid in the form of potassium and magnesium salts. Since aspartic acid is relatively nontoxic, studies are now in progress to elucidate its pharmacological and therapeutic roles.

SECTION SIX

Threonine Amino Acids

THREONINE
The Immunity Booster

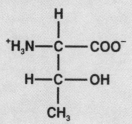

SERINE
The Potentiator of Madness

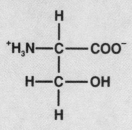

GLYCINE
The Wound Healer

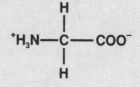

ALANINE
The Helper for Hypoglycemia

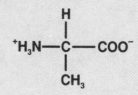

CHAPTER THIRTEEN

Threonine:
The Immunity Booster

Threonine is a little-known essential amino acid that is a necessary building block for all protein, especially for tooth enamel, collagen, and elastin. It promotes the growth of the thymus, a small gland that regulates many of the hormones and cells vital to immune defense. Even a moderate reduction in dietary intake of threonine can produce a profound depression in immune response.

FUNCTION

Threonine is the precursor of glycine and serine, two other amino acids in the threonine group. It is present in the heart, central nervous system, and skeletal muscle. Threonine has been identified as being one of the essential agents that protect against mental instability, irritability, and "difficult" personalities.

Intravenous administration of threonine increases glycine and threonine concentration in the spinal cord and brain. This method of increasing glycine in the brain is of importance because glycine, which acts as a sedative in the brain, may not enter the brain well. Large doses of glycine, 30 g for example, are necessary to produce glycine's sedative effect.

Just as the neurotransmitters acetylcholine, serotonin, catecholamines, and histamine have been demonstrated to be dependent upon the availability of dietary precursors, it appears that neurotransmitter concentrations of glycine may be dependent on dietary sources of threonine as well as on glycine. Glycine can be made by the body from glucose and other energy sources, but it has generally been assumed that dietary intake of glycine is relevant to its concentration and synthesis. Yet a deficiency of threonine dehydratase, the enzyme that breaks down threonine, has been thought to be a cause of hyperglycinemia (elevated glycine levels). This suggests that threonine is converted to glycine and glycine to threonine and that these amino acids are often therapeutically interchangeable. The conversion rate may, however, be slow.

Threonine can help to stabilize blood sugar since it can be converted into glucose in the liver by gluconeogenesis (formation of glucose from noncarbohydrate substances such as amino acids). Low levels of threonine can result in hypoglycemic conditions, especially if accompanied by low levels of serine or glycine.

Threonine has been shown to be useful in indigestion and to improve intestinal absorption. It helps to metabolize fat and acts as a lipotropic in controlling fat buildup in the liver.

Threonine also seems to benefit people who have been burned, wounded, or undergone surgery. In such trauma, threonine appears in higher than normal levels in urine. This suggests that threonine is released from the tissue following trauma to aid in the healing process. Threonine also appears to help in the formation of cyanocobalamin (vitamin B_{12}), a substance essential for the metabolism of the sulfur amino acids.

METABOLISM

Threonine, like all amino acids, requires adequate amounts of pyridoxine (vitamin B_6) to be metabolized properly. It is broken down primarily by the enzyme threonine dehydratase. The activity of this enzyme decreases with age.

In addition to serving as a precursor of glycine and serine, threonine can be degraded into propionic acid and methylmalonic acid as can methionine and valine.

REQUIREMENTS

Threonine is an essential amino acid, and so cannot be manufactured in the body from other amino acids. It is therefore critical that sufficient amounts be included in the diet. Like the needs for most essential amino acids, requirements for threonine appear to decrease with age. Infants four to six months old require 68 g a day, while children aged four to twelve need only 28 g, and adults seem to require just 8 g per day.

In animal studies, seventeen experimental kittens on threonine-deficient diets developed neurological dysfunction and lameness; the symptoms were resolved with dietary supplements of threonine.

The relatively low requirement estimated for adults has been challenged by several studies that suggest that adult requirements for threonine and several other essential amino acids are underestimated. More realistic approximations suggest an average adult male needs 15 mg/kg of threonine per day.

Aging individuals require more threonine supplementation under stress. In our plasma amino acid survey of 100 patients, we found no significant difference between baseline threonine levels in different age groups, however, there is no question that threonine requirements increase during stress.

FOOD SOURCES

Good levels of threonine can be found in most animal proteins, cottage cheese, and wheat germ. There is substantially less threonine content in grains; therefore, vegetarians are more likely than others to have deficiencies if the diet is not supplemented. Other potential nonmeat sources of this amino acid include beans, brewer's yeast, nuts, seeds, soy, and whey.

TABLE 13.1. THREONINE LEVELS IN FOOD		
FOOD	AMOUNT	CONTENT (GRAMS)
Avocado	1	0.13
Cheese	1 ounce	0.25
Chicken	1 pound	1.00
Chocolate	1 cup	0.36
Cottage cheese	1 cup	1.37
Duck	1 pound	1.35
Egg	1	0.30
Granola	1 cup	0.40
Luncheon meat	1 pound	2.40
Oatmeal	1 cup	0.43
Pork	1 pound	3.40
Ricotta	1 cup	1.27
Sausage meat	1 pound	1.15
Turkey	1 pound	1.50
Wheat germ	1 cup	1.35
Whole milk	1 cup	0.36
Wild game	1 pound	4.00
Yogurt	1 cup	0.32

FORM AND ABSORPTION

Dietary and supplemental sources of threonine occur in the L- form. To utilize threonine optimally, pyridoxine (vitamin B_6), magnesium, and niacin are needed. Valine, isoleucine, and leucine are also suggested to assure that maximum effects can be achieved.

CLINICAL USES

The amino acids in the threonine group have simple chemical structures. Glycine is the cornerstone of each amino acid in this group. It works as an amino sugar and allows all the amino acids in this group to function as sugar exchangers. Therapeutically, they function as brain stimulants and immune controllers.

Depression

At our clinic, we have found 1 g of L-threonine in the morning and in the evening to be a useful adjunct therapy in agitated depression and manic depression. Threonine levels normalize on this therapy.

Of our first 100 depressed patients administered plasma amino acid profiles, fifteen showed low threonine levels. All fifteen patients had either primary or secondary diagnosis of severe depression. This group also included two patients with epilepsy, one with phenylketonuria, two with chronic schizophrenia, one with folliculitis (a bacterial infection of the hair follicle), and one with multiple myeloma (a cancer of the bone marrow). Several of these depressed patients responded to threonine therapy.

Of the first 128 depressed patients we tested, three had elevated threonine levels. Two patients were taking tryptophan, cysteine, and other amino acids, and one was taking the asthma medication theophylline (Theo-Dur).

Immune Stimulation

Interest in threonine has been aroused by studies conducted on the effect of dietary threonine and lysine on the immune response. Rats fed diets containing wheat gluten, supplemented with threonine and lysine, were found to significantly increase thymus weight as well as increase immunoglobulin response. The results showed that the influence of threonine in the system was real and not related to an increase of body weight. Other studies suggest that a high number of accepted allografts, transplants that are successful because of immunosuppression, occur in threonine-supplemented rats. Overall, most studies find that threonine is an immunostimulant.

A moderate reduction of dietary threonine produced a profound depression of the immune response or antibody production (a protein created by the

---

Threonine Helps Patient
Gain Control of Depression

A sixty-two-year-old man with severe psychotic depression, peptic ulcer, spastic colon, and high blood pressure came to us desperate for relief. The patient did not improve on antidepressants. He had extremely low threonine levels—43 percent of normal. One 500-mg capsule of L-threonine in the morning and in the evening led to gradual control of his depression within one month.

immune system capable of destroying or neutralizing a foreign organism or toxin) against tumor growth in mice. It is not surprising that glycine also has immunostimulant properties, since threonine is metabolized into glycine.

Lotan and colleagues suggest that the effects of threonine relate to a specific requirement by the thymus for this amino acid.

We have found threonine given orally to be of some value in patients who are extremely sensitive to wheat gluten. Doses of 2 to 4 g of threonine per day allow these patients to safely add some wheat to their diets.

Muscle Spasticity

Using threonine supplements to increase brain glycine levels stimulated pilot studies using threonine supplementation in human muscle spasticity. Barbeau and colleagues used 1 g of L-threonine in patients suffering from multiple sclerosis (MS) and familial spastic paraplegia (a group of disorders characterized by progressive stiffness or spasticity of the legs with varying degrees of weakness). The result showed an overall improvement in spasticity and mobility of lower limbs by 25 percent.

In another study, 500 mg of L-threonine was administered two times a day for twelve months to six patients with genetic spasticity syndrome, followed by a four-month observation period. All six patients showed partial improvement of spasticity, with an increase in intensity of knee jerks but a decrease in intensity of muscle spasms. Measurement of upper limb showed 29 percent improvement and a 42 percent improvement in lower limb measurements; the range of overall improvement was 19 to 35 percent. No toxic, clinical, or biochemical changes were reported.

These results warrant a controlled trial in well-defined, preferably genetic cases of spasticity.

Plasma Levels in Clinical Syndromes

Alcohol ingestion causes histidine levels to decline significantly and threonine levels to increase substantially in the plasma of normal adults. We frequently find deficient levels of threonine in epileptic and depressed patients, occasionally in association with low plasma glycine levels.

Threonine levels increase in animals treated with sedative anticonvulsants. The lowest threonine levels we found were in a twenty-eight-year-old patient with epilepsy who had been on the anticonvulsant phenytoin (Dilantin) and phenobarbital (Solfoton) for ten years.

THREONINE LOADING

We asked volunteers to take 5 g of L-threonine after they fasted. At two hours, threonine levels were five times normal, and four times normal at four hours.

Generally, peak absorption is at two hours. Levels of the amino acids valine, isoleucine, leucine, and tryptophan decreased, and glutamine increased. Other biological parameters such as chem screen, polyamines, and trace metals did not change.

High dose therapy of 5 g of L-threonine daily most likely does not alter the plasma amino acid levels until more than two weeks after initiation of therapy. We gave one patient daily oral doses of 5 g for two weeks and did not observe any change in plasma amino acids except in threonine, which increased from low to normal to high levels.

SUPPLEMENTATION

At present, there is no known therapeutic use for threonine in the brain. However, it may be beneficial in providing biochemical support for people with genetic spasticity disorders and multiple sclerosis.

Deficiency Symptoms

There are no known signs or symptoms of threonine deficiency.

Availability

Free-form L-threonine is available in 500 mg capsules.

Therapeutic Daily Amount

Suggested doses for therapeutic purposes range from 300 to 1,200 mg a day. To utilize threonine optimally, pyridoxine (vitamin B_6), niacin (vitamin B_3), and magnesium are needed. Valine, isoleucine, and leucine are also recommended to assure maximum effect.

Maximum Safe Level

Not established.

Side Effects and Contraindications

None known.

THREONINE: A SUMMARY

Threonine is an essential amino acid in humans. It is abundant in human plasma, particularly in newborns. Severe deficiency of threonine causes neurologic dysfunction and lameness in experimental animals.

At our clinic, we frequently find low levels of threonine and glycine in depressed patients. These patients respond to 1 g of threonine in the morning and in the evening. Plasma levels of threonine are a useful way to monitor treatment.

Threonine is an immunostimulant that promotes the growth of thymus gland. It also can probably promote cell immune defense function. This amino acid has been useful in the treatment of genetic spasticity disorders and multiple sclerosis at a dose of 1 g daily.

Threonine may increase glycine levels. It is highly concentrated in meat products, cottage cheese, and wheat germ. Additional important uses of threonine as a useful therapeutic agent are likely to be found as studies continue.

CHAPTER FOURTEEN

Glycine:
The Wound Healer

Glycine is a nonessential amino acid with the simplest structure of all the amino acids. It serves as the cornerstone of each amino acid in the threonine family of amino acids. Because of glycine's high concentration in the skin and connective tissues, it is especially valuable for repairing damaged tissues and encouraging healing.

FUNCTION

Glycine is important in the control of gluconeogeneis, the formation of glucose from noncarbohydrate substances such as amino acids. Glycine, in fact, derives its name from glucose (blood sugar) because it has the sweet taste of sugar. Glycine is one of the few amino acids that can spare glucose for energy by building up glycogen levels (glycogen is the stored form of glucose). If a starved animal is fed quantities of glycine, glycogen is stored in the liver. By increasing the body's stores of glycogen, glycine frees up glucose for energy needs.

Glycine is also known to serve as a source of nitrogen for the manufacture of many other nonessential amino acids. It is utilized in the synthesis of hemoglobin, glycerol, phospholipids, cholesterol conjugates, skin proteins, collagen, and glutathione. It is essential in the manufacturing of creatine, a substance found in muscle tissue that is used to make DNA and RNA, the body's carriers of genetic information.

Glycine is required by the body for the maintenance of the central nervous system. Glycine, like taurine and GABA, functions as a major inhibitory neurotransmitter that can calm the body. In animals, glycine receptors exist throughout the central nervous system, spinal cord, and brain stem areas, and are uniformly distributed throughout the brain. Glycine may increase neurotransmission of GABA and acetylcholine (a neurotransmitter involved with memory made from choline) in the hippocampus, the memory center of the brain.

Glycine is also important in the photochemical action of the retina, as is taurine and is thought to be involved in behaviors related to convulsions and retinal function.

METABOLISM

Glycine can be derived from several amino acids. The major pathways of glycine production are thought to occur by way of the transamination of glyoxylate, a form of glyoxylic acid and an important intermediate compound in metabolism and the conversion from the amino acid serine. Its conversion from serine is neither rapid nor abundant, however. Human volunteers receiving 15 g of serine show an 800 percent increase in serine level, whereas glycine levels increase by only 33 percent. If necessary, glycine can be converted into serine.

Glycine may also be manufactured from threonine through a metabolic process called degradation. In rats, one-third to one-fifth of ingested threonine is converted to glycine, and 2 g of L-glycine is synthesized per kilogram of body weight per day. Another source for glycine is choline betaine of dimethylglycine (vitamin B_{15}).

Glycine breaks down rapidly in the body. The body converts approximately 1 g of protein per kg of body weight a day.

REQUIREMENTS

There is no RDA for glycine. Glycine is a nonessential amino acid that can be easily made from numerous other amino acids within the body. It is an extremely abundant amino acid in the body and is as common as glucose. The daily intake of glycine in the average adult in the United States is 3 to 5 g. Glycine is required for optimum growth and for creatinine synthesis in experimental animals. It is conceivable that under some conditions, glycine might become essential in humans.

FOOD SOURCES

Glycine is highly concentrated in protein foods and is found naturally in beans, brewer's yeast, dairy products, eggs, fish, legumes, meats, nuts, seafood, seeds, soy, sugar cane, whey, whole grains, and gelatin, which is 33 percent glycine.

FORM AND ABSORPTION

Dietary and supplementary glycine occurs in the L- form. Because of its simple molecular structure, glycine is quickly absorbed. In persons with inborn errors of glycine metabolism, the amount of glycine increases ten to seventeen times in the cerebrospinal fluid, indicating that glycine readily passes the blood-brain barrier. (Some patients with abnormalities in glycine metabolism also have abnormalities in metabolism of the amino acid valine.)

TABLE 14.1. GLYCINE LEVELS IN FOOD		
FOOD	AMOUNT	CONTENT (GRAMS)
Avocado	1	0.17
Cheese	1 ounce	0.12
Chicken	1 pound	1.60
Chocolate	1 cup	0.17
Cottage cheese	1 cup	0.70
Duck	1 pound	2.70
Egg	1	0.20
Granola	1 cup	0.60
Luncheon meat	1 pound	3.90
Oatmeal	1 cup	0.40
Pork	1 pound	3.13
Ricotta	1 cup	0.70
Sausage meat	1 pound	1.87
Turkey	1 pound	2.00
Wheat germ	1 cup	2.02
Whole milk	1 cup	0.17
Wild game	1 pound	5.40
Yogurt	1 cup	0.19

Dipeptide amino acid forms, and possibly tripeptides, seem to be better absorbed than monopeptides. Glycine dipeptides (glycine-glycine) may be better absorbed than single glycine molecules. Some studies suggest that leucine or isoleucine may inhibit glycine absorption. However, when leucine and isoleucine were given with dipeptide glycine, no inhibition of glycine absorption occurred.

TOXICITY

Takeuchi and colleagues explored the toxic effects of high-glycine diets fed to experimental animals. Diets containing 7 percent glycine resulted in growth depression brought about by glucagon and glucocorticoid deficiency. High toxic doses of glycine, as is frequently the case for other nutrients, produce the opposite effects of normal glycine nutrition. However, this effect could be reversed by supplementing with L-arginine and L-methionine. Toxicity from glycine therapy in humans has not been described. High levels of L-glycine supplementation can be toxic, similar to sugar, in causing vision problems.

The Many Uses of Glycine

Glycine has many practical applications in pharmaceuticals and food. It is an agent in several types of pharmaceuticals; ferrous glycinate preparations use glycine as an iron binder; certain aluminum antacids and painkillers contain glycine. It has been suggested that antacids containing 30 percent glycine and 70 percent calcium carbonate are superior because this combination increases the buffer action of glycine and the neutralizing action of calcium carbonate.

Glycine's sweet, cool taste is often used to mask bitterness and saltiness. It can disguise the bitter taste of potassium chloride and may be useful in making this essential salt substitute more palatable. Glycine is used as a sweetener with citrate or sodium succinate.

In food, glycine is used as a preservative and an antimicrobial agent. It has been used to prevent rancidity of fats and to stabilize emulsions of mono- and diglycerides and ascorbic acid preparations. Glycine plus citric acid can markedly increase the shelf life of salad dressing. It is also effective, as is ascorbic acid, in the preservation of foods against spore-forming microbes, and is mildly bacteriostatic in custard pies and fillings.

Combining a salt of glycine with aspirin decreases the harmful effects of aspirin. The proper ratio of glycine to aspirin is probably fifty-fifty.

CLINICAL USES

Although glycine has important functions within the body, as the following wide range of its clinical uses shows, it is extremely abundant in the body and is as common as glucose. Therefore, there are presently few therapeutic uses for glycine.

Benign Prostatic Hypertrophy

Glycine has been used in combination with alanine and glutamic acid to improve the symptoms of benign prostatic hypertrophy (BPH) and delayed variation by decreasing the amount of residual urine. It appears that glycine may be required for the health and proper functioning of the prostate.

Cholesterol

Glycine is a hypolipidemic agent that can lower triglycerides and cholesterol. A 30 g loading dose of glycine decreased cholesterol approximately by 5 percent and triglycerides by 20 percent.

Detoxification

Glycine alleviates the toxic damage of several substances such as phenol, benzoic acid, and methionine. It relieves the nutritional anemia caused by excess methionine given to rats. After two months of feeding 2.5 percent L-methionine to rats, a moderate degree of anemia was present. The toxicity of excess methionine seems to be directly related to the blocking of hemoglobin synthesis. Glycine accelerated methionine oxidation, lowered blood methionine levels, and promoted appetite in the rats.

Glycine's detoxification of benzoic acid is important, since benzoate derivatives are common in food additives. Glycine conjugates benzoic acid to hippuric acid, which is excreted.

Other claims for detoxification by glycine relate to its ability to stimulate the synthesis of glutathione, the most important antioxidant detoxification system of living things including humans. Cysteine is usually the most important element in this process, but glycine can also stimulate glutathione metabolism. When glycine is deficient and glutamic acid and cysteine are abundant, this could occur in collagen disorders.

Epilepsy

In the treatment of epilepsy, data about glycine seem to be similar to those on taurine, with increased levels of glycine in the brain, particularly at the epileptic site. The brain naturally accumulates more glycine at the seizure site to protect itself. Low levels of glycine in epileptic individuals have not been identified. The anticonvulsant valproic acid (Depakene) elevates plasma glycine, which is its probable major mode of action. Strychnine—a poison that causes seizures—is known to abolish the inhibition of spinal reflexes, induce convulsions, and block the action of glycine in the central nervous system.

Gout

Some claims for glycine's therapeutic properties have focused on its relationship to purine metabolism and uric acid. Purines are organic compounds that contribute to uric acid production. Uric acid is the end product in the metabolism of purines normally excreted in urine. Excess blood levels of uric acid are found in gout.

Glycine taken orally increases the renal clearance of uric acid, thereby lowering the serum urate concentration. In low concentrations, glycine also inhibits purine biosynthesis. However, increased amounts of glycine are likely to stimulate purine biosynthesis. A high-purine diet, normally obtained from a substantial meat intake, increases urinary uric acid by 0.5 to 0.75 mg/ml of ingested purine. Glycine and other amino acids such as alanine, aspartic acid, and glutamic acid seem to decrease the reabsorption of uric acid by the kidney.

How much glycine is necessary to lower serum uric acid levels is still not known. Following 30 g of L-glycine loading, serum uric acid level decreased by

33 percent in the first three hours, but in the fourth hour, it rose above the initial level. Glycine may be a useful adjunct in the therapy of gout. Further studies are needed.

Growth Hormone Stimulant

In doses of 4 to 8 g, L-glycine is important in pituitary function because it increases serum growth hormone. Doses of 12 g of L-glycine increase the hormone prolactin in serum. As a potent stimulant of the secretion of glucagon, glycine may also raise blood sugar. The most significant hormonal effects in glycine therapy are the increase in growth hormone and glucagon. Our clinical trial with 30 g of L-glycine orally induced a rise in growth hormone levels ten times greater than baseline (the starting point) at two hours after ingestion. Measuring growth hormone an hour earlier might have detected an even greater rise. Further studies are needed.

Hypothermia

The inhibitory amino acids—glycine, taurine, GABA, and possibly tryptophan and alanine—have been found to be elevated in the brains of hypothermic (low body temperature) and hibernating animals. These nutrients may have mild antithyroid effects as well.

Kidney Disease

Creatinine is formed from creatine, an energy-producing substance present in muscle tissue, and creatine is formed from glycine and arginine in the kidney. The study of blood creatinine levels is particularly useful in diagnosing kidney disease. The amount of creatinine excreted in the urine by healthy individuals is independent of the amount of protein, food, or total nitrogen in the urine. Children and poor muscularly developed individuals have frequently low creatinine in the serum and may be relatively deficient in glycine.

Manic Depressive Disorder

Glycine is thought to be an important factor in psychiatric disorders. Rosenblat and colleagues measured the concentration of twenty amino acids in erythrocytes (red blood cells) and plasma of thirteen female bipolar (manic depressive) patients and ten female healthy controls. The concentration of glycine in the erythrocytes was significantly elevated in the manic depressive group. No differences were found in plasma levels. Preliminary findings indicated high glycine levels for patients who had manic depression, but who were now in remission, and were previously unresponsive to electroshock therapy. It is not known whether the increase of glycine found in erythrocytes is also found in the brain of the depressive patients.

The increase in erythrocyte glycine without significant changes in other amino acids is surprising, since glycine shares a carrier-mediated transport system with proline and alanine. The elevation of glycine was not attributed to diminished synthesis or increased degradation of glutathione in erythrocytes, because the tripeptide concentration was not decreased in these depressed patients. The manic depressive group was treated with lithium, which is known to elevate plasma glycine levels.

Deutsch and colleagues from the Department of Psychiatry at New York University confirmed that glycine increased in the erythrocytes of individuals with bipolar disorders. They suggested that this was due to lithium. No such abnormalities were found in patients with unipolar depressive disorders. Furthermore, elevated glycine did not correlate with the mood state. This effect is probably due to lithium, and may or may not relate to its therapeutic mode of action. We have not seen any elevations in plasma glycine in the dozens of people taking lithium at our clinic.

We have tried large doses of 15 to 30 g of L-glycine in two manic individuals during acute attacks. Calmness and cessation of the manic episode occurred within one hour; indeed, depression can be induced. Further clinical trials are warranted.

Metabolic Disorders

Glycine appears to be involved with several branched-chain amino acids and their metabolism. It may be useful for acute management of isovaleric acidemia, an inherited disorder of leucine metabolism. Glycine seems to bind with isovaleric acid, a toxic substance, to form isovalerylglycine, which is less toxic.

In patients with acidosis, an abnormal state of reduced alkalinity of the blood and body tissues, glycine improves even comatose episodes. High doses of glycine (175 mg/kg in a normal adult, or 12 to 14 g in a 150 lb man) must be administered rectally because it may cause vomiting when taken orally. However, at our clinic, we have used as much as 30 g of glycine orally in adults, and the only side effect experienced was loose stools.

Painkiller Interaction

The painkilling effect of morphine is antagonized by injection into the brain of glycine and other inhibitory amino acids. Excitatory amino acids such as glutamate or aspartate do not have this effect.

Muscle Spasticity

Studies of glycine and spasticity are particularly significant. Glycine is reduced by 30 percent in ventromedial, central, and dorsal areas of the spinal cord in spastic animals; abnormal levels of glycine in blood have been found in patients with spastic disorders. Spasticity seems to be associated with postsynaptic inhibition (the uneven transference of nerve impulses) in the spinal cord, with a decrease of glycine activity in certain regions of it. With doses of 50 mg/kg per day, or 3.5 g for an average 150-lb male, improvement was shown in human spasticity. Glycine was also effective when used in dogs to reduce extensor and abductor spasms.

Seven human subjects have been treated at our clinic with 3 g of L-glycine daily with the alleviation of spasticity. Glycine administration is accompanied by an increase in glycine content in the brain. Glutamate content of the brain also can be significantly elevated in glycine-treated animals.

Myasthenia

Studies of myasthenia, a muscle disorder, have suggested that manganese, glycine, and vitamin E could be useful in its treatment. However, these reports had not been properly documented. The response to these agents was actually diagnostic. Myasthenia in many ways resembles the collagen diseases of dermatomyositis and scleroderma. Glycine supplements were thought to be of value because myasthenia patients have high creatinuria, or loss of creatinine in the urine, and creatine is synthesized from glycine. Vitamin E is also thought to reduce the excretion of creatinine. However, the therapeutic benefits of glycine for myasthenia is purely speculative.

Glycine has also been used in the treatment of muscular dystrophy with some undocumented success.

Plasma Levels and Clinical Syndromes

The measurement of glycine levels is becoming increasingly more available to doctors and nutritionists for study. Glycine levels are sometimes found to be increased in patients on lithium and anticonvulsants, or patients suffering from starvation, renal oxalate stones, rickets, and various metabolic diseases. At our clinic, we have found low plasma glycine levels in two epileptic patients and in dozens of depressed patients. Plasma glycine levels are likely to be useful for the diagnosis of various clinical syndromes and as a guide in glycine therapies.

Sedation

Studies have shown that 3 to 10 g of L-glycine can have sedative effects and when used with inositol helps in reducing aggression. All inhibitory amino may have this effect in large doses.

Wound Healing

Along with zinc, glycine is one of the most prevalent nutrient ingredients in ointments and creams used for wound healing. Collagen, a protein and a substance rich in glycine, proline, and arginine, is essential for wound healing in humans. Collagen is the richest source of dietary glycine available, and in a predigested form, it is found to be the best way for glycine to be absorbed. Patients who benefit the most from this type of therapy are postoperative burn and trauma patients.

Diets high in glycine and proline, with arginine present, can also contribute to wound healing. Glutamic acid, a precursor of proline, is a good source of proline. However, serine, which can be converted to glycine, is not a good source of glycine; therefore, it must be obtained from other sources (see Table 14.1 on page 211). In studies of experimental animals, wound healing was accomplished best by supplementing with a combination of glycine, proline, and arginine.

Diets supplemented with glycine and arginine in experimental animals result in increased nitrogen retention (for example, better absorption of amino acids), following femur fracture under ether anesthesia. Diets supplemented with glycine and arginine improved growth of cells before and after trauma and improved nitrogen retention. Posttrauma nitrogen retention can be increased to 60 to 70 percent with diets heavily supplemented with glycine.

Arginine was found to improve growth in the posttrauma period, while glycine alone was actually found to depress nitrogen retention before and after trauma. Hence, this clearly suggests that for the healing effects of glycine to be beneficial, arginine also must be administered to traumatized animals. This may be true for all wound healing.

Many hypotheses exist to explain the effective role of glycine and arginine in wound healing. It has been shown that arginine and glycine are both required for optimum growth and for proper creatinine synthesis in experimental animals, particularly chickens. Both amino acids are detoxifying: Arginine detoxifies ammonia, and glycine detoxifies benzoic acid by binding with it to form hippuric acid. Glycine may also play a part in the repair of muscle fibers.

Gelatin, a protein that contains 33 percent glycine, is useful in wound healing. Gelatin products have been used for many years as a glycine supplement to help the growth of nails, which are made of glycine-rich keratin. Excessive estrogens tend to cause nails to peel, and the best remedy is adequate zinc and manganese along with dietary protein.

Another interesting study revealed that glycine, cysteine, and threonine in combination are useful in the healing of leg ulceration, although these amino acids were of no use in the healing of blisters. The effects of these amino acids individually have not been established.

DIMETHYLGLYCINE: A MIRACULOUS METABOLITE?

Dimethylglycine (DMG) is a derivative of glycine and a normal compound found in low levels in cereal grains, seeds, and meats. DMG serves as a building block for many important compounds, including methionine, choline (a B vitamin derivative important to the synthesis of the neurotransmitter acetylcholine), hormones, and DNA. The quantities of DMG in the body are almost too small to measure except by special techniques, yet it can have a wide range of beneficial effects.

DMG was originally manufactured *in vitro* through a Russian patent as part of a formula known as calcium pangamic acid, incorrectly referred to as "vitamin B_{15}." Calcium pangamate is the ester formed between DMG and calcium gluconate. The formula contained significant amounts of DMG, and the calcium gluconate was found to rapidly hydrolyze to DMG when given orally. Hence, it was deduced that the active effects of pangamic acid were due to DMG, not the calcium gluconate, though common usage has led to the acceptance of the term "vitamin B_{15}." This DMG-based formula demonstrated to aid cardiovascular function by reducing angina and high triglyceride and cholesterol levels and improving oxygen utilization by the body. It was also found to improve liver function.

Research begun in 1975 in the United States began to support many of the health benefits found in the Russian studies. Many claims have been made about DMG for strengthening immune response; boosting physical and mental performance in athletes and older people; and enhancing cardiovascular function in people with arrhythmia, circulatory problems, angina, blood pressure, and elevated triglycerides. Additional research indicates that DMG can protect the liver, aid in detoxification, reduce seizure activity in some individuals, promote improvement in children and adults with autism; increase stamina and sex drive; and aid in the treatment and prevention of hypoglycemia, lupus, fatigue, diabetes, allergy, muscle cramps, arthritis, pain, and melanomas.

Claims for DMG are mostly attributed to its conversion to glycine. In the body, DMG is produced in the one-carbon transfer cycle from choline via betaine in an enzyme-controlled transmethylation reaction. Sequentially, choline is converted to betaine, DMG, sarcosine (a sweet, crystalline amino acid), and finally glycine. DMG functions as an intermediate in this process. By being metabolized, DMG acts as a methyl donor that assists in methylation similar to the metabolic pattern of betaine, methionine, and folic acid. DMG's effects generally could also be attributed to methionine glycine by themselves.

In this breakdown process, DMG generates two carbon molecules, including sarcosine, glycine, serine, and the ethanolamines, all of which are beneficial to the cell. It also stimulates oxidative enzyme activities that may help protect DNA from mutation and inhibits enzymes for cholesterol and triglyceride synthesis, thereby lowering cholesterol and triglycerides in serum. The increase of oxidative enzymes is brought about by certain nutrients such as copper, and the lowering of cholesterol is done by glycine, lecithin, or choline. DMG may prolong the effects of choline by slowing its breakdown. Hence, we see that the effects of DMG are probably those of a composite of nutrients, including copper, methionine, glycine, choline, or lecithin. The possibility exists, however, that DMG in therapy may have properties greater than the sum of its parts.

Studies on the use of nutritional supplements in racehorses, including DMG; vitamins A, E, and D; and the minerals iron, copper, and manganese, have found that beneficial effects occurred after one month of therapy with 1,200 mg of DMG per day. The study is difficult to evaluate because the horses were being given many other nutrients as well. However, the authors suggest DMG could lower blood lactic acid levels, make the horses more aggressive, and improve their appetites.

Many pharmacological actions of DMG have been identified. Some of the most interesting have been the creation of increased reserves of glycogen, creatinine phosphate (a high-energy phosphate molecule used in muscle and central nervous system tissues), and phospholipid in skeletal and cardiac muscle fibers. DMG's reported benefits in aging may also be due to glycine. DMG, like glycine, probably contributes to the synthesis of glutathione, an important antioxidant made primarily from cysteine. Also, as people age, methyl groups can decrease. DMG acts as an antidote in its role as a methyl donor.

Other reported effects of DMG relate to glycine as an osmoprotectant in plant life, like betaine and proline. That is, as salt levels increase, glycine, as well as betaine and proline, increase. They are useful amino acids, protecting life from the stress of deficient amounts of water. For this purpose, DMG would have no advantage over glycine.

Thus, many of the effects of DMG can be attributed to glycine. An average person ingests 3 to 5 g of glycine daily. DMG is available in 100 mg to 125 mg tablets. Although DMG is very effectively absorbed from the digestive tract, data further suggest current dosing of DMG is far too small to expect any positive effects. The recommended dose of DMG can range from 125 mg to over 1,000 mg a day, depending upon the condition being treated.

Ironically, we have tried doses of 3 g in fasted human controls, with no elevation in plasma glycine levels or change in amino acids. Even if the DMG were converted to glycine, this would not be enough of a dose to raise glycine levels acutely. DMG in these large doses may produce depression.

DMG may have many interesting effects. The most interesting effects of DMG are its possible role in controlling autism and epilepsy and a more likely role as an immunostimulant. However, it might be cheaper and easier to obtain these effects from supplementation with glycine, choline, and methionine.

Autism

There is a growing body of evidence that DMG is beneficial for people with autism. Autism is a biological brain disorder of unknown causes marked by a broad range of puzzling social and personal behaviors. Studies and hundreds of clinical reports have demonstrated that DMG can improve the behavior, social interaction, verbal communication, and disturbing activities of children with autism. In one study, 39 autistic children, age three to seven, were given 125 to 375 mg of DMG per day, for a three-month trial period. Based on evaluations from parents and teachers in a number of critical areas, 80 percent of the children improved significantly.

Epilepsy

Interest in DMG as a treatment for epilepsy relates to the role of glycine as a neurotransmitter. One report in the *New England Journal of Medicine* found that 100 mg of DMG reduced medication-resistant epilepsy in one patient from seventeen seizures to one seizure per week. Several studies since have found no effect of DMG in epilepsy. In our opinion, the doses tested have been ridiculously low. At present, there is no serious information to use in evaluating DMG and epilepsy. All the reports are at doses too low to be meaningful.

Immunity

Persons receiving 120 mg of DMG for ten weeks in a double-blind study compared with twenty healthy volunteers showed a fourfold increase in antibody response to pneumococcal vaccine. It seems that DMG enhanced both antibody and cell-mediated immune response by stimulating white blood cell metabolism. This claim has not yet been made for glycine, and it remains to be seen whether this report can be duplicated. Another report suggested that immunological suppression in x-ray irradiated guinea pigs could be reversed by injections of DMG. DMG as an immunological adjunct holds promise. Again, in the case of immune function, the sum of the effects of DMG's biochemical parts may not be as great as the effects of the whole.

GLYCINE LOADING

The disappearance of glycine from plasma has been observed during our loading studies. Thirty grams of oral L-glycine given to human volunteers peaks at four hours at four times the normal value. The plasma concentration of serine, which can be made from glycine, increases about threefold. In contrast, the conversion of serine to glycine is slower than the conversion of glycine to serine based on our results of a serine loading. Glycine levels rise and fall no more than 33 percent following a 15 g serine load; glycine concentration was observed to peak at two hours after the serine was administered. Branched-chain amino acids inhibit the change of glycine to serine in certain human cell types.

SUPPLEMENTATION

At present, we advocate no role for supplemental glycine in healthy individuals. Glycine is extremely abundant in the body, virtually as common as glucose, which makes it difficult to raise glycine levels, and thus create a therapeutic effect. Glycine administered intravenously in high doses of 15 to 30 g may be of benefit as an antipsychotic or as a calming agent in some individuals.

Deficiency Symptoms

There are no known signs of glycine deficiency.

Availability

Free-form L-glycine is available in 500 mg capsules.

Therapeutic Daily Amount

Doses ranging fom 2 g to 60 g per day have been used for therapeutic purposes in clinical trials.

Maximum Safe Level

Not established, however, no serious adverse effects from using glycine have been seen even with doses as high as 60 g a day.

Side Effects and Contraindications

May produce nausea in excessive doses.

GLYCINE: A SUMMARY

Glycine is a simple, nonessential amino acid, although experimental animals show reduced growth on low-glycine diets. The average adult ingests 3 to 5 g of glycine daily. Glycine is involved in the body's production of DNA, phospholipids, and collagen, and in release of energy. Glycine levels are effectively measured in plasma in both normal patients and those with inborn errors of glycine metabolism. Glycine is probably the third major inhibitory neurotransmitter of the brain; glycine therapy readily passes the blood-brain barrier.

Reports of possible therapeutic uses are varied. Glycine is probably effective in calming the manic episodes of manic depression, and in the treatment of spasticity and epilepsy, because of its sedative properties. Depressed and epileptic patients often have low glycine levels.

Gout, myasthenia, muscular dystrophy, benign prostate hypertrophy, and high cholesterol may respond to glycine therapy. The data supporting these claims are optimistic but not well documented. However, it is well documented that glycine releases growth hormone when administered in high doses.

Glycine is a very nontoxic amino acid. We have done studies with 30 g of glycine without producing any side effects. Some manic-depressive patients have benefited from its effects. We often use threonine as an alternative source of glycine therapy.

Dimethylglycine (DMG) is an intermediate in the metabolism of choline and glycine. DMG's effects are mostly attributed to its conversion to glycine. The most interesting effects of DMG are its possible role in controlling epilepsy and a more likely role as an immunostimulant.

CHAPTER FIFTEEN

Serine:
The Potentiator
of Madness

S erine is a nonessential amino acid that is manufactured from the amino acids derived from threonine and glycine. It is a component of the protective myelin sheaths that surround nerve fibers and of proteins in the brain. One such serine compound is phosphatidylserine, a substance especially abundant in nerve cells that is widely used to treat depression and dementia as well as normal age-related memory loss. Too-high levels of serine in the body, however, may have a detrimental effect on the immune system and can be neurotoxic.

FUNCTION

Serine is a highly reactive amino acid that is found in high concentrations in all cell membranes. It is a hydroxy-amino acid with glycogenic qualities, which enables it to play an active role in the metabolic pathways involved in the proper metabolism of carbohydrates, and fats and fatty acids.

Serine is important in the manufacture of creatine, porphyrins (nonprotein nitrogenous tissues constituents), and purines and pyrimidines (essential constituents in DNA synthesis), and serves as a supplier of methyl groups when needed for DNA synthesis. Serine helps in the formation of ethanolamine, choline, phospholipids, and sarcosine, substances that are needed to produce neurotransmitters and cell membranes, and aids in the production of immunoglobins and antibodies, substances that are essential to maintain a healthy immune system.

Serine can be converted to pyruvate, a common compound in carbohydrate metabolism, which enables it to contribute to the breakdown of carbohydrate for energy and to the exchange of glycogen to glucose in the process of gluconeogenesis. Serine also combines with carbohydrates to form glycoproteins, which help to build basic structural proteins such as hormones, enzymes, and immunologically active molecules. Serine proteases, including trypsin and chymotrypsin, are catalysts for the hydrolysis of peptide bonds in proteins, and assist in the process of digestion.

Serine can also be reconverted to glycine, and from glycine to amino levulinic acid (ALA). ALA is a precursor of porphyrins and hemoglobin, and in addition, has been found to be a useful, nontoxic weed killer that can be sprayed at dusk and works with the following day's sunlight. A role for serine as a pesticide, however, has not yet been explored. Serine is included as a natural moisturizing agent in many cosmetic and skin care formulas.

Low to average concentrations of serine are found in muscle compared to other amino acids.

METABOLISM

Serine can be made in the body from threonine and glycine. Its conversion from glycine, however, requires adequate quantities of pyridoxine (vitamin B_6), niacin (vitamin B_3), and folic acid. The critical enzyme involved in this conversion is serine hydroxymethyl transferase, which utilizes pyridoxine and niacin. Glycine is also a precursor to serine, and the two are interconvertible.

Proper metabolism of serine to phosphatidylserine is dependent upon sufficient levels of folic acid and methionine in the brain. Folic acid increases the buildup of serine, while methionine decreases the serine by working it into membranes. A high serine-to-cysteine ratio (cysteine is formed from methionine) may be indicative of membrane disturbance and has been reported to occur in patients with psychosis.

REQUIREMENTS

There is no RDA for serine. However, like all the amino acid building blocks of protein, serine can become essential under certain conditions, and therefore is important in maintaining health and preventing disease.

FOOD SOURCES

Serine is available from dietary protein, but it must first be converted from glycine by glycolysis before it can be used by the body. The best sources for serine are meat, especially pork, and gelatin, as well as many foods that often cause allergic reactions, such as wheat gluten, peanuts, and soy. These allergic reactions can also manifest in the brain. Cerebral allergies cause the lining of the brain to swell and can result in symptoms as diverse as recurrent headaches, to schizophrenic, violent, or aggressive actions. Many poor-quality foods such as luncheon meats and sausage are high in serine.

TABLE 15.1. SERINE LEVELS IN FOOD		
FOOD	AMOUNT	CONTENT (GRAMS)
Avocado	1	0.16
Cheese	1 ounce	0.40
Chicken	1 pound	0.90
Chocolate	1 cup	0.50
Cottage cheese	1 cup	1.70
Duck	1 pound	1.40
Egg	1	0.50
Granola	1 cup	0.50
Luncheon meat	1 pound	2.40
Oatmeal	1 cup	0.50
Pork	1 pound	3.00
Ricotta	1 cup	1.40
Sausage meat	1 pound	1.12
Turkey	1 pound	1.50
Wheat germ	1 cup	1.50
Whole milk	1 cup	0.50
Wild game	1 pound	3.70
Yogurt	1 cup	0.50

FORM AND ABSORPTION

Serine is not a well-absorbed amino acid. In dietary protein, L-serine must first be converted to glycine to be used. In supplement form, it is available as L-serine, but most often it is used in the form of its derivative phosphatidyl serine. The D- and DL- form of serine may promote growth and formation of tumors. It appears that D-serine may work by inhibiting the absorption of L-serine.

CLINICAL USES

Presently, there are few therapeutic roles established for serine. This amino acid is primarily used as a diagnostic tool.

Cancer

Serine-phosphorus compounds are involved in many biochemical pathways. D-serine is an immunosuppressive agent and has been noted to promote the growth of some experimental tumors. The DL- form of serine promotes various forms of tumor formation. D-serine probably works by inhibiting the absorption of L-serine. Thus, L-serine should be tested as an anticancer agent, and D-serine should be tested as an antipsychotic agent.

Hypotension

The serine analog DL-threo 3, 4 dihydroxyphenylserine (threo-serine) raises blood pressure in patients with orthostatic hypotension (a sudden fall in blood pressure that occurs when assuming a standing position) that occurs secondary to familial amyloidosis (an inherited condition marked by dizziness upon standing, numbness and tingling in the arms and legs, and possibly diarrhea). This analog increases urinary excretion of the neurotransmitters norepinephrine and adrenaline, and decreases serine's conversion to norepinephrine. This modified amino acid was ineffective in patients with orthostatic hypotension of unknown causes. Serine itself in large doses does not raise blood pressure, either. Phosphatidyl serine is worth investigating for use in low blood pressure.

Pain

Phosphatidylserine and certain enzymes increase opiate binding action in neurons. Serine enhances the effects of opiates such as morphine; therefore, serine supplements may be useful for augmenting pain-relief therapies, especially in cases of chronic pain.

Plasma Levels in Clinical Syndromes

We have had six patients at our clinic with low serine levels. Two patients had hypertension, two were depressed, one had allergies, and one showed high triglycerides. The finding of two hypertensive patients with low serine is of interest since drugs that inhibit serine metabolism have been used experimentally to control blood pressure. Threonine and glycine are frequently also low in low serine patients.

Recent research suggests a link between low levels of serine and conditions of chronic fatigue syndrome (CFS), a mysterious and sometimes debilitating condition characterized by weakness and lack of energy, and hyperoxalemia, an abnormally high accumulation of oxalates in the urine, associated with the formation of kidney stones.

We have seen two patients with elevated serine levels. Both were women in their twenties, who were plagued by allergies. One was taking theophylline (Aerolate) and the other was on thyroid medication; both patients restricted gluten from their diets with good results. Elevated serine has been found in the brains of animals prior to induced convulsions.

Psychosis

Waziri and colleagues at the University of Iowa studied fifty-one psychotic patients and twenty-seven healthy controls. Significantly high serine-to-cysteine plasma ratios of 1.5:1 were found in the psychotic patients compared to 1:1 in the controls. The ratio in the psychotic group varied upward with the severity of the psychosis. It is thought that elevated levels of serine result in suppression of dopamine excess. Reports have identified four psychotic patients who developed a short-lasting exacerbation of psychosis following serine administration. This did not occur with methionine or glycine, derivatives of cysteine and serine, respectively.

In another study, Waziri and colleagues demonstrated serine metabolism defects with loading doses of approximately 30 g of L-serine orally in psychotic patients and healthy individuals. Plasma serine levels were significantly elevated in the psychotic patients in response to this dose of serine, yet the serine did not exacerbate their symptoms. Thus, serine levels may be an important lead in understanding the biochemistry of psychosis.

Serine enzymes are involved in the metabolism of alkaloids, naturally occurring amines that display pharmacological activity. Serine has been known to induce catalepsy (a trancelike state that may occur in schizophrenia or epilepsy in which the muscles are more or less rigid) in animal models of psychosis. This information has not been entirely supported by research in humans, but more studies are underway.

Cycloserine, a serine analog and an antibiotic that inhibits pyridoxine and serine metabolism, has been reported to produce psychosis in some individuals. The experimental carcinogen azaserine, a modified form of serine, will not cause cancer during pyridoxine deficiency, because this vitamin is essential in metabolizing the serine to which the carcinogen is attached. Serine-excess psychosis may occur only in pyridoxine-deficient psychotic persons.

Psychotic individuals with elevated serine in their plasma have been documented to have deficiencies of pyridoxine and the manganese-dependent enzyme serine hydroxymethyltransferase. These patients correspond to the pyroluric patients described by Pfeiffer and colleagues in which there is a genetically determined chemical imbalance involving an abnormality in hemoglobin synthesis. The treatment of these patients, pioneered by Dr. Pfeiffer at the Brain Bio Center in Princeton, New Jersey, is based upon high doses of pyridoxine, zinc, and manganese. Furthermore, metabolism of the antipsychotic chlorpromazine (Thorazine) inhibits serine transport in experimental models, suggesting that antipsychotic drugs may act by inhibiting serine metabolism.

Aboaysha and Kratzer showed that growth retardation caused by high-serine diets in children could be prevented by daily oral doses of 5 mg of pyridoxine. Furthermore, pyridoxine supplements can reverse the growth-stunting effects of high-serine diets even after they have occurred. Pyridoxine is essential for conversion of phosphatidylserine to phosphatidylcholine, a critical metabolite in brain metabolism, associated with memory. Studies of serine loading in proto-zoans (primarily single cell organisms) resulted in most of the serine becoming incorporated into membrane phospholipids.

Unfortunately, we have been unable to confirm the high-serine psychosis hypothesis at our clinic. However, the method we employed for measuring amino acid levels is different from the methods used by the scientists who made these observations.

Suspiciously high blood concentrations of certain amino acids are often found in schizophrenic patients and individuals with slight neuropsychological alterations. It appears that N-methyl-D-aspartate receptors are activated in schiz-ophrenia as they are after stroke. Thus, there may be some parallels in the bio-chemistry of schizophrenia and stroke. We find glycine elevated in individuals with paranoid or undifferentiated schizophrenia. We may see higher glutamic and aspartic acid levels, but research suggests that serine exerts a more signifi-cant role here. Either too much serine is being produced or there are not enough antioxidants present to counterbalance the serine. Excess serine lacks the destructive clout of the glutamic and aspartic acid cascade following stroke, but it nevertheless appears to have a neurotoxic effect. Thus, in addition to being treated for the presence of autoimmune imbalances, many schizophrenic patients may also need to receive treatment similar to that of stroke victims. (See "Stroke" on page 178.)

One should use supplemental serine with caution because of this neurotoxic potential and possible contribution to psychotic behavior. It should probably not be used by individuals with borderline psychosis. In cases where serine is used, it is advisable to administer antioxidants with it.

Foods high in serine should be restricted in the diets of psychotics or indi-viduals prone to psychotic reactions (see Table 15.1 on page 225).

Tubular Necrosis

Serine supplements have been noted to cause psychotic reactions. In another study, a large dose of serine, 80 mg per 100 kg in animals, (equivalent to 60 g in a 150-lb adult male) caused some acute tubular necrosis at the proximal tubule of the kidney. Tubular necrosis is a kidney disorder involving damage to the renal tubule cells, resulting in acute kidney failure.

IMPORTANT METABOLITES

Modifications of serine metabolism in the brain hold much promise. The two most interesting compounds derived from serine are phosphatidylserine, a sub-stance classified as a phospholipid, and cycloserine, an antibiotic used in trans-plant procedures to protect against organ rejection.

Phosphatidylserine

It has been shown that blocking serine metabolism generates an antipsychotic effect. Building serine up can help relieve the depression that can accompany Alzheimer's disease.

Now an impressive volume of research shows that phosphatidylserine, a phosphorus-containing lipid derived from serine, not only benefits individuals with Alzheimer's disease, but can also benefit people with other memory disorders and depression. In our clinic, we use phosphatidylserine for many Alzheimer's patients. A substantial number of caregivers report improvements, particularly in the areas of memory and depression. At PATH, we believe phosphatidylserine has merit as part of a multimodal approach to this illness. Although the brain normally makes sufficient quantities of phosphatidylserine, its production decreases as we age, which may result in deficiency.

Phosphatidylserine is especially abundant in nerve cells and is active throughout the brain, with particular effect apparently in the hippocampus, the memory center of the brain. Recent studies show that phosphatidyl serine may work by stabilizing choline in this area. Consistent oral administration of 3.5 g of phosphatidylserine daily, improved spatial memory and passive avoidance retention in aged rats. Translated to humans, extremely high dosages may be necessary. Supplemental phosphatidylserine is widely used in Europe, and is available only in 100- to 200-mg potency in the United States. Some individuals with senility may need numerous pills to replicate the type of memory benefits achieved with laboratory animals. However, due to biochemical individuality, there will likely be individuals who can benefit from as little as 200 to 400 mg, that is, one-eighth or less of the amounts the rodents received.

Phosphatidylserine is recommended in our clinic when we identify memory disorders, early senility, depression, and slow P300 brain wave in BEAM testing (see page 59 to learn more about this diagnostic method). An increase in serine and glycine is thought to potentially speed the processing of the evoked potentials in brain maps (a visual/spectral analysis of brain waves). These amino acids may improve brain metabolism. Multiple sclerosis patients also have abnormal brain maps. They may respond to phosphatidylserine as well.

Cycloserine

Cycloserine (Spiramycin) is a modified amino acid and antibiotic approved for use in transplant procedures as a protective agent against rejection.

Cycloserine blocks serine metabolism and also causes serious suppression of amino acid metabolism in general. While this activity negatively affects the immune system, it may serve to counteract autoimmune activity. An immune system attack of brain tissue is involved in some cases of schizophrenia. Similar pathology is known to occur also in lupus erythematosus (a chronic inflammatory disorder of the connective tissue) and rheumatoid arthritis. Blocking serine metabolism with cycloserine may have benefits not just for autoimmune schizophrenia but for other disorders as well.

This theory is interesting; however, it will take research to determine how best this medication can be used for treatment-resistant schizophrenia. The suggested dosage of cycloserine is about 50 mg. Cycloserine is available as an intravenous or oral solution, or in soft-gel capsules, by prescription only.

SERINE LOADING

Serine loading of 15 g raised serine levels to nine times normal at two hours and four and a half times normal at four hours. Glycine levels also increased significantly, about one and a half times normal. The levels of branched-chain amino acids decreased, but this effect occurs in almost all loading studies and is apparently due to the stress of fasting. Other biological parameters—polyamines, chem screen, and trace metals—were not affected.

SUPPLEMENTATION

At present, serine supplementation has no proper therapeutic purpose. One should use supplemental serine with caution because of this neurotoxic potential and possible contribution to psychotic behavior.

Deficiency Symptoms

There are no known signs of serine deficiency.

Availability

Although not readily available, free-form L-serine is available in 500 mg capsules.

Therapeutic Daily Amount

Not applicable.

Maximum Safe Level

Not established.

Side Effects and Contraindications

Excessively high doses may cause immune suppression, psychotic reactions, and possibly elevated blood pressure. One should use supplemental serine with caution because of this neurotoxic potential and possible contribution to psychotic behavior. It should probably not be used by individuals with borderline psychosis. In cases where serine is used, it is advisable to administer antioxidants with it.

SERINE: A SUMMARY

A high serine-to-cysteine plasma ratio is a potential clinical marker for psychosis, which in turn corresponds to pyroluria as a marker for pyridoxine and zinc-dependent psychosis. Many poor-quality foods, such as luncheon meats and sausage, are high in serine. Foods that cause cerebral allergy—for example, gluten, soy, and peanuts—are also high in serine. Serine supplements may cause such adverse effects as psychotic episodes and possibly elevated blood pressure.

Low serine levels can occur in hypertensive patients, and high serine levels can occur in allergy patients. Therapeutic applications of how to apply this knowledge to treatment are presently under investiagation.

Serine is also immunosuppressive, which makes it a harmful agent in cancer patients but potentially useful in autoimmune diseases. A serine analog (threo-serine) may raise blood pressure in people with hypotension. A role for serine may develop in pain relief, but at present serine supplementation has no proper therapeutic purpose. D-serine should be tested as an antipsychotic agent.

CHAPTER SIXTEEN

Alanine:
The Hypoglycemia Helper

A lanine is a nonessential amino acid that is made in the body from the conversion of pyruvate, a common compound in carbohydrate metabolism, or the breakdown of DNA and the dipeptides carnosine and anserine. Alanine aids in the metabolism of glucose, yet it can also be broken down quickly into glucose and used as an energy source when needed by the muscle, brain, and central nervous system.

FUNCTION

Alanine is largely concentrated in muscle and only slightly in blood, liver, kidney, and brain. A variety of studies suggest that alanine, like glutamine, is one of the most important amino acids released by muscle as a form of circulating energy in the body. It is the primary amino acid that transports nitrogen from muscle to the liver, and thereby guards against the accumulation of toxic substances that may occur during aerobic exercise when muscle protein is quickly degraded to meet energy needs. Alanine may also build muscle.

Alanine can be swiftly converted by the liver into usable glucose. It contributes to the regulation of blood sugar levels, especially important in conditions such as hypoglycemia and diabetes; and, like glycine, GABA, and taurine, it functions as an inhibitory neurotransmitter. The amino acid phenylalanine is mediated through an alanine-GABA cycle.

Beta-alanine, a form of alanine found in bacteria, is a constituent of pantothenic acid (vitamin B_5) and coenzyme A, two substances critical to many metabolic processes involved in the conversion of fats, carbohydrates, and protein to energy.

Alanine improves immune response by helping to produce antibodies and assist in the metabolism of organic acids. Without alanine, growth hormone, glycemic control, and the immune system can become compromised.

METABOLISM

Alanine is one of the simplest amino acids. Little is known about the metabolism of alanine. Normal alanine metabolism, like that of other amino acids, is highly dependent upon enzymes that contain pyridoxine (vitamin B_6).

Alanine is manufactured from pyruvate and from the breakdown of DNA, and the dipeptides carnosine (a small molecule made from alanine and the amino acid histidine) and anserine. These dipeptides are not usually detectable in the plasma of healthy individuals; but, when consumed in considerable amounts in chicken or turkey, they can then be detected in the urine. Their breakdown into alanine depends on an enzyme that utilizes the trace metal zinc.

When alanine is formed by the breakdown of carnosine, it results in the production of alanine and histidine. Isoleucine, one of the branched-chain amino acids, can also stimulate its release from the muscle. Alanine can be converted quickly in the liver to usable glucose, which suggests that there may be a valuable glucose-alanine cycle between the muscle and liver.

REQUIREMENTS

There is no RDA for alanine. Because the body can easily manufacture alanine from a variety of sources, deficiency states seldom occur.

FOOD SOURCES

The best food sources for alanine are meat products and other high-protein foods like wheat germ and cottage cheese.

FORM AND ABSORPTION

The L- form of alanine is the most common type and is the form in which alanine is incorporated into the body's protein. D-alanine analogs have been found to have antibacterial activity.

NUTRIENT INTERACTIONS

Alanine in very large dosages seems to be a pharmacological antagonist of taurine transport and inhibits the uptake of taurocholate, the taurine bile acid in rat liver. In very low doses, alanine inhibits taurine transport and seems to share similar mechanisms with taurine in the brain. Chemically similar amino acids inhibit transport of like amino acids. GABA also inhibits taurine transport.

TOXICITY

No toxic effects were found when a 20 percent alanine diet was fed to rats. This alanine intake increased urinary alanine one hundredfold to a thousandfold, and serum alanine fiftyfold without toxic side effects. Plasma pyruvate and ammonia

TABLE 16.1. ALANINE LEVELS IN FOOD		
FOOD	AMOUNT	CONTENT (GRAMS)
Avocado	1	0.24
Cheese	1 ounce	0.20
Chicken	1 pound	1.46
Chocolate	1 cup	0.30
Cottage cheese	1 cup	1.60
Duck	1 pound	2.23
Egg	1	0.35
Granola	1 cup	0.62
Luncheon meat	1 pound	3.30
Oatmeal	1 cup	0.47
Pork	1 pound	4.10
Ricotta	1 cup	1.22
Sausage meat	1 pound	1.70
Turkey	1 pound	2.15
Wheat germ	1 cup	2.11
Whole milk	1 cup	0.30
Wild game	1 pound	5.20
Yogurt	1 cup	0.34

(breakdown products of carbohydrate and protein metabolism) were slightly increased in males but not in females. Toxicity with elevated alanine levels in humans has not been described.

CLINICAL USES

The amino acids in the threonine group have simple chemical structures. Glycine is the cornerstone of each amino acid in this group. It works as an amino sugar and allows all the amino acids in this group to function as sugar exchangers. Alanine appears to be the most critical for maintaining blood sugar levels.

Athletic Recuperation

The ketosis that may occur as a result of strenuous aerobic exercise may be reduced by alanine therapy. Ketosis is a process whereby the body burns stored fat for fuel. Post-exercise ketosis following aerobic exercise may be treated by alanine supplements. Ketosis, which speeds up weight loss, is inhibited by alanine. The role of alanine in the treatment of the athlete should be explored further.

Cholesterol

The effect of large doses of alanine on cholesterol levels was assessed during the trial mentioned briefly above in which no toxic effects were observed when a 20 percent alanine diet was fed to rats. Alanine intake increased urinary alanine one hundredfold to a thousandfold and serum alanine fiftyfold without toxic side effects, yet cholesterol levels decreased in males and was unchanged in females. Hence, alanine in large doses may join the numerous other amino acids that can lower cholesterol.

Epilepsy

Alanine, like taurine, is an inhibitory neurotransmitter and may act as such in the brain. The actions of alanine are antagonized by the convulsants picrotoxin and strychnine. The alanine effect parallels the antiepileptic effect of GABA and taurine, and it may have an important future in the treatment of epilepsy.

Hepatitis

A low ratio of serum alanine to the enzyme aspartate amino transferase is typical of patients with alcoholic hepatitis. The metabolism of alanine is impaired in alcoholics because the active form of pyridoxine, pyridoxal phosphate, is diminished in these patients. Pyridoxine deficiency is probably the cause of many of the low alanine plasma levels we see in patients.

Hypoglycemia and Diabetes

The relationship of insulin to alanine and other amino acids suggests an amino acid involvement in hypoglycemia. When insulin rises, the level of alanine drops, as do the levels of methionine, tyrosine, and phenylalanine. We do not understand clearly how insulin affects amino acids, but it appears that low levels are an indication of hypoglycemia.

Alanine deficiencies have been found in patients with hypoglycemia. Alanine levels in plasma correlate to degrees of hypoglycemia that are common during fasting. Alanine stimulates an increase in blood sugar, triggering the release of the hormone glucagon, which releases glucose. Thus, alanine may be a useful therapy in hypoglycemics, particularly if they show tremors, rapid heartbeat, and anxiety as a symptom.

There is also evidence for an alanine-ketone cycle. Ketones are any one of a number of compounds containing a ketone group (CO) that occur from incomplete catabolism, or breakdown, of fatty acids. Alanine is antiketogenic, meaning alanine may prevent ketosis and reduce elevated triglycerides, a common problem in diabetes, and for this reason, its use in diabetes is under investigation. Alanine suppresses ketogenesis in humans by direct effect on the liver, independent of insulin. Ketone bodies made in people with diabetes inhibit the breakdown of protein and the release of alanine from the liver. When sugar levels increase in diabetics with low insulin levels, alanine increases, which may result in ketoacidosis. If not properly treated, this dangerous condition can lead to loss of consciousness and coma. Alanine levels may parallel blood sugar levels both in patients with hypoglycemia and in those with diabetes. High-protein diets have been used successfully to stabilize blood sugar levels.

Immunostimulation

Alanine seems to be a singularly important amino acid in the body's reproduction of lymphocytes. Lymphocytes are substances that are responsible for building immunity in the body. Alanine contributes to thymus growth, which increases the division of lymphocytes in human blood. Alanine may be an important therapy to consider in immune-deficient individuals. Amino acid profiles may have an important role in the investigation of immune deficiency.

Infectious Diseases and Acute Infections

Elevated serum alanine occurs in patients with acute infections and in some infectious diseases. Preliminary studies suggest amino acid imbalances may be present in Epstein-Barr virus (EBV). EBV is a member of the herpes family, and it causes mononucleosis. People with chronic fatigue syndrome (CFS) carry high levels of EBV antibodies and elevated levels of alanine in their blood. Both conditions are associated with elevated levels of alanine and low levels of tyrosine and phenylalanine. The implications, however, are not well understood.

One therapeutic role on the horizon for this amino acid is the addition of alanine to oral hydration solutions for individuals with diarrhea caused by infections. Glutamine and glycine have also been suggested.

D-alanine analogs have been found to have antibacterial activity and are currently being investigated.

Kidney Stones

Alanine can promote phosphate and oxalate stone breakdown in experimental animals. High-alanine diets may eventually have a role in kidney stone prevention. Pyridoxine helps metabolize alanine. A diet deficient in pyridoxine can raise oxalates, leading to increased possibilities of kidney stones.

Plasma Levels in Clinical Syndromes

Elevated levels of alanine are found in individuals with arginosuccinate deficiencies. Arginosuccinate is one of the enzymes required to break down arginine. We have found deficiencies of alanine levels occasionally in patients with branched-chain amino acid deficiencies. A ratio of low serum alanine to aspartate enzymes occurs in alcoholic hepatitis.

We have on occasion seen patients with elevated alanine levels in plasma. Patients with agitated depression often have low levels of glycine, threonine, and alanine; unipolar depression often shows low beta-alanine levels. The significant uses of alanine are under evaluation.

Of the first 100 patients in whom we measured plasma amino acid levels, 14 percent were low in alanine. Thirteen of these were women; four had inborn errors of metabolism such as phenylketonuria (PKU) or hypothermia, and seven had some form of psychotic depression either as a primary or secondary diagnosis. Low alanine levels also occurred in a patient with severe anorexia, in one patient with folliculitis, in two patients with severe allergies, and in one patient with severe kidney disease (glomerulonephritis). One male with low plasma alanine levels was healthy, but had a very slight build. The implications of these data are unclear.

Treatment of other more primary amino acid defects, for example, low tryptophan, in one of these patients elevated the alanine levels. Eventually we may try to use alanine therapy directly at our clinic, but we haven't yet seen severe isolated alanine deficiency. Alanine deficiency is treated with multiple amino acid formulas.

Only two other patients have shown elevated alanine levels. Both of these patients were taking other amino acids, for example, taurine and tryptophan, or tryptophan, tyrosine, and methionine. A high dose of any amino acid will eventually elevate alanine levels, probably by transamination (the process of transferring amine groups from one amino acid to another).

In general, alanine depletion can be seen in individuals with hypoglycemia. It is also typically present in people who have low growth hormone, and low levels of taurine and branched-chain amino acids.

SUPPLEMENTATION

To date, we have not used L-alanine therapeutically. Eventually we may try to use alanine therapy directly at our clinic, but we have not yet seen severe isolated alanine deficiency. Low levels of alanine are often manifested by low blood sugar levels. Typically, we treat this condition using either a multiple amino acid formula, or a high-protein diet, in combination with the mineral chromium and the herb *gymna sylvestre.*

Deficiency Symptoms

Signs and symptoms of alanine deficiency may include hypoglycemia, fatigue, muscle breakdown and wasting, elevated insulin and glucagon levels, and low growth hormone level.

Availability

Although not readily available, free-form L-alanine is available in 500-mg capsules.

Therapeutic Daily Amount

Dosages range from 500 to 1,500 mg a day depending upon the condition being treated.

Maximum Safe Level

Toxicity with elevated alanine levels in humans has not been described.

Side Effects and Contraindications

None known.

ALANINE: A SUMMARY

Alanine is a nonessential amino acid made in the body from the conversion of the carbohydrate pyruvate or the breakdown of DNA and the dipeptides carnosine and anserine. It is highly concentrated in muscle and is one of the most important amino acids released by muscle, functioning as a major energy source. Plasma alanine is often decreased when the BCAAs are deficient. This finding may relate to muscle metabolism. Alanine is highly concentrated in meat products and other high-protein foods like wheat germ and cottage cheese.

Normal alanine metabolism, like that of other amino acids, is highly dependent upon enzymes that contain pyridoxine. Alanine, like GABA, taurine, and glycine, is an inhibitory neurotransmitter in the brain. These inhibitory agents may be a useful therapy for some epileptic patients.

Alanine is an important participant as well as a regulator in glucose metabolism. Alanine levels parallel blood sugar levels in both diabetes and hypoglycemia, and alanine reduces both severe hypoglycemia and the ketosis of diabetes. It is an important amino acid for lymphocyte reproduction and immunity. Alanine therapy has helped dissolve kidney stones in experimental animals.

At our clinic, we have often found patients with decreased plasma alanine levels who also show low glycine and taurine. The significance of this data to alanine therapy is under study. Toxicity with alanine therapy has not been reported.

SECTION SEVEN

Branched-Chain Amino Acids

ISOLEUCINE, LEUCINE, AND VALINE
The Stress Relievers

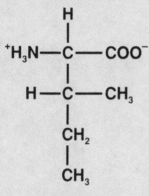

ISOLEUCINE

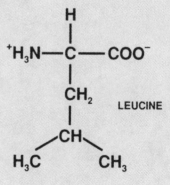

LEUCINE

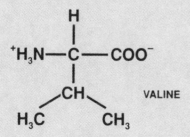

VALINE

CHAPTER SEVENTEEN

Isoleucine, Leucine, and Valine: The Stress Relievers

Isoleucine, leucine, and valine are members of the branched-chain family of amino acids. Each is considered an essential amino acid and a necessary building block for protein. They are called "branched-chain" amino acids because their carbon structures are marked by branched points. Together, they work to protect muscle during stress or during high-energy states and act as fuel for muscle metabolism.

FUNCTION

Among amino acids, the branched-chain amino acids (BCAAs) are the most essential for maintaining muscle and skeletal health. In tissue, leucine accounts for an astounding 8 percent of the amino acids of body proteins. In muscle, leucine is the fourth most concentrated amino acid, following glutamic acid, aspartic acid, and lysine. Valine and isoleucine trail closely behind leucine. The strong concentration of these amino acids in muscles is not surprising, since that is where they are primarily used.

Glucose that is not needed for immediate energy production is converted into glycogen in the liver. It is stored either in the liver or in the muscles and is converted back into glucose when needed by the body. BCAAs are great sources and producers of energy for muscle under many kinds of severe stress. They are thought to be the major fuel involved in anabolic reactions—the building phase of metabolism in which substances are combined to form complex compounds. They stimulate protein synthesis, increase the re-utilization of amino acids, and decrease the breakdown of protein under stress. Furthermore, leucine is the only amino acid that can substitute for glucose in fasting states, and is an important source of calories and fuel for the body. (There are many other glucose-producing amino acids, but leucine appears to be the most able to maintain proper blood sugar levels.) This makes the BCAAs particularly useful in stress states such as surgery, trauma, cirrhosis, infections, fever, starvation, and muscle training and weight lifting, which require proportionally more BCAAs than other amino acids.

In people undergoing and recuperating from surgery and in some cases of severe trauma, the BCAAs, particularly leucine, are being used to create a more ideal standard hospital intravenous solution to help the body recover. In athletic training, BCAAs have been proven to enhance muscle-protein metabolism, decrease exercise-induced degradation of proteins, and play a part in the oxidative metabolism in the muscle during strenuous exercise. For bodybuilders, weight lifters, and athletes, BCAAs provide a viable alternative to steroids.

In disease conditions affecting movement and muscles, BCAAs are gaining a reputation for decreasing muscle wasting. They are being used to help astronauts withstand the rigors of space travel and show potential for treating symptoms of amyotrophic lateral sclerosis (ALS, also known as Lou Gehrig's disease), a severe neuromuscular disease that results in paralysis. When BCAAs are depleted from the body, a "wearing-out" syndrome can occur, resulting in decreased muscle mass and bone density.

In the brain, BCAAs function as constituents of neuropeptides (nerve proteins, or biochemicals, that send chemical messages from the brain to receptor sites in cell membranes) and as neurotransmitters capable of producing a calming and pain-relieving effect.

METABOLISM

BCAAs are metabolized primarily by muscle. Despite their structural similarities, the branched-chain amino acids have different metabolic routes. The breakdown of leucine is accomplished solely through fat pathways, valine solely through carbohydrate pathways, and isoleucine through both. Their different metabolisms account for different requirements for these essential amino acids, different symptoms of deficiency, and not surprisingly, different applications in medicine.

The first reaction in normal BCAA metabolism requires pyridoxine (vitamin B_6) to activate transaminase enzymes, the enzymes primarily responsible for BCAA metabolism. The next oxidative reaction depends on thiamine (vitamin B_1), and thereafter, copper and riboflavin (vitamin B_2) derivatives are required as cofactors. Biotin, magnesium, and alpha-ketoglutarate, which is made from glutamic acid, are also required to metabolize the BCAAs properly.

BCAA transaminases are unique in that they are distributed predominantly in skeletal muscle and in much smaller amounts in the liver. These enzymes metabolize leucine about five times as fast as they do valine. In contrast, the dehydrogenase enzymes—enzymes also typically involved in metabolism—are more concentrated in the liver than in skeletal muscle. In the metabolism of BCAAs, the overall cooperation between the muscles and the liver is evident.

Many types of inborn errors of BCAA metabolism exist and are marked by various abnormalities. The most common form is branched-chain ketoaciduria (often referred to as maple syrup urine disease) in which keto acids are excreted, creating a characteristic urine odor. There are several forms of this disease, which can be marked by a tenfold elevation of valine, a fifteenfold elevation of iso-leucine, and a twentyfold elevation of leucine. Many other amino acids are reduced in this metabolic condition, including alanine, asparagine, cysteine, glu-tamic acid, proline, and taurine.

Maple syrup urine disease can produce ataxia, convulsions, or coma when high blood levels of BCAAs are present. Most forms of this disease can be treated simply by dietary restrictions of BCAAs. Reducing one's intake of BCAAs, espe-cially of isoleucine, however, can cause the occurrence of hypoglycemic episodes. Dietary management can also create a folic acid deficiency and, there-fore, should be attempted only under the supervision of a healthcare practitioner.

REQUIREMENTS

Isoleucine, leucine, and valine are essential amino acids, and so cannot be manufactured by the body from other amino acids. It is, therefore, critical that sufficient amounts of these amino acids be included in the diet. BCAAs make up approximately 40 percent of the total minimum daily requirement for essen-tial amino acids. According to Harper and colleagues of the University of Wis-consin, the BCAAs make up 50 percent of the indispensable amino acids in the daily food supply.

A deficiency in valine results in disaccharidase enzyme deficiency in the gut of experimental animals. During valine deficiency, as with deficiencies of other essential amino acids, dietary nitrogen or dietary protein is not well absorbed. Cusick and colleagues of the Department of Food Science at the University of Illi-nois found that when valine was withdrawn from the diet of weaning rats, the animals developed a unique pattern of neurological symptoms, marked by head retraction, staggering, and aimless circling. Myelin degeneration was found in the region of the brain called the medial longitudinal fasciculus, where the facial and vestibular nerves were degenerated. Removal of valine from the diet also caused damage to the nuclei of the brain and the chief protein-synthesizing machinery of the cells.

Isoleucine deficiency has been less studied than valine deficiency. It is marked by tremors and twitching of the muscles of the extremities in experimental ani-mals. To our knowledge, no attempts to study leucine deficiency in experimen-tal animals have been made.

Of all other amino acid groups, the BCAAs are more sensitive to fluctuations in calorie or protein intake. Fasting for even twenty-four hours will increase the plasma concentration of all three BCAAs in humans and rats, while most other amino acids decline. Starvation beyond one week, or kwashiorkor (protein-calorie malnutrition), lowers the BCAAs to below normal levels. Following a protein meal, blood levels of BCAAs increase to a much greater extent than other amino acids because the liver extracts little of them from the blood. Muscle tissues reuse most BCAAs in contrast to the liver, which does not store them.

The current minimum daily requirements established by the National Academy of Sciences for the BCAAs are as follows: for infants, 83 mg/kg of body weight for isoleucine, 92 mg/kg for valine, and 135 mg/kg for leucine; for children ages ten to twelve, 28 mg/kg for isoleucine, 25 mg/kg for valine, and 42 mg/kg for leucine; and for adults, 12 mg/kg for isoleucine, 14 mg/kg for valine, and 16 mg/kg for leucine, or 840 mg, 980 mg, and 1,042 mg respectively.

Cheraskin and colleagues of the University of Alabama have gone over these data and have studied ideal consumption diets in a variety of normal populations and suggested that these minimum daily requirements may be five to ten times less than what is actually needed. The optimal dose could be up to 5,000 mg of each BCAA under conditions of stress.

FOOD SOURCES

Leucine is more highly concentrated in foods than are isoleucine and valine. A cup of milk contains 800 mg of leucine and only 500 mg of isoleucine and valine combined. A cup of wheat germ has about 1.6 g of leucine and 1 g of isoleucine and valine combined. The ratio evens out in eggs and cheese. One egg and an ounce of most cheeses each contain about 400 mg of leucine and 400 mg of valine and isoleucine combined. The ratio of leucine to other BCAAs is greatest in pork, where leucine is 7 to 8 g and the other BCAAs combined are only 3 to 4 g.

Other good sources of leucine include brown rice, beans, nuts, and soy flour. Relatively high sources of isoleucine and valine are nuts, chicken, chickpeas, lentils, liver, rye, and soy protein.

FORM AND ABSORPTION

Dietary protein and supplements are made from the L- form of the branched-chain amino acids. In both of these sources, L-isoleucine is the best absorbed of the group. Few data are available on oral supplementation, though we do know that supplements of individual BCAAs are occasionally used by healthcare practitioners. In general, however, the BCAAs should always be taken in balance with one another.

Isoleucine and leucine compete with valine for transport and can block out valine when competing for entry to the brain. BCAA therapy is frequently administered intravenously in total parenteral nutrition (TPN) to malnourished patients and in cases of severe trauma. The best solutions are probably those with the highest concentration of leucine compared to isoleucine and valine. Typically,

TABLE 17.1. BRANCHED-CHAIN AMINO ACID LEVELS IN FOOD				
FOOD	AMOUNT	CONTENT (GRAMS)		
		ISOLEUCINE	LEUCINE	VALINE
Avocado	1	.14	0.20	0.20
Cheese	1 ounce	.35	0.60	0.42
Chicken	1 pound	1.24	1.80	1.20
Chocolate	1 cup	0.48	0.78	0.53
Cottage cheese	1 cup	1.82	3.20	1.90
Duck	1 pound	1.54	2.60	1.76
Egg	1	0.38	0.53	0.44
Granola	1 cup	0.53	0.90	0.68
Luncheon meat	1 pound	2.30	4.08	2.80
Pork	1 pound	3.43	5.90	3.89
Ricotta	1 cup	1.45	3.00	1.70
Rolled oats	1 cup	0.50	0.83	0.54
Sausage meat	1 pound	1.10	2.03	1.23
Turkey	1 pound	1.70	2.60	1.76
Wheat germ	1 cup	1.20	2.20	1.63
Whole milk	1 cup	0.49	0.79	0.54
Wild game	1 pound	4.35	7.00	4.40
Yogurt	1 cup	0.43	0.79	0.65

such solutions contain up to 20 g of leucine and as much as 14 to 16 g of the other BCAAs combined.

Although BCAAs compete with one another for absorption, the competition for transport to the brain is more intense between the BCAAs and tyrosine, phenylalanine, tryptophan, and methionine. BCAAs themselves may be important neurotransmitters and are constituents of neuropeptides, which have neurotransmitter functions. Many enkephalins (pain-relieving peptides) contain large amounts of leucine and may lower brain levels of serotonin and dopamine.

In the future, a form of BCAA supplementation known as keto-analogs may prove a useful form for increasing absorption of BCAAs by the body; however, more trials measuring significant metabolic parameters for possible changes need to be undertaken before we can recommend keto-analogs.

The D- form of leucine has been shown to have a similar effect to that of D-phenylalanine in preventing the breakdown of endorphins and enkephalins, natural painkillers in the body.

CLINICAL USE

Branched-chain amino acids have many useful applications. Stress states, surgery, trauma, cirrhosis, infections, fever, and starvation or fasting states require proportionally more BCAAs than other amino acids.

Anorexia Nervosa

Low levels of valine and isoleucine, as well as tryptophan, have been found in people who have anorexia nervosa, a disorder characterized by an abnormal fear of weight gain and a consequent refusal to eat. In our clinic, we have consistently found low plasma BCAAs in anorexic patients. The deficiency of these BCAAs probably contributes to muscle loss in these patients.

Fasting produces a short-term decline in plasma BCAAs in the first four hours, and then a rise peaking at seventy-two hours. Subsequently, a final decline occurs. Anorexia in some ways resembles a prolonged fasting state.

A fifty-five-year-old woman came to us for help. She had anorexia, which had developed for no apparent reason. While living in Europe, her appetite had gradually decreased and her weight had declined from 130 to 100 pounds in six months. Since she was five feet nine inches tall, this amounted to emaciation. All of the physicians she had seen attributed her severe anorexia to cancer. She underwent liver and bone CAT scans, and dozens of blood profiles. Finally, desperate and nearing the need for a feeding tube in the hospital, she came to us. The most striking results of her tests were low plasma BCAAs. She was immediately started on a supplement rich in BCAAs. After two and a half months of therapy, she had reached 125 pounds.

Endocrine Function

The endocrine system is made up of a set of glands that secrete hormones into the bloodstream. Among these glands are the pancreas and thyroid. BCAA levels are elevated in humans and animals with diabetes. The pancreas secretes the hormone insulin in response to high sugar levels; a state that frequently occurs in diabetes. In diabetic rats, BCAAs and their enzymes are elevated along with low concentrations of insulin. Low insulin levels reduce the absorption of BCAAs by muscle, which may cause other plasma amino acids to rise. People with diabetes tend to lose muscle mass and require more BCAAs in their diets, as do older adults and people with cancer ataxia or cirrhosis of the liver.

Various stress rates are marked by low insulin and glucagon ratios, further supporting the role of BCAAs, particularly leucine, in hypercatabolic, or highly stressed physiological states.

The hormone thyroxin increases the transport of leucine. When given to certain types of rats, thyroxin has been found to result in an increase in transport in BCAA-like systems. Hence, thyroid is a protagonist of rapid BCAA metabolism.

The bodies of people with hyperthyroidism (overproduction of thyroid hormone) probably use BCAAs too rapidly.

The BCAAs have also been found to cause a slight, temporary elevation in growth hormone production. The amount of growth hormone secreted is not significant enough to counteract the loss of growth hormone that occurs with aging, but it may be beneficial in athletic training. (See "Muscle Building" on page 251.) Of the BCAAs, leucine has the greatest effect on the release of growth hormone. This may be because leucine functions as the trigger of muscle growth in the body.

Huntington's Chorea

Several individuals with Huntington's chorea, a Parkinson's disease–like condition, have been found to have low levels of BCAAs. In addition, proline, alanine, and tyrosine are often low. There is no doubt that there are neurotransmitter abnormalities in Huntington's chorea, as in Parkinson's disease, which might be marked by dopamine deficiency or other neurotransmitter deficiencies.

At least 5 percent of people with Parkinson's disease have olivopontocerebellar atrophy (a group of hereditary ataxia disorders). Early clinical trials suggest these patients do well with 10 g of L-leucine a day. They may benefit from isoleucine and valine as well.

Liver Disease

People with cirrhosis, an advanced form of liver disease that is commonly caused by long-term alcohol abuse, have decreased levels of BCAAs. Cirrhosis of the liver is a degenerative inflammatory disease that results in scar tissue and the inability of the liver to function properly. Protein formulas high in BCAAs and low in aromatic amino acids (phenylalanine, tyrosine, and tryptophan) and methionine have been documented to be useful during liver disease. BCAAs have been found to make the liver more able to handle amino acid metabolism. They tend to slow down the delivery of the aromatic amino acids to the liver.

This altered ratio of serum BCAAs to aromatic amino acids in cirrhosis occurs for several reasons. BCAAs and aromatic amino acids compete for transport into the brain. Increases in ammonia that commonly occur in liver disease alter the brain's permeability levels, greatly enhancing the entrance of aromatic amino acids over BCAAs. Branched-chain amino acids are metabolized in muscle, while aromatic amino acids are metabolized in the liver, which adds to the altered ratio of serum amino acids. Certain studies have found that supplemental pyridoxine can lower the ratio of aromatic amino acids to BCAAs in liver disease. BCAAs can also reverse the catabolic state of cirrhotic individuals, that is, prevent the breakdown of muscle for energy.

When toxins that would be detoxified by a healthy liver accumulate in the brain, hepatic encephalopathy can develop. This condition is characterized by a decline in brain function manifested as speech difficulties, disrupted sleep, tremors, and other symptoms. Low levels of BCAAs to high aromatic amino acids are commonly found in people with this condition. A reduction by BCAAs of the increased urinary excretion of 3-methylhistidine, a marker of protein metabolism used to assess the occurrence of muscle wasting in cirrhotic persons, has suggested an anticatabolic effect of these amino acids. The greater the excretion of urinary 3-methylhistidine, the better the protein balance in the body.

Hepatic coma, the end stage of liver disease, is characterized by an increase of ammonia and tryptophan or tyrosine in the brain. It has reportedly been reversed using 5 mg of L-valine per kg of body weight. Administering this therapy in the average cirrhotic patient, blood levels of valine increase to eight times normal. Raising valine levels causes less tryptophan and tyrosine to enter the brain, due to competition with the valine. Valine may also be more effective than the other BCAAs, possibly because it is more easily converted to glucose and can be more readily used in brain metabolism. Leucine may also be effective under some circumstances since it inhibits the transport of tryptophan in the brain and excess leucine can decrease the buildup of brain serotonin.

In addition to oral BCAA therapy, a 40-g protein diet high in BCAAs, or a diet containing 4 percent BCAAs, with a restriction of aromatic amino acids, has been found to be effective in treating advanced liver disease. BCAA supplements are effective in hepatic coma, which also may be benefited by the high levels of the amino acid ornithine, which is also needed in higher amounts when the liver is not functioning properly.

A decrease in BCAAs and an increase in aromatic amino acids is only one factor in hepatic encephalopathy. This is a diverse metabolic disorder, marked by decrease in protein synthesis, ammonia excess, and abnormal fatty acid metabolism. BCAAs can also prevent the coma sometimes produced by excess methionine given to patients with severe liver disease.

Individuals with other disorders of liver metabolism—such as portacaval shunt (a type of liver disease involving portal hypertension) and extrahepatic biliary atresia (a rare gastrointestinal disorder in newborns that destroys the bile ducts outside the liver that carry bile from the liver to the intestines)—have problems similar to patients with hepatic coma and may also benefit from BCAA therapy.

Children with extrahepatic biliary atresia, like those with severe liver disease, have low BCAA to aromatic liver disease ratios. Methionine levels and aromatic amino acid levels are significantly elevated. Plasma amino acids ornithine and threonine are also significantly elevated while taurine is significantly decreased. This further emphasizes that the need for BCAAs is immediately increased in highly stressed physiological states.

Muscle Building

Branched-chain amino acids have proven useful for bodybuilding and athletic activity. The BCAAs are thought to enhance energy, increase endurance, and contribute to the health and repair of muscle. We have been impressed over many years by the number of well-muscled patients who claim that BCAA supplements, ranging in dosages from 5 to 10 g a day, contributed to muscle gain.

The anabolic effect of the BCAAs, while not in the same league as steroids, is nevertheless much safer. BCAAs stimulate protein synthesis directly in muscle. Of the three BCAAs, leucine may be the major fuel involved in anabolic reactions and therefore is of major importance in protein storage. It may stimulate insulin release; in muscle and other tissues, insulin not only stimulates protein synthesis but also inhibits protein breakdown. Leucine, by itself or with other BCAAs, promotes protein synthesis. Suboptimal intakes of protein increase the efficiency of leucine, while an excess of protein increases the channeling of dietary protein to leucine pools where it is stored.

Athletes also require increased BCAAs while under stress. BCAAs can increase the reutilization of amino acids and decrease the breakdown of protein under stress. Working at Burke Rehabilitation Center in White Plains, New York, Albanese found significantly decreased serum isoleucine and leucine levels in athletes during intense physical stress. The amino acids phenylalanine, cystine, and tryptophan have been found to decrease as well during intense physical stress; valine was not measured.

When taking BCAAs to repair or build muscle, it is important to keep in mind the concept of amino acid balance. When BCAA intake increases, the entry of phenylalanine and tyrosine into the brain is impaired, which may inhibit overall brain function temporarily. Therefore, use BCAAs prudently. We recommend taking BCAAs before a workout and supplementing with some of the brain-stimulating amino acids such as phenylalanine and tyrosine after a workout. To avoid imbalances, we strongly recommend dosages be individually tailored by a nutritionally oriented health professional who can strategize with a patient based on blood level testing, diet, workload, and performance goals.

At PATH Medical, we have formulated a balanced multinutrient supplement called Fast Path that includes the BCAAs and targets both the brain and the body of fitness enthusiasts and athletes. Fast Path contains the following:

Arginine: 86 mg	Cysteine HCl: 73 mg
Isoleucine: 73 mg	Leucine: 98 mg
Lysine: 73 mg	Methionine: 61 mg
Phenylalanine: 49 mg	Threonine: 49 mg
Tyrosine: 49 mg	Valine: 86 mg

We believe that BCAAs are superior to steroids as a therapy for muscle building and to aspirin for control of hypercatabolic states that occur with intense physical stress. Aspirin and other nonsteroidal anti-inflammatory drugs have been thought to be useful in stopping the muscle ache, inflammation, and fever that may occur after certain physiological stressful states. But these drugs also have harmful effects; for instance, they inhibit interleukin, immune system chemicals that aid in fighting infection and are essential for recovery from catabolic states. Indeed, a little fever is good for you, and the benefits of aspirin are probably outweighed by its interference with the body's normal defense mechanisms. For adults, BCAA supplements, particularly leucine, may replace aspirin as the initial treatment for fever of less than 101°F.

Plasma BCAA Levels in Clinical Syndromes

Isoleucine and leucine have been found to be deficient in some individuals suffering from many different psychological and physical disorders. We have had ten patients at our clinic with low leucine levels. The patient with the lowest levels, 3 g/100 ml, was a fifty-year-old depressed diabetic man who had recently undergone neurosurgery and suffered from hypertension. He had significant control of his depression following therapy with an amino acid supplement containing leucine. The cause of his low leucine levels was probably surgery combined with diabetes. The other patients with low leucine levels had low amino acids in general: Three patients had been chronically hospitalized, two patients had kidney disease, and four patients had severe chronic depression. Two of the four patients with severe chronic depression had been in and out of psychiatric hospitals.

We also found thirteen patients with low isoleucine levels. One chronic schizophrenic patient had undetectable plasma isoleucine. A thirty-year-old chronic schizophrenic patient made a remarkable recovery on niacinamide and niacin therapy, with relief of hallucinations. Patients with low isoleucine levels may have an increased need for niacin, as do pellagra patients. Other patients with low isoleucine levels included three institutionalized patients, five depressed patients, one patient with grand mal seizures, another with petit mal seizures, and one patient with folliculitis.

Low valine levels have been found in five depressed patients under stress, three institutionalized patients, one patient with thought disorder (a state characterized by an inappropriate interpretation of a one's environment, or nonreality-based thinking), and one patient with cardiomyopathy. A thirty-five-year-old man with severe cardiomyopathy experienced tremendous improvement following a high-protein diet and supplement program. The increase in valine in his diet may have been a factor in his improvement.

We found the highest leucine levels in patients with depression; one patient had extremely low magnesium levels. The same patients with high leucine levels had high to normal levels of isoleucine and valine. One patient—a fifty-year-old woman suffering from severe psychotic depression who was resistant to drugs and nutrients—had valine levels that were 25 percent greater than normal. The significance of these findings is unclear.

Protein Intolerance

Some individuals with food allergy and/or an intolerance to certain types of protein have high serum valine levels. Abnormalities in these people include urine excesses of beta-aminoisobutyric acid, GABA, and occasionally taurine and beta-alanine. In some individuals, dietary valine may lead to these maladaptive reactions, but in general, valine is not the actual culprit; rather it is the subnormal levels and coenzyme activity of the pyridoxine enzyme involved in the breakdown of valine. Treatment possibilities include low-protein diet, pyridoxine, magnesium, and in some cases alphaketoglutaric acid, a precursor of glutamic acid. At this time, the role of errors in valine metabolism in protein intolerance and allergy remains speculative.

Psychosis

Low levels of isoleucine and leucine, as well as methionine, have been identified in some children with psychosis. Other studies have shown that, in some individuals, high levels of leucine can contribute to psychosis, particularly in pellagra. In reviewing the literature, Abram Hoffer said that high-corn diets, which cause pellagra, are rich in leucine compared to isoleucine and can be associated with psychotic behaviors. Psychotic people have low levels of tryptophan and niacin. Hoffer also found that leucine increased the loss of niacin in the urine, while isoleucine stops it. Leucine worsens the psychotic symptoms of pellagra, while isoleucine may reverse them. We have documented low isoleucine levels in some chronic schizophrenic patients; these patients often have low blood histamine and respond to niacin.

Ten years ago, Hoffer conducted pilot studies using 3 g a day of isoleucine with niacin, which rapidly cleared the psychosis in a few acute schizophrenic outpatients. Hence, he has proposed that an isoleucine-niacin formula be utilized for treating certain forms of schizophrenia. Further testing and measuring of plasma amino acids is needed to substantiate this hypothesis.

BCAAs may prevent some of the hallucinations experienced by people with schizophrenia by balancing tyrosine-to-tryptophan ratios. This is a hypothesis that has not been proven yet. Nevertheless, oral BCAAs remedy the hallucinatory effects of hepatic encephalopathy brought on by alcoholism and liver or spleen failure. Such psychotic behaviors respond dramatically to BCAAs. This is a prime example of a toxic liver psychosis responding to an amino acid preparation.

Stress

The effects of stress on the body are similar regardless of the type of stress experienced. As stress increases, total caloric needs go up, primarily because the body's protein-calorie needs increase. Thirty percent of the diet ideally should be amino acids when the body is under severe stress, because stress causes protein to break down faster.

Many amino acids have been found to be useful during stress. BCAAs have regulatory effects on overall protein metabolism and, when given as supplements, decrease the rate of breakdown and utilization of other amino acids. A higher degree of stress requires more nutrients and, specifically, more BCAAs and pyridoxine.

Several studies have suggested that starvation or fasting states, injury, surgery, or infection require more BCAAs than other amino acids. Nitrogen retention in critically ill patients seems to be proportional to the amount of BCAAs in the diet. Some researchers have actually found BCAAs elevated in the serum of septic or grossly infected patients. In fact, BCAA supplements seem to correct most of these high-stress physiological states. It is possible that, under certain conditions, BCAAs cannot be utilized properly; however, evidence is overwhelming that BCAAs can be quite useful in reversing most stressful states. Cerra reported that in trauma cases when BCAAs are given intravenously at 0.5 g per kg a day, equivalent to 35 g of BCAAs in a 150-pound man, the catabolic state can be physiologically overcome.

As might be expected, serum levels of virtually all amino acids are decreased following major surgery. Recovery with low-calorie (IV fluid) regimens requires at least four days before BCAA levels return to normal. Intermediate regimens of 3,000 calories containing 66 g of amino acids result in the return to normal BCAA levels in four days, while full total parenteral nutrition (TPN) feeding with 3,000 calories containing 32 g amino acids takes two days for BCAAs to normalize. This study by Moss of Rensselaer Polytechnic Institute was done on cholecystectomy patients to whom BCAAs were fed into the intestine via a tube. It has become standard surgical therapy to give TPN to patients with low serum albumin (the principal protein in blood) as much as a month prior to surgery. These TPN solutions are very rich in BCAAs and contain as much as 4,000 calories and 200 g of protein a day.

In our opinion, BCAAs ensure fast-track recovery from surgery. Over the years, numerous people who have taken BCAAs have reported recoveries from major operations that have astounded their surgeons. For a week before and up to a week after surgery, we recommend BCAAs along with zinc, antioxidants, and other nutritional factors. BCAAs and zinc are the core ingredients; a typical recommendation involves 1 to 2 g of BCAAs and 30 to 100 mg of zinc daily. Using high doses of amino acids after surgery is most important. Most individuals are able to stop this particular program about three days after their operation.

The metabolism of branched-chain amino acids changes under stress. There may be a BCAA-alanine cycle that supplies calories and nitrogen to peripheral tissues. In fact, leucine actually makes a contribution to alanine formation, and alanine is a major source of energy to skeletal muscles. BCAAs are used to synthesize alanine as well as other branched-chain amino acids. Glutamine released to the blood from the liver can make a contribution in the synthesis of glucose. Glutamine is more commonly used in the kidneys, and alanine is used in the muscles. BCAAs can be transferred for use by either of these intermediary amino acids.

We could say that BCAAs are protein-sparing and help save muscle protein. For instance, in trauma and sepsis, skeletal muscle takes over the role of the liver and other organs in metabolism, becoming a major regulatory organ, and develops a requirement for increased BCAAs and alanine. Of the three BCAAs, leucine seems to produce the greatest effect when acting alone.

We know that there is increased oxidation and destruction of BCAAs under stress, particularly the stress caused by starvation or fasting. A greater caloric or metabolic contribution is made by BCAAs in diabetes, exercise, sepsis, surgical injury, trauma of any kind, and liver disease than in nonstress states, which is why branched-chain amino acids are often referred to as the "stress amino acids."

BCAA LOADING

Ten grams of L-valine given orally to normal subjects raised blood levels of valine to six times normal. Amino acids, chemical screen, polyamines, zinc, copper, and iron did not change significantly. Astonishingly, L-valine raised growth hormone levels to ten times normal.

Oral loading of 10 g of L-isoleucine resulted in an increase in isoleucine to fifteen times normal and a 50 percent increase of alanine; iron increased slightly. Further studies are needed, but it appears that L-isoleucine is the best absorbed of the BCAAs.

Oral L-leucine loading of 10 g resulted in a threefold increase in leucine levels in plasma, with a slight increase in iron. Other chemical screen biological parameters are not affected by leucine loading. No side effects were experienced with any of the BCAAs at doses of 10 g.

SUPPLEMENTATION

BCAA supplementation as therapy, both oral and intravenous, in human health and disease holds great promise.

Deficiency Symptoms

There are no known deficiency symptoms for leucine and valine. However, a severe deficiency of isoleucine can produce symptoms similar to hypoglycemia. Aging, injury, and surgery increase the body's needs for BCAAs.

Availability

BCAAs are best absorbed when taken together. Formulas that contain a combination of up to 1,000 mg of L-isoleucine, L-leucine, and L-valine are available in either powder or capsule form.

Therapeutic Daily Amount

The therapeutic dose of BCAAs is 1 to 5 g a day depending upon requirements.

Maximum Safe Level

Not established. When taken in excess, BCAAs are simply converted into other amino acids, and thus are generally regarded as safe, even in large doses.

Side Effects and Contraindications

Side effects may include upset stomach, dizziness, or vomiting when beginning supplementation or when taken at high doses of 5 g or more.

BRANCHED-CHAIN AMINO ACIDS: A SUMMARY

Valine, isoleucine, and leucine are the branched-chain essential amino acids. Despite their structural similarities, the branched-chain amino acids have different metabolic routes, with valine going solely to carbohydrates, leucine solely to fats, and isoleucine to both. The different metabolism accounts for different requirements for these essential amino acids in humans: 12 mg/kg of valine, 14 mg/kg of leucine, and 16 mg/kg of isoleucine. Furthermore, these amino acids have different deficiency symptoms. Valine deficiency is marked by neurological defects in the brain, while isoleucine deficiency is marked by muscle tremors.

Many types of inborn errors of BCAA metabolism exist, and are marked by various abnormalities. The most common form is the maple syrup urine disease, marked by a characteristic urine odor. Other BCAA metabolic abnormalities are associated with a wide range of symptoms, such as mental retardation, ataxia, hypoglycemia, spinal muscle atrophy, rash, vomiting, and excessive muscle movement. Most forms of BCAA metabolism errors are corrected by dietary restriction of BCAAs and at least one form is correctable by supplementation with 10 mg of biotin daily.

BCAAs are useful because they are metabolized primarily by muscle. Stress states—for example, surgery, trauma, cirrhosis, infections, fever, and starvation—require proportionately more BCAAs than other amino acids and probably proportionately more leucine than either valine or isoleucine. BCAAs and other amino acids are frequently fed intravenously to malnourished surgical patients and in some cases of severe trauma.

BCAAs, particularly leucine, stimulate protein synthesis, increase re-utilization of amino acids in many organs, and reduce protein breakdown. Furthermore, leucine can be an important source of calories, and is superior as fuel to the ubiquitous intravenous glucose (dextrose).

Leucine also stimulates insulin release, which in turn stimulates protein synthesis and inhibits protein breakdown. These effects are particularly useful in athletic training. BCAAs should also replace the use of steroids as commonly used by weight lifters. Huntington's chorea and anorexic disorders are characterized by low serum BCAAs. These diseases, as well as some forms of Parkinson's disease, may respond to BCAA therapy. BCAAs, and particularly leucine, are among the amino acids most essential for muscle health.

BCAAs are decreased in patients with liver disease, such as hepatitis, hepatic coma, cirrhosis, extrahepatic biliary atresia, or portacaval shunt; aromatic amino acids (tyrosine, tryptophan, and phenylalanine), as well as methionine, are increased in these conditions. Valine, in particular, has been established as a useful supplemental therapy to the ailing liver. All the BCAAs compete with aromatic amino acids for absorption into the brain. Supplemental BCAAs with pyridoxine and zinc help normalize the ratio of BCAAs to aromatic amino acids.

The BCAAs are not without side effects. In high doses, leucine, for example, exacerbates pellagra and can cause psychosis in pellagra patients by increasing excretion of niacin in the urine. Leucine may lower brain serotonin and dopamine. A dose of 3 g of isoleucine added to the niacin regimen has cleared leucine-aggravated psychosis in schizophrenic patients. Isoleucine may have potential as an antipsychotic treatment.

Leucine is more highly concentrated in foods than other amino acids. A cup of milk contains 800 mg of leucine and only 500 mg of isoleucine and valine combined. A cup of wheat germ has about 1.6 g of leucine and 1 g of isoleucine and valine combined. The ratio evens out in eggs and cheese. One egg and an ounce of most cheeses each contain about 400 mg of leucine and 400 mg of valine and isoleucine combined. The ratio of leucine to other BCAAs is greatest in pork, where leucine is 7 to 8 g and the other BCAAs combined are only 3 to 4 g.

In serum, BCAAs, particularly leucine, are great producers of energy under many kinds of severe stress, such as trauma, surgery, liver failure, infection, fever, starvation, muscle training, and weight lifting. BCAA supplements, while now used only preoperatively for malnourished patients and in intravenous solutions after surgery, should be used in all stress situations. In sum, BCAA therapies have great potential in the medicine of the future, which seeks better health by imitating natural body processes.

SECTION EIGHT

Amino Acids with Important Metabolites

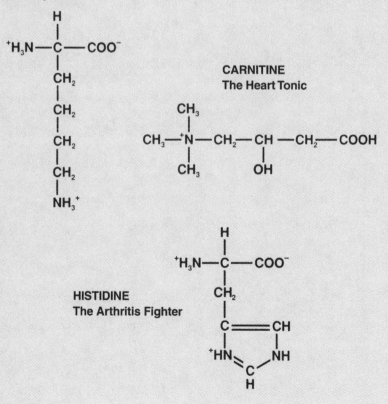

LYSINE
The Herpes Killer

CARNITINE
The Heart Tonic

HISTIDINE
The Arthritis Fighter

CHAPTER EIGHTEEN

Lysine:
The Herpes Killer

L ysine is an essential amino acid that is needed for proper growth and development in children and to help maintain a proper balance of nitrogen in adults. Lysine is well known for its usefulness in fighting cold sores and herpes virus infections—viruses that until now have resisted most forms of therapy. Since then, lysine has been found to have broader immune-enhancing capabilities.

FUNCTION

In addition to slowing viral growth and reproduction, lysine has been shown to increase growth of the thymus and stimulate the growth of thymus factors. The thymus gland is the primary site for the maturation of T cells, which secrete interleukin and interferon, and B cells, which produce antibodies—all substances that support proper functioning of the immune system. It aids in the production of human growth hormone and enzymes, and in the formation of collagen, the protein that forms the matrix of bone, cartilage, and connective tissue. Lysine also appears to impact bone health by improving calcium absorption and retention. Lysine may assist with weight loss.

Lysine is the precursor for several important amino acids. It is the parent molecule from which carnitine is made; carnitine is effective for the prevention of a range of ailments that affect the heart and circulatory system. (Carnitine is discussed in Chapter 19.) Lysine is one source for the manufacture of citrulline, an amino acid mentioned in Chapter 9 that transports the toxic byproducts of protein metabolism from the body and functions as a diuretic, tonic, and immune-system enhancer. Metabolism of lysine also creates amino caproic acid; this metabolite has been useful in the prevention of blood clotting in patients with bleeding conditions or fibrolysis. It is used to irrigate catheters following surgery and in cases of diffuse intravascular coagulation, which commonly occurs in advanced infection and cancer.

Lysine is found in large quantities in muscle tissues. Only glutamic acid and aspartic acid are as concentrated as lysine is in muscle.

METABOLISM

Lysine is degraded into various important metabolites during its metabolism, and not surprisingly, it is metabolized through many different pathways.

Lysine is degraded principally to acetyl CoA, a form of coenzyme A, a vital catalyst in the body and a critical nutrient in carbohydrate metabolism.

During its metabolism, lysine also assists in transamination (the transfer of amino groups) by forming the linkage, or peptide bond, between transaminase enzymes such as SGPT and SGOT, and pyridoxal phosphate, the coenzyme needed for this activity to occur. Lysine is able to do this because it is constructed of two amino groups: one connects to the transaminase enzyme while the other joins with pyridoxal phosphate. Enzymes performing these reactions have been found present in tissues of the liver, kidney, heart, adrenal gland, thymus gland, brain, and skin (in order of decreasing activity).

When some lysine is broken down into citrulline, which is needed in the body for normal protein metabolism, minor amounts of lysine also enter into the homocitrulline, homoarginine, and pipecolic acid pathways of metabolism (pipecolic acid, a neurotransmitter, is found to be highly concentrated in the brain when lysine is given intravenously).

Lysine and arginine share a common transport system that, because of their various chemical properties, can make them antagonistic. An excess of arginine can lead to a depletion of lysine, and an excess of lysine can lead to a depletion of arginine. This metabolic antagonism between lysine and arginine can be useful in treating illnesses related to excessive lysine levels in the body, as we'll discuss later in the chapter.

Lysine's successful conversion to these metabolites along these different metabolic pathways primarily requires pyridoxine (vitamin B_6), riboflavin (vitamin B_2), and niacin (vitamin B_3). Vitamin C and iron help increase absorption and utilization of lysine by the body. Metabolism of lysine is particularly sensitive to the presence of viral infections, stress, and aging.

REQUIREMENTS

Lysine is an essential amino acid that cannot be made by the body from other amino acids. Lysine's essentiality to the body became evident when researchers at Kansas State University found that a diet deficient in lysine results in depressed growth when fed to experimental animals. This lysine-deficient diet when fed to three consecutive generations of animals resulted in persistent differences in the animals' growth. The offspring of these three generations continued to show the effects of lysine deficiency for several more generations and the increased require-ment for the amino acid.

How much lysine does the body actually need? The National Academy of Sci-ences recommends 12 mg/kg of lysine a day for adults, equivalent to 840 mg a day for a normal male adult. Children and infants need considerably more lysine for proper growth and development. It is recommended that children ten to twelve years old receive 44 mg/kg a day and that infants three to six months old receive up to 99 mg/kg a day.

Commonly used supplements of 500 mg of L-lysine represent more than half the daily requirements of 840 mg for adults. Yet, in actuality, most adults ideally consume 8,400 mg, ten times the minimum recommendation. Young at Massa-chusetts Institute of Technology showed that an adult's intake of lysine ranges from 1 to 24 mg/kg daily (up to 15 g).

The relatively low requirement estimated for adults has been challenged by several studies that suggest that adult requirements for lysine and several other essential amino acids are underestimated. More realistic approximations suggest an average adult male needs 35 mg/kg of lysine a day.

FOOD SOURCES

Lysine is high in foods such as wheat germ, cottage cheese, and chicken. Among meat products, wild game and pork have the highest concentration of lysine. Other good sources of lysine include eggs, fish, soy products, and yeast. Fruits and vegetables contain little lysine, except avocados.

Lysine in sweet potatoes and other vegetables is often the limiting amino acid in these foods, that is, the amino acid in lower amounts and therefore the first to become deficient, whereas arginine is high in vegetables in proportion to lysine. Gustafson and colleagues have suggested that lysine deficiency within a protein is not as critical as other amino acid deficiencies, such as methionine and threonine, especially concerning weight gain and food intake.

FORM AND ABSORPTION

Dietary and supplemental lysine occurs in L- form. In both diet and supplement forms, lysine's primary antagonist is the amino acid arginine. Both lysine and arginine compete for transport through the intestinal wall and have various chemical properties that can make them antagonistic. An excess of arginine antagonizes lysine; therefore, if using L-lysine therapeutically, it is best to avoid foods high in arginine such as carob, chocolate, coconut, dairy products, gelatin, meat, oats, peanuts, soybeans, walnuts, white flour, wheat, and wheat germ. Ornithine may also lead to the depletion of lysine. Likewise, lysine, and possibly ornthine, can inhibit arginine metabolism and absorption.

TABLE 18.1. LYSINE LEVELS IN FOOD			
FOOD	AMOUNT	CONTENT (GRAMS)	ARGININE TO LYSINE RATIO
Avocado	1	0.20	.65
Cheese	1 ounce	0.55	.40
Chicken	1 pound	2.00	.80
Chocolate	1 cup	0.65	.50
Cottage cheese	1 cup	2.50	.60
Duck	1 pound	2.60	.85
Egg	1	0.40	.95
Granola	1 cup	0.50	1.85
Luncheon meat	1 pound	4.00	.80
Oatmeal	1 cup	0.60	1.0
Pork	1 pound	7.10	.75
Ricotta	1 cup	3.30	.50
Sausage meat	1 pound	2.25	.80
Turkey	1 pound	3.00	.80
Wheat germ	1 cup	2.10	1.3
Whole milk	1 cup	0.65	.45
Wild game	1 pound	7.00	.75
Yogurt	1 cup	0.70	.35

TOXICITY

In animal studies, large doses of lysine (1.9 g/kg, equivalent to 140 g in humans) administered intravenously seem to increase the kidney toxicity of aminoglycoside-based antibiotics. Large intravenous doses of lysine without antibiotics do not appear to be toxic to the kidneys. Lysine toxicity has not occurred with oral doses in humans.

CLINICAL USES

Medicine has yet to discover lysine's full therapeutic range. Lysine is particularly useful for treating marasmus (a wasting condition) and herpes simplex, but in large part, lysine dosages are too small and may fail to reach the concentrations necessary to prove its potentially diverse therapeutic applications.

Immunological Support

Contradictory results have been reported in studies of the effects of lysine deficiency on the immune system. Lysine, added to a wheat-gluten diet, had no effect on antibody concentration in experimental animals. Another study found that lysine deficiency slightly depressed the immune response. Lotan and colleagues, working at the University of Houston, found that lysine deficiency suppressed the immune system in the same proportion that overall body growth was suppressed. Resupplementing with lysine resulted in increased growth of thymus and improved immune-system parameters.

Herpesvirus Infections

Herpesviruses are a group of viruses that cause painful fluid-filled blisters or sores that may also itch, burn, and tingle. These blisters or sores are highly infectious until they are completely healed. The herpes simplex virus 1 (HSV-1) is the virus that causes cold sores or blisters around the edges of the lips or nose. Herpes simplex virus 2 (HSV-2) is the virus that causes similar symptoms but in the genital area. HSV-2 is the most prevalent sexually transmitted disease in the United States, affecting one out of every five people. Herpes zoster, the varicella-zoster virus, causes chickenpox and shingles. Herpesvirus infections have until now been resistant to most forms of therapy. They have gained much public attention due to increases in HSV-2 to almost epidemic proportions.

Does lysine effectively fight herpesvirus infection? Studies have demonstrated that it may have some antiviral effect in both HSV-1 and HSV-2. Unfortunately, consistent replication of the results from the study in which lysine gained its notoriety for blocking the virus has not been documented. One study, in fact, found the opposite.

Our experience at PATH Medical is that lysine, along with other factors, can be beneficial. For the treatment of herpes, we use a combination of lysine along with zinc, acyclovir (Zovirax), and acyclovir cream. In addition, we address the patient's level of stress, which we find often triggers repeated herpes outbreaks. Many people have underlying depression and other disorders that also must be treated. Our multiple approach to stress includes multivitamins and minerals, amino acids, cranial electrical stimulation (CES), and analyses of personality traits and lifestyle. This complementary program has helped many individuals; our remission rate is quite high.

Griffith and colleagues, working at Indiana University Medical School, found that supplemental lysine suppressed the clinical manifestations of herpesvirus infections. In this study, oral doses of 312 to 1,200 mg a day of L-lysine given to forty-five patients, sometimes in repeated doses, resulted in accelerated recovery from herpes simplex infection and suppression of recurrence. Additional studies of the herpesvirus in tissue culture have demonstrated that a high arginine-to-lysine ratio promotes the virus's growth, whereas a high lysine-to-arginine ratio suppresses or "blocks" viral growth. Studies by Milman and colleagues found that 100 mg daily of L-lysine resulted in significantly fewer recurrences in some people. Yet overall, the rate of recurrence was not changed; the dose given was probably too low.

Based on these data, lysine has been extensively used clinically. Even recipes that use ingredients high in lysine and low in arginine have been developed. Studies conducted by the *Saturday Evening Post* show that 1,500 to 3,000 mg of L-lysine or more are safe and effective. Toxicity levels are probably far from being reached. Among the 1,500 people who purchased lysine during this study and whose average daily intake was 900 mg, 88 percent said this amino acid had helped them. Lysine, they said, seemed to reduce the severity of cold sore attacks and accelerated the healing time.

Other nutrients, such as 600 mg or more of both vitamin C and bioflavonoids, also help reduce the duration of cold sores. Blister formation was severely inhibited by this concentration. Zinc (25 mg) and vitamin C (250 mg) have also been used successfully against oral herpes. Wahba, working at Hadassah University Hospital, Jerusalem, found that 4 percent zinc sulfate solutions were useful when applied to herpes sores. All eighteen patients treated were found to have pain, tingling, and burning that were relieved within twenty-four hours by zinc therapy. Crusting (a sign of healing) occurred within one to three days, and no adverse effects were observed. Zinc, vitamin C, bioflavonoids, and L-lysine are now the foundations of the nutrient therapy of herpes.

Other treatments, such as dyes, 2 deoxyglucose, or acyclovir, may be useful under certain conditions for genital herpes (HSV-2). Fitzherbert used zinc sulfate topically against genital herpes in women. Zinc collagen sponges have been helpful, and zinc douches also may be of value. The degradation of lysine is increased by the zinc antagonist copper. Lysine oxidase is a copper-dependent enzyme, and high levels of copper in the body may even promote herpes growth and lysine degradation.

Herpes simplex virus is suspected of causing and promoting a variety of diseases as the inset "Possible Diseases Caused by Herpes Simplex Virus 1 and 2" on page 268 illustrates. HSV-2 has definitely been identified as one of the causes of cervical cancer, and herpesviruses are similar to the Epstein-Barr virus, which has been found to cause lymphoma. Ironically, previous treatments of herpes with red dye and phototherapy were cancer causing. In contrast, nutrient treatments have few side effects and no known cancer-causing effect, although abnormalities in lysine transport in various tumors has been identified.

Herpesvirus Recurrence

Once a patient recovers from the primary outbreak of herpes simplex viral infection, the virus settles in the nearby nerves and spinal ganglia, where it is protected from circulating antibodies and can remain dormant for varying amounts of time. Because herpes reactivation and growth always begin in the ganglion cells, every case of recurrent herpes simplex viral infections is a ganglionitis. The virus then passes down the nerves to induce the formation of the herpetic blister in the skin or mucous membranes, but this represents only the "rim of the volcano." This means that every time a person has a cold sore on his or her lip, the base of the brain, where cranial nerves exist, may also be involved. Herpes simplex is considered a chronic disease of the nerves that periodically spreads to the skin.

Adour and colleagues have suggested that herpes simplex viruses may be the causative agent in many cranial nerve syndromes including migraine headache, acute vestibular neuronitis, globus hystericus (a transitory sensation of a lump in the throat, often accompanied by emotional or acute anxiety), carotidynia (a pain along the length of the carotid artery), Bell's palsy, and Ménière's disease. When a drop of blister fluid from a human cold sore is put into the eye of a laboratory rodent, the animal will die within a month of fatal herpes encephalitis.

Marasmus

Marasmus, a wasting condition in young children usually due to starvation, became a familiar picture to many in the 1980s due to news coverage of famines in Africa. Children suffering from marasmus do not always respond to simple protein-calorie supplements, and extra lysine has been found to promote more rapid recovery. Lysine enrichment of wheat is probably necessary in the areas of the world where wheat is the basic source of protein. A high lysine-to-tryptophan ratio is particularly important. Grains with higher lysine content are constantly being hybridized.

Osteoporosis and Aging

With aging, calcium is lost from the bones, often resulting in osteoporosis. This condition in which the bones become porous and brittle and, as a result, more likely to break, is particularly prevalent in women, although older men, too, lose bone calcium. One factor in this condition may be a relative lysine deficiency. Wolinsky and Fosmire, working at the University of Houston, found that a deficiency of lysine increased the loss of calcium in urine by mice. Lysine therapy may be a useful adjunct to calcium therapy for weakened bones in older people.

Extra lysine may be desirable in the elderly since it has been shown to fight toxicity from lead and other heavy metals that accumulate in aged individuals and to increase trypsinogen, a digestive stimulant. This latter claim has yet to be substantiated clinically.

Plasma Levels in Clinical Syndromes

We have had nine patients at our clinic with low lysine levels. One was a sixty-

Possible Diseases Caused by Herpes Simplex Virus 1 and 2

The herpes simplex virus is suspected of causing the diseases listed below. Control of the herpesvirus by lysine therapy could be a major health achievement toward helping to prevent the occurrence of these conditions.

Skin

• Vesicular skin eruption (a rash consisting of superficial cavities containing fluid)

• Eczema herpeticum (a herpes-like skin condition such as Kaposi's varicelliform eruption that often affects infants and young children)

• Traumatic herpes (a herpes-like skin condition such as "herpes gladiatorum" that appears on the face, neck, and shoulders)

• Herpetic whitlow (a herpes-like skin condition that affects the fingers and toes)

Mucous Membranes

• Acute gingivostomatitis (a herpes-like condition involving the lips, gums, and the adjacent oral mucosa common in young children)

• Recurrent stomatitis (an inflammation of the mucous tissue of the mouth, also known as canker sores)

• Cervicitis (an inflammatory condition of the uterine cervix)

Mucocutaneous Junction

• Herpes labialis (fever blisters)

• Herpes progenitalis (genital blisters)

• Vulvovaginitis (an inflammatory condition of the vagina or vulva)

Eye Conditions

• Conjunctivitis (an inflammatory condition of the mucous membrane lining the inner surface of the eyelids, or conjunctiva)

• Keratoconjunctivitis (an inflammatory condition of the cornea and conjuntiva)

year-old man with severe Parkinson's disease, who was resistant to any treatment and had the lowest lysine levels of any of our patients—almost undetectable. This patient showed clinical improvement in response to lysine and other nutrients, but the exact effect of the lysine therapy is difficult to evaluate. Among the other patients with low lysine, four had severe psychotic depression, one had hypothyroidism, one had kidney disease, and one had severe asthma and was taking theophylline (Aerolate).

Central Nervous System Disorders

• Meningoencephalitis (an inflammatory condition of both the brain and membranes enclosing the brain and spinal cord)

• Myelitis (an inflammatory condition of the spinal cord associated with motor and sensory dysfunction)

• Radiculitis (an inflammatory condition involving a spinal nerve root)

• Trigeminal neuralgia (painful attacks of pain that radiate along the trigeminal facial nerves involving the eyes, forehead, lips, nose, cheeks, and tongue)

• Tic douloureux (a brief, extremely painful attack of trigeminal neuralgia)

• Bell's palsy (a transient or permanent paralysis of the facial nerves)

Systemic Infections

• Acute respiratory disease (any type of pulmonary failure characterized by large amounts of fluid in the lungs)

• Tracheobronchitis (an inflammatory condition of the trachea and bronchi)

• Pneumonia (an inflammatory condition of the lungs)

• Early disseminated disease (a condition in newborns marked by red lesions and high fever, and associated with cardiac and neurologic complications)

• Hepatitis (an inflammatory condition of the liver)

• Cystitis (an inflammatory condition of the bladder)

Hypersensitivity Reactions

• Erythema multiforme (a skin condition characterized by erythematous and vesicula lesions typically involving the palms and soles, and mucous membranes)

Malignancies

• Cervical cancer (an abnormal, and potentially fatal, growth of tissue on the cervix)

• Oral cancer (an abnormal, and potentially fatal, growth of tissue on the lip or in the mouth)

High to normal lysine levels have been found in the same patients who had elevations in other amino acids. These patients were often on amino acid therapy.

Loading several grams of the L-lysine metabolite carnitine to normal subjects can raise lysine in plasma by as much as 20 percent. The significance and confirmation of this finding is unclear.

We have seen one case of elevated lysine levels in a patient with Reye's syndrome, a rare, serious disease that affects many internal organs, particularly the brain and liver, and which usually occurs in children given aspirin or aspirin-containing medications for viral infections. Elevated lysine levels have been reported in infantile spasms and following phenobarbital (Solfoton) administration. Levels of lysine have been noted to fall with prolonged stress.

Amino Adipic Acid

Of the twelve patients that we have had with detectable amino adipic acid (a metabolite of lysine), most were taking L-tryptophan. Furthermore, tryptophan loading raised amino adipic acid levels rapidly. The significance of the interaction of this lysine metabolite with tryptophan is not clear, and further research is necessary to confirm these observations.

Hydroxylysine

We have found detectable levels of hydroxylysine, a breakdown product of protein and connective tissue, in seventeen patients. The patient with the highest level (twenty times the group's average) was on warfarin (Coumadin), a blood thinner that results in various kinds of bruising and tissue breakdown. Other conditions found associated with very high levels of hydroxylysine were anorexia, severe Parkinson's disease, cerebellar degeneration, and infertility. Elevated hydroxylysine levels probably can occur with any chronic degenerative disease, and even with severe depression or psychosis. Among the patients who had lower but still detectable hydroxylysines were one with hypothyroidism, one with cardiomyopathy, one with delayed maturation, one with narcolepsy, one with rheumatoid arthritis, one with severe asthma, and one with epilepsy.

The treatment for high levels of hyroxylysine is unclear. Large doses of vitamin C have been suggested. In fact, hydroxylysine levels normalized in several of the seventeen patients on follow-up who were taking a gram or more of vitamin C daily.

Stress

Lysine is one of several amino acids that are sacrificed in stressful situations. Hale and colleagues, working at the United States Air Force School of Aerospace, studied changes in amino acid excretion after forty-eight hours of simulated airplane piloting. After two days, levels of lysine in the urine decreased significantly, as did levels of tyrosine, phenylalanine, cysteine, citrulline, and aspartic acid. In contrast, Albanese and colleagues, working at the Burke Rehabilitation Center in White Plains, New York, found no significant change in serum lysine levels in young, healthy adults following physical exercise. The stress that occurs as a result of physical exercise affects the body very differently than that resulting from psychological or mentally stressful situations.

LYSINE LOADING

Large oral doses of 8 g a day of L-lysine are commonly used to fight cold sores with positive results. We have studied 8 g of L-lysine in healthy adults. In these trials, lysine levels rose four times normal after two hours without any elevation of lysine metabolites such as amino adipic acid or hydroxylysine. Lysine metabolites and other plasma amino acids were not significantly changed. Biological parameters, chem screen, trace metals, and polyamines also remained stable.

SUPPLEMENTATION

At present, typical lysine dosages may be too small to be therapeutically effective. Oral doses of L-lysine over 8 g a day for adults have not yet been tested for safety. Doses of 20 to 30 g of L-lysine may be necessary for lysine to prove therapeutically useful. Proper use of this nutrient requires further research. Experiments evaluating the biochemical nature of polylysine (several lysines hooked together) are underway in several laboratories.

Deficiency Symptoms

Signs and symptoms of lysine deficiency include fatigue, decreased concentration, irritability, hair loss, poor appetite, weight loss, anemia, enzyme disorders, and abnormalities in gastric functioning, including the absorption of calcium.

Availability

Supplemental L-lysine is available in 500-mg capsules.

Therapeutic Daily Amount

Dosing has not been adequately studied, but some beneficial effects occur in doses ranging from 100 mg to 4 g a day.

Maximum Safe Level

Not established; however, lysine supplements should not be taken longer than six months without supervision of a physician, as prolonged use may cause an imbalance of arginine.

Side Effects and Contraindications

People who are allergic to eggs, milk, or wheat should not take lysine supplements.

LYSINE: A SUMMARY

Lysine is an essential amino acid. Experimental animals on a lysine-deficient diet showed depressed growth and altered immune-system function for several generations.

Normal requirements for lysine have been found to be about 8 g a day or 12 mg/kg in adults. Children and infants need more—44 mg/kg a day for children ten to twelve years old, and 97 mg/kg a day for children three to six months old.

Compared to most other amino acids, lysine is highly concentrated in muscle. Lysine is high in foods such as wheat germ, cottage cheese, and chicken. Of meat products, wild game and pork have the highest concentration of lysine. Fruits and vegetables, except avocados, contain little lysine.

Normal lysine metabolism is dependent upon many nutrients, including niacin, pyridoxine, riboflavin, vitamin C, and iron. Excess arginine antagonizes lysine.

Lysine is particularly useful in therapy for marasmus (wasting) and herpes simplex. It stops the growth of herpes simplex in tissue culture, and has helped to reduce the number and occurrence of cold sores in clinical studies. Dosing has not been adequately studied, but beneficial clinical effects occur in doses ranging from 100 mg to 4 g a day. Higher doses may also be useful, and toxicity has not been reported in doses as high as 8 g per day. Diets high in lysine and low in arginine can be useful in the prevention and treatment of herpes. Some researchers think herpes simplex virus is involved in many other diseases related to cranial nerves such as migraines, Bell's palsy, and Ménière's disease.

Lysine also may be a useful adjunct in the treatment of osteoporosis. Although high-protein diets result in loss of large amounts of calcium in urine, so does lysine deficiency. Lysine may be an adjunct therapy because it reduces calcium losses in urine. Lysine deficiency also may result in immunodeficiency. Requirements for this amino acid are probably increased by stress.

Lysine toxicity has not occurred with oral doses in humans. Lysine dosages are presently too small and may fail to reach the concentrations necessary to prove potential therapeutic applications. Lysine metabolites, amino caproic acid and carnitine, have already shown their therapeutic potential. Thirty grams daily of amino caproic acid has been used as an initial daily dose in treating blood-clotting disorders, indicating that the proper doses of lysine, its precursor, have yet to be used in medicine.

Low lysine levels have been found in patients with Parkinson's disease, hypothyroidism, kidney disease, asthma, and depression. The exact significance of these levels is unclear, yet lysine therapy can normalize lysine levels and has been associated with improvement of some patients with these conditions.

Abnormally elevated hydroxylysines have been found in virtually all chronic degenerative diseases and during warfarin (Coumadin) therapy. The levels of this stress marker may be improved by high doses of vitamin C.

CHAPTER NINETEEN

Carnitine:
The Heart Tonic

C arnitine is not classified as an essential amino acid since it can be synthesized in the body. Yet this amino acid is so important in providing energy
to all muscles—including the heart—that many healthcare professionals
now recommend carnitine supplements in the diet, particularly for people who
do not consume much red meat, the main food source for carnitine.

Even the *Physician's Desk Reference,* the resource guide to therapeutic substances for conventional medicine, gives indication for carnitine supplements as
"improving the tolerance of ischemic heart disease, myocardial insufficiencies,
and hyperlipoproteinemia (abnormally high cholesterol or triglyceride levels, or
both). Carnitine deficiency is noted in abnormal liver function, renal dialysis
patients, and severe to moderate muscular weakness with associated anorexia."

Carnitine has been described as an amino acid, a vitamin, and a metabimin
(an essential metabolite). Yet, in the strictest sense, it is neither an amino acid
nor a vitamin. Unlike true amino acids, carnitine is not used by the body in the
construction of protein or as a neurotransmitter. Yet, like other amino acids
employed or manufactured by the body, carnitine is an amine, specifically a
trimethylated carboxy-alcohol, which gives it a chemical structure similar to that
of an amino acid. Therefore, carnitine is usually considered among the amino
acids.

A vitamin, on the other hand, is defined as a substance that is essential to the
body but which the body cannot manufacture itself. Like the B vitamins, carnitine
contains nitrogen and is very soluble in water. One early study found that the yellow mealworm could not grow without carnitine in its diet. However, as it turned
out, almost all other animals, including humans, do make their own carnitine in
small amounts; thus, carnitine is no longer considered a vitamin.

However, in certain circumstances—such as may occur with deficiencies of
carnitine's precursors methionine and lysine, or its cofactor vitamin C, or as a

result of kidney dialysis—carnitine shortages develop. Under these conditions, carnitine must be absorbed from food, and for this reason, it is sometimes referred to as a "metabimin" or a conditionally essential metabolite.

FUNCTION

Carnitine is an unusual amino acid that has different functions than most other amino acids. In 1959, it was discovered that when carnitine from muscle is added to liver tissue, it increases the rate at which the liver oxidizes fats, thereby increasing the amount of energy available. It was found that carnitine acts by carrying fat, specifically long-chain fatty acids, across the cell membrane to the mitochondria (the site of energy production within the cells). The more carnitine available, the faster these fats are transported and the more fat is oxidized for energy. This energy is then stored—not as fat—but as adenosine triphosphate (ATP). ATP is an intermediate compound that supplies energy to cells and serves as a trigger for many of the body's activities, including muscle contraction. Thus, carnitine's primary role seems to be to regulate fat metabolism and increase its use as an energy source.

Carnitine's ability to speed fat oxidation suggests that it may be valuable to people on weight-loss diets. Not only does carnitine increase the rate in which fat is burned, but it also makes it possible to exercise longer without fatigue. This may make it easier for those who want to improve their chances of losing weight by exercising.

Carnitine has another function directly related to energy availability. It helps the body to oxidize amino acids when necessary. Amino acids are not a primary source of energy, but when a person exercises for a long time, the limited carbohydrate stored in the muscles may all be used up, and fat may not be immediately available. Or when someone fasts (whether deliberately or involuntarily, as during famine), the muscles may begin to consume branched-chain amino acids for fuel. Carnitine may make this substitution possible.

Carnitine may also have some involvement in prostaglandin metabolism. Prostaglandins contribute to the functioning of smooth muscle. It regulates fat burning in the heart (whose main source of energy may be fat) and in skeletal muscles; it helps to change branched-chain amino acids into fuel for the skeletal muscles when necessary; and it plays some role in prostaglandin metabolism in smooth muscles.

In addition, carnitine has been found to reduce ketone levels in the blood. Ketones are the result of incomplete oxidation of fats, and are often found to be in excess in the blood of people with diabetes (ketosis). Diabetic hearts metabolize carnitine abnormally. Ketosis may also occur from high-protein or high-fat diets, and tends to make the blood overly acidic; symptoms such as bladder problems and irritable bowel syndrome, insomnia, water retention, arthritis, migraine headaches, abnormally low blood pressure, and more are associated with too much acidity in the body.

Carnitine's location in the body has given researchers additional clues about its functions and, therefore, possible therapeutic uses. Carnitine is most highly concentrated in the heart (particularly the sarcoplasmic reticulum), the organ to which fat oxidation is most crucial for energy. The heart contains more carnitine than any other organ, and some of carnitine's most important therapeutic uses are for the prevention and treatment of ailments that affect the heart and circulatory system.

Carnitine is also found in sperm, where it helps to provide the energy for their motility. Since sperm motility is necessary for fertility, it should not be surprising that infertile men tend to have lower levels of carnitine in their sperm than others. Carnitine is also strongly concentrated in human breast milk and colostrum, which is not surprising since infants' muscles and brains are growing so quickly.

Although the brain depends exclusively on glucose for energy, carnitine is also found there, especially in the cerebellum. Carnitine's role in the brain, however, is dwarfed by its derivative N-acetyl-carnitine. This important modified amino acid is able to cross the blood-brain barrier more effectively than carnitine, where it has significant effects on healthy neurological function, especially age-related changes involving degeneration of the brain and nervous system.

METABOLISM

Carnitine can be manufactured in the body if sufficient amounts of the essential amino acids lysine and methionine are available. The synthesis of carnitine also requires the presence of adequate levels of vitamin C; the B vitamins pyridoxine, niacin, and thiamine; and the minerals iron and possibly manganese. A shortage of any of these nutrients can lower carnitine levels.

This is known to be the case with lysine and vitamin C. It is not clear what percentage of lysine, on the average, is made into carnitine, but it seems to have an enhancing effect on the level of carnitine present. Some of the symptoms of vitamin C deficiency, such as muscle weakness and high blood triglycerides, are similar to those of carnitine deficiency. Likewise, carnitine may be necessary for adequate treatment of scurvy.

REQUIREMENTS

At present, there is no is no daily estimated requirement for carnitine. The average adult male consumes approximately 50 mg of carnitine a day through diet; however, there is substantial evidence that for optimal health, we should be getting at least 250 to 500 mg in our diet daily. Animal studies have shown that males have considerably more carnitine in their red blood cells than females, an indication that carnitine requirements for men may be greater than those for women. A high-fat diet has also been associated with low carnitine levels.

Many cases of carnitine deficiency are found in genetic errors, resulting from an inherited defect in carnitine synthesis. Other factors known to cause a carnitine deficiency include several neuromuscular disorders, such as Duchenne-type muscular dystrophy, kidney failure, cirrhosis, pregnancy (possibly owing to the large requirements of the growing fetus), preterm infancy, intake of carnitine-deficient soy formula, total parenteral nutrition (TPN), kwashiorkor, hyperlipidemia, heart muscle disease (cardiomyopathy), and propionic or organic aciduria (acid urine resulting from genetic or other anomalies). In all of these conditions and in the inborn errors of carnitine metabolism, carnitine has proven essential to life.

FOOD SOURCES

The root of the word "carnitine" is like that of "carnivore" and "carnal," because carnitine was first found in meat. Since carnitine helps supply animal muscles with energy for motion, it is found in nature primarily concentrated in muscle meats, especially beef, pork, and lamb. Because of this, there is some danger that vegetarians and those on low-protein diets may be at risk for carnitine deficiencies. Lysine and methionine, the two essential amino acids from which carnitine is made, are not easily obtainable in sufficient amounts from vegetable sources. Of the common vegetable protein, corn, wheat, and rice are low in lysine; beans are low in methionine. By combining these vegetables appropriately, vegetarians can help guard against carnitine deficiency. Or, to be certain, they may supplement their diets with L-carnitine.

Table 19.1 on page 277 shows the number of milligrams of carnitine present in 3.5 ounces of food. Most vegetables contain no carnitine at all.

FORM AND ABSORPTION

Carnitine is best absorbed in its L- form found naturally in foods or as a supplement form. Only the L- form of supplemental carnitine should be taken. Although D- and DL- forms of carnitine are available, there is evidence that D-carnitine may cause toxicity and muscle weakness, and could actually inhibit L-carnitine's action. Therefore, D-carnitine and the less expensive DL-carnitine are *not* recommended.

Supplementation with N-acetyl-carnitine is another option. Doses as high as 2 g are well absorbed. This form of carnitine has been found to cross the blood-brain barrier more efficiently and to more readily relieve carnitine tissue deficiency.

CLINICAL USES

Carnitine is useful for treating a wide variety of clinical conditions and improving functions, including those discussed below.

TABLE 19.1. CARNITINE LEVELS IN FOOD		
FOOD	AMOUNT	CONTENT (MG)
American cheese	3.5 ounces	3.70 mg
Asparagus	3.5 ounces	.195 mg
Bacon	3.5 ounces	23.3 mg
Beef steak	3.5 ounces	95.0 mg
Chicken breast	3.5 ounces	3.90 mg
Cod fish	3.5 ounces	5.6 mg
Cottage cheese	3.5 ounces	1.10 mg
Egg	3.5 ounces	0.0121 mg
Ground beef	3.5 ounces	95.0 mg
Ice cream	3.5 ounces	3.70 mg
Macaroni	3.5 ounces	.126 mg
Orange juice	3.5 ounces	.0019 mg
Peanut butter	3.5 ounces	.083 mg
Pork	3.5 ounces	27.7 mg
Rice (cooked)	3.5 ounces	.0449 mg
White bread	3.5 ounces	.147 mg
Whole milk	3.5 ounces	3.30 mg
Whole wheat bread	3.5 ounces	.360 mg

Athletic Performance

Carnitine speeds the oxidation of fats. Fats, in contrast to carbohydrates that burn quickly, are the primary energy source for long-sustained exercise. Because carnitine plays such a critical role in fat-burning, it probably has a role to play in improving endurance.

It is known that carnitine improves muscle strength in those with neuromuscular disorders (see "Neuromuscular Disorders" on page 281); that muscle carnitine levels increase with exercise; and that carnitine improves stress and exercise tolerance. It has been suggested that supplemental carnitine might improve athletic performance. Recent clinical studies of carnitine showed that body-fat percentage and total pulse recovery are improved in wrestlers and runners on carnitine.

Cirrhosis

Cirrhosis is a disease in which fibrous tissue replaces healthy liver tissue, and liver functions are compromised. One of these liver functions happens to be the last step in the biochemical synthesis of carnitine, and it should not be surprising that people with cirrhosis show significant reductions in blood carnitine.

What is quite interesting, however, is that when carnitine is given to alcohol-dependent rats, the expected fat accumulation in the liver seems to be prevented and blood lipid levels also remain normal. It is not yet known whether this phenomenon applies to humans as well.

Carnitine also seems to have a role in the liver's ability to metabolize protein and decrease hyperammonemia (excessive ammonia buildup) in mice. It may also reduce liver toxicity that can result from the antiseizure drug valproate (Depakote).

Heart Disease

Carnitine is critical for the health of the heart. It is one of the most important compounds for the prevention and treatment of ailments that affect the heart and circulatory system. A lack of carnitine in the body usually affects the heart first.

High blood triglycerides, like high cholesterol, are a risk factor for coronary artery disease. Carnitine supplementation can lower blood triglycerides and increase the blood levels of high-density lipoprotein (HDL) cholesterol, the only type of cholesterol that actually lowers the risk of coronary artery disease. In general, people who receive adequate carnitine do not show elevated blood triglycerides. Carnitine in dosages of 500 to 1,000 mg has also effectively lowered blood cholesterol levels, triglyceride levels, and the risk index (the ratio of total cholesterol to HDL cholesterol) in individuals with hyperlipoproteinemia.

In addition to reducing dangerous fats in the bloodstream, carnitine helps regulate heart rhythm. It has been shown to improve heart arrhythmias in both hemodialysis and ischemic heart disease patients (see "Kidney Disease" on page

Carnitine Treats Sky-High Triglycerides

A seventy-seven-year-old diabetic woman came to our clinic stating that she had high triglycerides. We measured her triglyceride level, which proved to be sky-high at 1,700 (type IV hyperlipidemia), and immediately began her on a program of primarily L-carnitine and niacin. The patient returned one month later for a follow-up visit. She had stopped taking the niacin because she was unable to tolerate the facial flush, a harmless side effect, but she had judiciously taken the 600 mg of L-carnitine three times a day. Her triglycerides after treatment were down to 400. Carnitine had done the job.

280), and to lower the frequency of angina attacks, increase stress resistance, lessen electrocardiogram abnormalities, and improve exercise tolerance in patients with coronary artery disease.

Animal studies underscore the potential of carnitine to alleviate the effects of cardiovascular disease. Several researchers have set up experiments in which heart attacks were artificially induced in laboratory animals by surgically reducing the blood supply to the heart. Under such conditions, the heart's carnitine storage is quickly depleted. Carnitine injections during the crisis, however, increased ATP (available energy) levels and heart rate and prevented, to some extent, heart fluttering and tissue damage. Carnitine may be a useful medicine in heart resuscitation procedures.

Additional studies have shown that during acute or chronic cardiac ischemia, fatty acids and acetyl-CoA-esters accumulate and precipitate myocardial damage. Carnitine forms esters with the fatty acid substances and decreases the potential necrotic damage.

In animals with diphtheria (an acute, toxin-mediated infectious disease), carnitine prolonged the survival time of those with fat accumulation and heart failure.

In healthy dogs, carnitine has been shown to act as a vasodilator, widening blood vessels for less resistance to the flow of blood. This suggests that carnitine may play a many-faceted role in preventing high blood pressure, not only by lowering blood lipids and preventing the buildup of fatty plaque on artery walls, but also by directly lowering peripheral resistance. Because carnitine, like arginine, may help dilate blood vessels, it may lower blood pressure.

Because of carnitine's ability for dilating blood vessels, it has been used in the treatment of circulation disorders such as claudication and peripheral vascular disorders and in vasospastic syndromes (abnormal vasoconstriction of the upper extremities after cold exposure) with good results. Two grams a day of N-acetyl-carnitine has been used effectively in vasospastic conditions.

The research on L-carnitine in heart disease strongly indicates that carnitine may be valuable in any form of heart disease. In sum, heart disease studies using carnitine suggest the following relationships: a deficiency of carnitine in patients with cardiomyopathy; vasodilator properties of carnitine in experimental coronary artery disease; a reduction in the necrotic area (tissue death) following heart attack with carnitine administration; improved oxygen delivery in diabetic hearts; and increased exercise tolerance in recovery from experimental heart disease.

Hypothyroidism

The thyroid gland controls the body's rate of metabolism. When the thyroid produces too much of the hormone thyroxine, the rate at which the body burns fuel and carries on other chemical reactions is speeded up (hyperthyroid); when it

Carnitine Calms a Fluttering Heart

A fifty-seven-year-old dentist came to our clinic after an episode of atrial fibrillation (incoordinate contraction of heart muscle fibers) and frequent supraventricular beats. An echocardiogram showed all heart dimensions were normal. The atrial fibrillation was well controlled with the beta-blocker atenolol (Tenormin). By adding 500 mg of L-carnitine three times a day, his supraventricular beats were completely eradicated. The patient had had a coronary angiogram that suggested blockage in at least one of the three coronary arteries, but he refused surgery; however, the angiogram did suggest that his arrhythmia could be on the basis of ischemia. For arrhythmia due to ischemia, carnitine may be an effective therapy.

produces too little, metabolism is slowed down (hypothyroid). Since both hypothyroid conditions and carnitine deficiency result in increased blood triglycerides, one group of researchers hypothesized that perhaps the two conditions were related. Their preliminary studies indicate that hypothyroid patients excrete less carnitine than normal; hyperthyroid patients excrete more than normal; and when thyroid hormone is prescribed for hypothyroid patients, their carnitine excretion levels return to normal.

Low serum carnitine has been found in some patients with subnormal thyroid, pituitary, and adrenal glands. Thyroxine's effect on metabolism may be mediated in part through carnitine. If so, carnitine might, in some cases, be an appropriate pharmacological adjunct to use with thyroid hormone or as a substitute for it. For example, carnitine might boost the effect of antidepressants or help in weight reduction, as does thyroxin. All these hypotheses remain to be tested.

Kidney Disease

After hemodialysis, one of two principal types of dialysis in which blood flows from a vein through a filtering machine and is then returned to the body, patients often suffer overall muscle weakness: Their grip is lost; their biceps cannot contract to lift weights; and they may have difficulty chewing and swallowing. Studies have shown that dialysis removes as much as 66 percent of blood carnitine, and chronic kidney patients' muscles are left with as little as 10 percent of normal carnitine quantities.

Kidney disease is often complicated by heart failure. When kidney patients are injected with carnitine after dialysis treatment, their blood and muscle levels of carnitine go up and their anemia steadily diminishes; more oxygen is available to tissues all over the body. Carnitine not only lowers high blood triglycerides, a dangerous side effect of dialysis, but it also increases blood levels of high-density lipoproteins (HDL), the protective cholesterol. Carnitine is also essential in renal Fanconi's syndrome, a heredity disorder of kidney function and cysteine metabolism.

Metabolic and Energy Expenditure in the Critically Ill

Considerable experience has now been accumulated using carnitine infusions. One and a half to two grams a day of L-carnitine infused intravenously results in a 50 percent increase in metabolic rate compared to fasting values. Energy expenditure increased by 15 to 25 percent after six to seven days of carnitine infusions. TPN (total parenteral nutrition) given together with carnitine infusions abruptly increased metabolic rate and raised body temperature by 1° to 2°C. This was accompanied by muscle shivering, hypertension, tachycardia (fast, abnormal heart rhythm), and increased respiratory rate. Lowering either TPN or carnitine reduced these effects, and morphine stopped them. Insulin doses in people with diabetes have been reduced by 70 percent after a twenty-four-hour infusion of 2 g of carnitine. Large doses (6 g) of carnitine may be an inotrope (substance that increases myocardial contractility) similar to digoxin, which stimulates the heart.

Neuromuscular Disorders

Some of the most important findings about carnitine have been discovered from studying the genetic disorders that prevent the formation of carnitine or of enzymes that use carnitine. "Lipid storage myopathy" causes extreme muscle weakness, muscle cramps, pain, fatigue, myoglobinuria (dark urine due to the breakdown of muscle tissue), and fat accumulation in the muscles. Lipid storage myopathy is aggravated by fasting or high-fat diets, which deplete carnitine.

It was found that carnitine supplements alone could completely cure this debilitating disorder in cases where the carnitine deficiency was caused by an inherited inability to manufacture carnitine. Subsequently, it has been found that carnitine supplements can help a number of other neuromuscular disorders associated with low carnitine excretion, presumably reflecting low levels of carnitine in the muscle.

Frascarelli and colleagues evaluated the effects of intravenous carnitine in a group of individuals with muscular dystrophy by means of analysis of electromyograms (EMG), a test for measuring muscle tension. Seven people out of the eleven tested showed a tendency toward normal electromyographic results between thirty-five and forty-five minutes after receiving carnitine.

Seizure and Psychotic Disorders

Much carnitine research in the United States has centered on the protective action of carnitine against valproate (Depakote) toxicity. This important pharmaceutical drug is used for seizure, anger, impulse, and manic-depressive disorders. However, divalproex sodium is known to cause potentially serious liver problems as a side effect. Carnitine protects the liver and prevents such damage. Pharmaceutical interests have sought—unsuccessfully—to capitalize on the protective action of carnitine by removing it from over-the-counter supplement status and making it a prescription item available only through physicians. In our clinic, we successfully utilize 500 mg to 1 g of L-carnitine along with antioxidants to avoid the side effects of divalproex sodium.

AN IMPORTANT METABOLITE

The majority of research on N-acetyl-carnitine, a carnitine derivative produced naturally in the body, has been conducted overseas, primarily in Italy. The best results have occurred with individuals taking massive doses of 1.5 g or more of N-acetyl-carnitine. N-acetyl-carnitine is expensive, however, and it is usually hard to convince individuals to take the high levels described in the literature. Research confirming its benefit over carnitine has yet to be performed in the United States.

Italian studies found N-acetyl-carnitine beneficial for angina and heart attack prevention, diabetic nephropathy (kidney damage), neuropathy (nerve damage), poor immune system function, and Alzheimer's disease. A low blood level of carnitine is a frequently associated with these problems. Unfortunately, its cardiac benefits require extremely high doses, ranging from 2 to 7 g. Therapeutic effectiveness of N-acetyl-carnitine at 1 to 1.5 g level was ambiguous. At 20 g per day, N-acetyl-carnitine may significantly increase high-density lipoproteins (HDL), the healthful or "good" form of cholesterol.

N-acetyl-carnitine, according to the research, may slow the progression of Alzheimer's disease. Carnitine appears to build up the neurotransmitters acetylcholine and possibly dopamine. This ability of carnitine once again confirms the benefit of amino acids on neurotransmitter systems and would warrant its use in treating patients with various degrees of Alzheimer's disease and other neuropsychological conditions.

One double-blind study showed some benefits for treating short-term memory loss. N-acetyl-carnitine may reduce the formation of lipofuscin, an age pigment or lesion, in brain cells. In our clinic, we have heard some positive reports from patients with moderate memory disorders using N-acetyl-carnitine.

N-acetyl-carnitine may be more effective than piracetam (Nootropil) in rebuilding the brain. Another form of carnitine, namely, acetyl levocarnitine, is thought to retard deterioration of some cognitive areas in patients with Alzheimer's disease. N-acetyl-carnitine has also been suggested for treating Down's syndrome.

N-acetyl-carnitine is a natural antidepressant. As such, it may reduce the depression common to Alzheimer's disease and the elderly in general. N-acetyl-carnitine may be one of a number of useful amino acids to be taken alone (for individuals who are reluctant to take medication) or in combination with medication. We believe the latter approach produces the best results. We recommend the inclusion of cranial electrical stimulation (CES) in the treatment program to further increase dopamine (see page 63 for more information on CES). N-acetyl-carnitine may also stimulate acetyl-choline production.

There is still no overwhelming evidence of a major impact on energy due to supplementation with N-acetyl-carnitine, although it is an idea worthy of further investigation.

CARNITINE LOADING

Therapy with 3 g of L-carnitine daily for ten days can raise free carnitine levels by 20 percent, N-acetyl-carnitine by 80 percent, and the total carnitine (a combination of free and protein-bound carnitine) by nearly 30 percent.

Another way to elevate carnitine is by lysine loading. Lysine is the primary source for carnitine. Five grams of lysine given to normal adults raises carnitine levels within six hours, followed by a further rise at forty-eight hours. Levels remain high for up to seventy-two hours. This conversion rate of lysine to carnitine can be impaired in states of malnutrition.

SUPPLEMENTATION

For maximizing brain health or correcting a deficiency of carnitine in tissue, N-acetyl-carnitine is the preferred form; otherwise L-carnitine may be used.

Deficiency Symptoms

Signs and symptoms of carnitine deficiency include confusion, muscle weakness, obesity, heart pain, and aging.

Availability

Supplemental free-form L-carnitine is available in 250- to 500-mg capsules and tablets. Large doses of carnitine must be obtained with a prescription. The D- and the DL- forms of carnitine are not recommended as they have an inhibitory effect on L-carnitine and may cause muscle weakness and toxicity.

Therapeutic Daily Dose

Depending on therapeutic use, doses of L-carnitine may range from 1 to 3 g a day.

Maximum Safe Levels

Doses up to 3 g have been used in clinical studies without adverse effects.

Side Effects and Contraindications

Doses of L-carnitine greater than 2 g a day cause no side effects other than occasional and temporary mild diarrhea. In individuals with uremia, a toxic condition caused by the accumulation of waste products in the blood, 3 g of L-carnitine a day has been found to affect triglyceride levels deleteriously; this unusual effect has not been reported in healthy people.

CARNITINE: A SUMMARY

Carnitine is an important amino acid made by the body from lysine and methionine. Its most important known metabolic function is to transport fat into the mitochondria of muscle cells, including those in the heart, for oxidation. Inborn errors of carnitine metabolism can lead to brain deterioration like that of Reye's syndrome, gradually worsening muscle weakness; Duchenne-like muscular dystrophy; and extreme muscle weakness with fat accumulation in muscles. Borum and colleagues have summed up the research by describing carnitine as an essential nutrient for preterm babies, patients with certain types of hypoglycemia (non-ketotic), kidney dialysis patients, patients with cirrhosis, and for patients with kwashiorkor, hyperlipidemia, heart muscle disease (cardiomyopathy), and propionic or organic aciduria (acid urine resulting from genetic or other anomalies). In all of these conditions and in the inborn errors of carnitine metabolism, carnitine is essential to life, and carnitine supplements are valuable.

Carnitine therapy may also be useful in a wide variety of clinical conditions. Carnitine supplementation has improved some patients who have angina. It may be worth a trial in any form of hyperlipidemia or muscle weakness. Carnitine supplements may be useful in protecting against valproate (Depakote) toxicity or metabolic liver disease and in cases of heart muscle disease. Hearts undergoing severe arrhythmia quickly deplete their stores of carnitine. Athletes, particularly in Europe, have used carnitine supplements for improved endurance. Carnitine may improve muscle building by improving fat utilization and may even be useful in treating obesity. Carnitine joins a long list of nutrients that may be of value in treating pregnant women and individuals with hypothyroidism, and in treating male infertility due to low motility of sperm.

CHAPTER TWENTY

Histidine: The Arthritis Fighter

istidine is an essential amino acid abundant in hemoglobin that is required for the growth and repair of tissue. It is also critical for the survival of premature babies. Children and adults can make small amounts of histidine in their bodies, but most of the histidine processed in the body must come from the diet. Inadequate levels of histidine are found in the blood of individuals with rheumatoid arthritis and in individuals with arthritic synovial fluid—the transparent, viscid, lubricating fluid secreted by joint membranes. Histidine is the only amino acid that is consistently found to be abnormal in this condition.

FUNCTION

Histidine level is a sensitive index of overall protein metabolism. It is a well-conserved amino acid in the body and serves as a reliable measure of protein availability. During severe stress, histidine is needed by the body more than any other amino acid. Histidine in the urine is an indication that it is being broken down and that muscle, rather than protein, is being used by the body for fuel.

Histidine has mild anti-inflammatory properties; it helps bind with trace minerals and copper, thus aiding their removal from the body; and it may help improve sexual functioning and pleasure. Histidine readily forms peptides with other amino acids. It may also be useful in hypertension because of its potential vasodilatory effects.

One of histamine's most important functions in the body is its conversion to histamine. Histamine is a molecule that is found everywhere in the body. It is a potent vessel dilator that plays a central role in allergic reactions and other functions of the immune system. It acts as a major neurotransmitter in the brain, especially in the hippocampus, and throughout the autonomic nervous system, and also as a stimulator to the secretion of pepsin and hydrochloric acid, which are important for digestion. Most histamine is stored in platelets, mast cells, and basophils; basophils are probably the greatest source of histamine. When allergens are present, histamine is released from these cells, resulting in inflammation, fluid production, and occasionally hives.

Histamine is also converted to several other amino acid metabolites: 3-methylhistidine; methylhistidine; single-molecule amino acids carnosine and anserine; and a form of alanine known as beta-alanine.

METABOLISM

Histidine may be manufactured in the liver from glutamic acid, and carnosine or possibly biotin (a member of the B family of vitamins). Histidine can also be produced as a result of muscle-protein breakdown and the conversion to 3-methylhistidine. However, these sources produce only small quantities of histidine. All these conversions require adequate levels of pyridoxine (vitamin B_6).

The metabolism of histidine in the human body is much better understood than its synthesis. Since the availability of histidine influences histamine production, the focus on histidine metabolism is in large part due to interest in histamine. Pyridoxine and niacin (vitamin B_3) are required for the transformation of histidine to histamine, yet other factors are involved that complicate their biochemical relationship.

Ishibashi of Rutgers University reviewed the complex relationship between dietary histidine and histamine. Dietary histamine does not always increase histamine in the brain, and further studies are needed to elucidate the relationship between supplemental histidine and histamine synthesis. Histidine loading may initially lower blood histamine levels by as much as 10 to 15 percent, while twenty-four hours later, histamine levels may rise as much as 20 percent. These paradoxical effects require further investigation.

Zinc and manganese have also been found to interfere with normal metabolism of histidine to histamine. Histidine may help transport copper and has a mild anti-inflammatory effect because of a histidine-copper-threonine complex that exists in the blood. Large doses of zinc (55 mg in liquid) cause a 10 to 20 percent decrease of serum histidine in humans due to its antagonist effect on copper. In contrast, a low dosage of zinc or prolonged zinc therapy will raise serum histidine and blood histamine levels. Hoekstra of the University of Wisconsin reviewed how zinc and/or manganese deficiency interferes with the normal metabolism of histidine to histamine. Histidine loading may lower serum zinc and raise serum iron. Vitamin E deficiency results in depletion of histidine from muscle. The significance of these findings is not clear.

REQUIREMENTS

Histidine is an essential amino acid. Although the body can produce it in small amounts, under certain circumstances—such as periods of rapid growth during childhood, after injury, or at other times of tissue formation and repair—the body does not supply enough to meet the demand. Therefore, it is vital that adequate amounts of histidine be included in the diet.

Infant requirements for histidine, like infant requirements for all the essential amino acids, are greater than those of adults. The histidine requirement estimated by the National Academy of Sciences for four- to six-month-old infants is 33 mg/kg. No definite need for histidine has been established for children and adults.

FOOD SOURCES

Most of the histidine processed in the body is derived from the diet. Natural sources of histidine include beans, dairy products, eggs, fish, meat, nuts, seeds, soy, and whey. Very little histidine is found in most cereals, grains, vegetables, fruits, and oils.

TABLE 20.1. HISTIDINE LEVELS IN FOOD		
FOOD	AMOUNT	CONTENT (G)
Cheese	1 ounce	0.25
Chicken	1 pound	1.70
Chocolate	1 cup	0.20
Cottage cheese	1 cup	1.00
Duck	1 pound	1.70
Egg	1	0.20
Granola	1 cup	0.25
Luncheon meat	1 pound	1.70
Oatmeal	1 cup	0.20
Pork	1 pound	3.30
Ricotta	1 cup	1.00
Sausage meat	1 pound	1.70
Turkey	1 pound	1.70
Wheat germ	1 cup	1.00
Whole milk	1 cup	0.20
Wild game	1 pound	0.40
Yogurt	1 cup	0.20

FORM AND ABSORPTION

Histidine is a well-absorbed and conserved amino acid. Like most amino acids, histidine is best absorbed from both food and supplements when in the L-form.

CLINICAL USE

Although it is known that histidine converts to histamine, it is still unclear how to use histidine as a treatment. There was hope that supplementation of histidine would allow the conversion to histamine and would help control many of the conditions discussed below. However, because of the complicated biochemical relationship involved in the conversion from histidine to histamine, treatment with histamine has yielded mixed results and requires further investigation.

Cataracts

Experimental animals missing either histidine or phenylalanine in their diets develop pre-cataract conditions, for example, widening of the sutures, separations of fiber cells, and haziness of the lens. Diets missing histidine will produce cataracts in three weeks. Diets lacking in leucine, threonine, isoleucine, valine, lysine, or sulfur amino acids also produce eye defects but do not produce blatant cataracts.

Plasma Levels in Clinical Syndromes

Low histidine and histamine levels tend to occur in rheumatoid arthritis patients, and in people with Parkinson's disease and some forms of psychiatric disturbances such as hyperactivity, mania, paranoia, and hallucinations. Elevated histamine and histidine levels have been found in patients with psychiatric disturbances such as depression, schizophrenia, compulsive personality, obsession, rituals, and phobias. Some 20 percent of people with schizophrenia are high in histamine.

Of the first 128 patients we studied at our clinic, twenty-six had low plasma histidine levels. More than 50 percent had severe depression, four were psychotic, two were mentally retarded and institutionalized, two had kidney disease, one had heart disease, one had phenylketonuria (PKU), one had cerebellar degeneration, and one had folliculitis (bacterial infection of the hair follicle).

The eleven highest histidine values were found in six patients with chronic psychosis, four depressed patients, and one healthy patient. Only one of these people was taking oral histidine; a controlled oral dose of 1 g in the morning and in the evening raised his histidine levels. This twenty-six-year-old man became less psychotic but remained dependent on histidine therapy. The patients with the highest histidine values were not taking histidine, but were taking different mega–amino acid therapy. It appears that mega–amino acid therapy can raise plasma histidine levels, but this elevation may indicate improved nutritional status.

Abnormalities of the histidine amino acid metabolites anserine and carnosine occur together, while beta-alanine abnormalities do not seem to correspond with histidine's metabolites. The interpretation of changes in beta-alanine, anserine, and carnosine levels remains unknown. Elevation of carnosine and anserine has been known to occur shortly after excessive or normal meat ingestion. Urinary beta-alanine is known to rise often after a kidney transplant.

We have also studied abnormalities in L-methylhistidine. Out of the 128 patients we studied, an elevation of this metabolite occurred in four patients with kidney disease, four with psychosis, and four with depression, and one healthy individual. The exact meaning of this elevation is unclear, but its correlation with kidney disease is of interest.

Rheumatoid Arthritis

Histidine in medical therapies originally had its most promising trials in rheumatoid arthritis. Of the many reported studies on amino acids in rheumatoid arthritis, histidine is the only amino acid consistently found to be abnormal in blood serum. Low histidine levels are also found in arthritic synovial fluid. Histidine levels in synovial fluid can be raised by oral D-penicillamine, an anti-inflammatory drug.

These observations led to the first clinical trials of histidine therapy. Patients with rheumatoid arthritis frequently have low blood histidine levels because histidine is removed more rapidly than average from their blood, as shown by abnormally low levels in histidine tolerance tests. Working at Downstate Medical Center in Brooklyn, Gerber treated several rheumatoid arthritis patients with 1 g or more of histidine daily and found improvement in grip strength and walking ability.

Gerber used serum histidine level measurements for diagnosing rheumatoid arthritis and determining the degree of degeneration caused by the disease. Histidine therapy raised some patients' serum histidine levels, but the statistical importance of the finding was lost once the patients took anti-inflammatory drugs. Patients who had high sed rates (erythrocyte sedimentation rate—a marker of inflammation) and great difficulty walking responded best to histidine therapy. Pinals and colleagues, working at Upstate Medical Center in Syracuse, effectively treated severely ill rheumatoid arthritis patients with a dosage of 4.5 g of histidine daily.

Unfortunately, the anti-inflammatory hopes we had for histidine in treating rheumatoid arthritis have not yet been substantiated by research. Some arthritis patients use histidine and report benefits; however, we do not actively recommend it. Anti-inflammatory prescription drugs chloroquine (Aralen) and D-penicillamine have an indirect preservation effect on histidine that may be related to their effectiveness in rheumatoid arthritis. Oral histidine supplementation in doses up to 4 and 5 g is certainly worth a trial in severe cases of rheumatoid arthritis.

The consumption of whiskey is found to lower plasma histidine levels significantly and increase threonine. This suggests that rheumatoid arthritis patients should avoid alcohol.

Stress

During stress, histidine is needed more than any other amino acid. Methylation of histidine in muscle fibers forms 3-methylhistidine. This 3-methylhistidine is excreted in measurable amounts in urine and is useful as an indicator of muscle mass and protein breakdown. Excretion of 3-methylhistidine decreases with age and also in stress states such as starvation or fasting when muscles slow their repair and breakdown processes. The ratio of 3-methylhistidine to creatine is believed to be an indicator of a catabolic (breakdown) or anabolic (buildup) state. Excretion of histidine is also affected by the amounts of various hormones in the body.

We found that patients with low 3-methylhistidine in plasma frequently have several low plasma amino acids, and we value this measure as an indication of protein nutrition.

Other Potential Uses

Allergy. Claims for histidine use in allergic disorders are contradictory. Theoretically, histidine should make allergic patients worse because of its role in histamine production. Histamines are released by the immune system in the presence of an allergen and cause a string of unpleasant reactions such as nasal congestion and mucus production. Allergy patients with high levels of IgE (antibodies produced by the immune system) have low blood histamine levels because of excess release of histamine.

Sexual Arousal. Clinical use of histidine for improved libido has been claimed. Histidine may raise histamine levels, and histamine does facilitate orgasm in both males and females.

Hypertension. Histidine has also been claimed for vasodilating and hypotensive effects due to its action in the autonomic nervous system. At present, these claims are speculative. However, we found that histidine loading tended to raise blood pressure.

Uremia. Some individuals with uremia, a severe kidney disease caused by the accumulation of waste products normally eliminated in the urine, have been found to have somewhat high phenylalanine concentrations but low serum tyrosine and histidine. Protein supplements may worsen uremic patients, but if protein is given, the supplement should be high in histidine and low in phenylalanine.

HISTIDINE LOADING

We have found basically two major side effects of histidine therapy: induction of depression with chronic therapy, and early induction of menstruation with histidine loading. These effects are rare and can be avoided, or possibly used constructively.

Histidine is a well-absorbed amino acid. Plasma levels increase by 225 percent two hours after loading with 4 g per 150 pounds and drop back to 150 percent of normal at four hours. Histidine loading may initially lower whole blood histamine levels by as much as 10 to 15 percent, while twenty-four hours later, histamine levels may rise by as much as 20 percent. Iron levels rise significantly with histidine loading, and zinc levels drop slightly. Valine is reduced by as much as 50 percent at four hours; other plasma amino acids are not affected.

SUPPLEMENTATION

Deficiency Symptoms

Signs and symptoms of histidine deficiency may include poor hearing and eczematous dermatitis, a skin condition that occurs in infants.

Availability

Supplemental free-form L-histidine is available in 500- to 600-mg capsules or tablets.

Therapeutic Daily Amount

Depending upon the condition, doses of histidine range from as little as 1 g a day to as much as 20 g a day.

Maximum Safe Level

Not established.

Side Effects and Contraindications

No significant side effects have been noted with large doses in adults when given for short periods of time. Chronic histidine therapy can induce depression and early induction of menstruation in rare cases. People with elevated histidine or histamine levels should not take supplemental L-histidine; these may include those with manic depression, schizophrenia, and chronic allergies.

HISTIDINE: A SUMMARY

Histidine is an essential amino acid for infants but not for adults. Infants four to six months old require 33 mg/kg of histidine. It is not clear how adults make small amounts of histidine, and dietary sources probably account for most of the histidine in the body. Inborn errors of histidine metabolism exist and are marked by increased histidine levels in the blood. Elevated blood histidine is accompanied by a wide range of symptoms, from mental and physical retardation to poor intellectual functioning, emotional instability, tremor, ataxia, and psychosis.

Histidine in medical therapies has its most promising trials in rheumatoid arthritis where up to 4.5 g daily have been used effectively in severely affected patients. Arthritis patients have been found to have low serum histidine levels, apparently because of too-rapid removal of histidine from their blood. Histidine has been shown to have anti-inflammatory properties. Histidine may accomplish this function through a complex interaction with threonine or cysteine and possibly copper. However, copper is usually elevated in rheumatoid arthritis patients and worsens the disease.

Other patients besides arthritis patients that have been found to be low in serum histidine are those with chronic renal failure. Histidine has been claimed to be useful in hypertension because of its vasodilatory effects. Claims of its use to improve libido and counteract allergy are without proof at present.

Histidine may have many other possible functions because it is the precursor of the ubiquitous neurohormone-neurotransmitter histamine. Histidine increases histamine in the blood and probably in the brain. Low blood histamine with low serum histidine occurs in rheumatoid arthritis patients. Low blood histamine also occurs in some patients with mania, schizophrenia, high copper levels, and hyperactivity with psychosis. Histidine is a useful therapy in all patients with low histamine levels.

Effective therapeutic doses of histidine may range broadly from 1 to 20 g per day. Therapy can be guided by measuring plasma histidine levels.

SECTION NINE

Putting It All Together

CHAPTER TWENTY-ONE

Multiple Amino Acid Abnormalities

In each of the previous chapters, we reviewed the conditions in which the individual amino acid levels were found to be abnormal. General categories of multiple amino acid abnormalities are also often found grouped in certain conditions. Several of the more common conditions in which this occurs are discussed in this chapter.

CLINICAL USES

Many of the conditions discussed below are accompanied by either elevations or deficiencies in several or more amino acids.

Aging

Amino acid plasma levels decline with age. Newborns, especially premature babies, have the highest plasma amino acid levels and the greatest requirements for amino acids. In children, the plasma amino acids and requirements fall; however, they are still higher than for adults. In adults, the plasma levels and requirements decrease further. Formal studies have not shown conclusively that plasma levels and requirements decrease even further in the elderly.

Individual amino acid requirements definitely change with age. In growing children, lysine makes up 23 percent of the total requirement of essential amino acids, while in adults, the lysine requirement declines to 11 percent. In growing children, the methionine-plus-cysteine requirements increase from 10 to 17 percent. Methionine and cysteine may be required in increased amounts with age, because they are part of the antioxidant glutathione. One study has suggested that plasma tryptophan may decrease in the elderly population. Significant changes in other amino acids probably occur with age, as well.

Cancer

Elevations in phenylalanine, tyrosine, glycine, asparagine, and valine have been found in some people with ovarian and uterine cancers. Increases in taurine, glutamic acid, and glutamine are found in some people with leukemia. Norton and colleagues have shown that patients with esophageal cancer have decreases in many plasma amino acids. Brenner and his researchers have attempted to correlate abnormalities in plasma amino acids in patients with gastric carcinoma or malignancies of the stomach.

Depression and Psychiatric Conditions

In general, low levels of tyrosine and phenylalanine coincide with fatigue-based depressions; decreased levels of GABA and glutamine are associated with anxiety-based depressions; and a deficiency in serotonin is associated with insomnia-based depressions. High levels of tyrosine and phenylalanine are associated with psychosis.

Different drugs are indicated for different forms of depression. Similarly, different amino acids are helpful for treating different kinds of depression. In our clinic, a person's type of depression is analyzed by a psychological test called the Millon. With this information and the results of amino blood assays, we are able to put together the most effective combination of medication and amino acids. Any uncertainties are cleared up by brain mapping—brain electrical activity mapping (BEAM)—a procedure that provides an assessment of the age and functional status of an individual's brain. (See "Brain Electrical Activity Mapping" on page 59 for more information about BEAM.)

Increasing evidence suggests that elevations in plasma tyrosine plus phenylalanine may contribute to hallucinations in people who are alcoholics and in people with schizophrenia. Studies by Bjerkenstedt and colleagues have shown that elevations in plasma alanine, taurine, methionine, valine, isoleucine, leucine, phenylalanine, and tyrosine can occur in some cases of schizophrenia, but we have not observed these effects in our practice. In contrast, elevations in plasma tryptophan and tyrosine have been correlated with the effectiveness of treatment with antidepressants. Serum deficiencies in essential amino acids—for example, tryptophan, tyrosine, methionine, GABA, taurine, and glycine—during clinical depression have been reported throughout this book.

Endocrine Conditions

Melatonin, tryptophan, and serotonin all have a role in neuroendocrinology. The precise nature of their influence is not clear at this time. More research is needed; however, we believe that brain chemistry should be considered in all endocrine problems. For instance, we know that levels of certain hormones are associated with serotonin levels in the brain. Low levels of testosterone and DHEA, for example, can be increased by raising dopamine levels. Many endocrine abnormalities are corrected by adjusting brain chemistry.

Food Allergies

Wunderlich and Kalita reported at least one case of food allergy in which serine, glutamic acid, and cysteine were decreased in urine and an excess in urine of carnosine (a peptide that breaks down into alanine) was found. Philpott and Kalita also found low levels of aspartic acid, glutamic acid, and cysteine in patients with food allergies. They corrected this problem with pyridoxine (vitamin B$_6$). They also found high amounts of amino adipic acid (a breakdown product of lysine), cystathione synthase (a pyridoxine-dependent enzyme), and methionine, which they postulate may indicate a pyridoxine utilization disorder.

Pangborn has suggested that low urinary levels of leucine, isoleucine, valine, and phenylalanine can be found in those people with food allergies. There are several different types of profiles that appear with food sensitivities. We feel that measurement of plasma amino acids is superior to measurement of urine levels, but have been unable to document any particular pattern of amino acids in allergy patients. Clearly, the evidence shows that there are multiple amino acid abnormalities in individuals with food allergies, and that plasma amino acids are a useful part of the biochemical workup.

High Amino Acid Levels

Elevated levels of amino acids accompany most genetic inborn errors in metabolism and are associated with a wide range of health problems. Table 21.1 on page 298 identifies a variety of clinical conditions in which amino acids are likely to be elevated in the urine. These include Fanconi's syndrome; anticonvulsant-induced rickets (vitamin D deficiency that may result in bone malformations); congenital ichthyosis (a hereditary skin disorder characterized by dry, flaky skin); mental retardation; use of outdated tetracyclines; fructose intolerance; galactosemia (elevated levels of galactose caused by the body's inability to convert lactose to galactose to glucose); hereditary macular degeneration; hyperthyroidism; ichthyosis vulgaris (dry, flaky skin); liver disease; nephrotic syndrome (damage to tiny blood-filtering units in the kidneys that results in the buildup of water); phenylketonuria (PKU); rickets; scurvy; tubular hypomagnesemia; vitamin D deficiency; cadmium, lead, or uranium intoxication; Wilson's disease (copper poisoning) and food allergies.

Typically, a generalized elevation in amino acids tends to show up in the urine.

Table 20.2 on page 298 lists the variety of clinical conditions associated with high blood levels of amino acids, or hyperaminoacidemia. We feel that amino

TABLE 21.1. CONDITIONS ASSOCIATED WITH AN ELEVATION IN URINARY AMINO ACIDS

CONDITION	AMINO ACID
Fanconi's syndrome, anticonvulsant-induced rickets, uranium intoxication	All elevated
Cadmium intoxication, congenital ichthyosis	All elevated
Mental retardation, use of outdated tetracyclines, fructose intolerance	All elevated
Galactosemia, hereditary macular degeneration	All elevated
Hyperthyroidism, ichthyosis vulgaris	All elevated
Lead intoxication, liver disease, nephrotic syndrome	All elevated
Phenylketonuria, rickets, Wilson's disease	All elevated
Food allergies	Amino adipic acid, methionine (Low: serine, glutamine, asparagine, cysteine)

TABLE 21.2. CONDITIONS ASSOCIATED WITH AN ELEVATION IN PLASMA AMINO ACIDS

CONDITION	AMINO ACID
Cushing's syndrome, glucocorticoid excess	Alanine
Diabetes	BCAAs
Duchenne's syndrome, myopathies	Glycine, glutamine, taurine
Familial pancreatitis	Lysine
Gout	Alanine, glutamine, leucine, isoleucine
Hyperactivity	Tyrosine
Liver failure	Tyrosine, phenylalanine, glutamine, glycine, asparagine
Lymphoma, hepatitis	All, except BCAAs
Migraine attack, use of migraine drugs	Tryptophan, GABA
Obesity, fasting	BCAAs
Phenylketonuria (PKU)	Phenylalanine
Prematurity and low birth weight	Tyrosine, proline
Renal failure	Cysteine
Rickets, muscular hypotonia	Glycine

acid measurements taken from blood are more likely to provide useful information about abnormalities with regard to specific amino acids. For example, we know that hyperalaninemia (an excess of alanine) can occur with excess production of the hormone glucocorticoid that can occur with high blood sugar or Cushing's syndrome; elevated glycine levels can occur in plasma with rickets, muscular hypotonia, and liver disease; and elevated lysine levels can occur with familial pancreatitis. Elevated proline, as well as elevated tyrosine, is common in premature infants. Persons with gout may show small plasma increases of alanine, leucine, isoleucine, serine, and glutamic acid, while glycine can be significantly decreased. In diabetes, there may be a two- to threefold increase in leucine, isoleucine, and valine.

Individuals with lymphoma and hepatitis may show increases in levels of all plasma amino acids, except for the branched-chain amino acids. In migraine headaches, GABA may be increased, and high plasma tryptophan has been reported a day before a migraine attack. In myopathies such as Duchenne's syndrome, increased glycine, glutamic acid, taurine, and the methionine byproduct, methionine sulfoxide, have been found. Obese persons may have a modest increase in the branched-chain amino acids. In rickets, generalized elevated blood levels of amino acids can occur.

Typically, elevated levels of an amino acid are treated by administration of its competing amino acid.

Low Amino Acid Levels

In a limited number of medical conditions, amino acids are consistently reduced in plasma, a condition known as hypoaminoacidemia. People showing these reduced levels include those with anorexia, cancer, folliculitis, alcohol abuse, or glucagonoma (overproduction of glucagon by a neuroendocrine tumor in the pancreas). Low plasma amino acids can probably occur temporarily during any severe stress. However, even malnutrition and kwashiorkor in children do not guarantee that all the plasma amino acids will be decreased. Fever and infectious diseases reduce most amino acids in serum; however, there is an increase in the phenylalanine-to-tyrosine ratio. Individuals with hypoglycemia can have low alanine levels. In renal failure, plasma tyrosine, phenylalanine, and methionine are often low; threonine, valine, isoleucine, leucine, lysine, and histidine may also eventually be reduced. Almost any medical condition may produce a reduction in plasma amino acids.

Individuals with pellagra show very low plasma tryptophan levels, and their plasma branched-chain amino acids may also be reduced. Rheumatoid arthritis is often accompanied by decreased plasma histidine. Low plasma amino acids have occurred in about 5 percent of our patients; these patients responded to a multi–amino acid formula.

Table 21.3 lists the wide range of clinical conditions in which amino acids are likely to be reduced in plasma.

TABLE 21.3. CONDITIONS ASSOCIATED WITH LOW PLASMA AMINO ACIDS

CONDITION	AMINO ACIDS DEFICIENT
Anorexia, cancer	All low (hypoaminoacidemia)
Depression	Tryptophan, taurine, tyrosine, phenylalanine
Fever, infection	All low, except increased phenylalanine
Folliculitis, alcoholism, stress	All low
Gout	Glycine
Ketotic hypoglycemia	Alanine
Pellagra	Tryptophan, sometimes BCAAs
Renal failure	Tyrosine, phenylalanine, methionine, and eventually all
Rheumatoid arthritis	Histidine
Scurvy	Threonine, lysine, glycine, histidine, arginine

Decreases in essential amino acids in plasma also occur with pregnancy, stress, exposure to organic solvents, sepsis, burns, ulcer disease, trauma, diphenhydramine (Benadryl) abuse, cancer, dialysis, zinc deficiency, and surgery.

Essential amino acid supplements may be of great value in treating many of these conditions. Our findings show that an increase in plasma amino acids can occur following high supplementations. Yet, very high doses that raise plasma levels of essential amino acids to five to twenty times normal may lower competing amino acids. Amino acid supplementation raises this to twice normal, and appears to raise other amino acids in plasma, which is useful in treating the conditions mentioned above.

Therapeutic effectiveness of antidepressants, migraine drugs, and D-penicillamine for rheumatoid arthritis has also been associated with increase in plasma amino acids.

Immune Response

We increasingly realize that viruses like HIV and Epstein-Barr generate their effects not only by damaging the immune system directly but also by damaging the brain. The field of psychoneuroimmunology has revealed that neurotransmitters, created by amino acids, govern the immune system. We don't know all the mechanisms, but we do know that much. As an example, norepinephrine, the neurotransmitter also known as adrenaline, helps curb autoimmune reactions. Tyrosine and DL-phenylalanine are major components of this neurotransmitter.

These two amino acids may be the most important of all the amino acids because of this connection.

TESTING FOR AMINO ACID LEVELS

As we increase our understanding of the fundamental importance of amino acids and their growing relevance in treatment programs, it is clear that blood amino acid measurement should be an integral part of the nutritional evidence gathered on those suffering from chronic illnesses. At PATH Medical, we recommended that all patients have an amino acid plasma test at least every two years. The assay provides invaluable information on the bodily status of the various amino acids, including the following:

- The presence of elevated homocysteine, an important and newly recognized risk factor for heart disease.

- Low branched-chain amino acids, an indicator of muscle weakness.

- Melatonin deficiency, commonly found in the elderly.

- Low alanine, an indicator of hypoglycemia.

- Low methionine, a factor in allergies and depression.

- Low cysteine and cystine, indicators of an antioxidant deficiency.

- Imbalances or deficiencies in phenylalanine, tyrosine, and tryptophan, often found in depression.

- Abnormalities of serine in patients with psychosis.

Such findings are extremely useful in guiding effective clinical therapy. For instance, a young woman with treatment-resistant seizures was referred to us by a nearby hospital. With the aid of the plasma amino acid test, we determined the presence of a metabolic abnormality of amino adipic acid. This situation was corrected, resulting in improved control of the patient's seizures.

We have used amino acid blood testing to closely monitor the absorption of amino acids in our therapy programs. Blood level readings can also help us determine whether psychiatric patients are taking their medication properly. Urine testing for amino acid levels also provides useful information, but we regard it as a test of second choice in most cases. We utilize urine testing primarily to help clarify ambiguous metabolic defects.

In general, levels of amino acids can be measured to better advantage in blood plasma than in urine. However, abnormalities in plasma levels are not always reflected in urine and vice versa. For example, scurvy patients may show a reduced concentration of threonine, glycine, lysine, histidine, and arginine in plasma, yet have normal urinary excretion of these amino acids. Excretion of hydroxyproline may be increased during laboratory-induced scurvy, yet hydroxyproline may remain normal in blood. The reason for these discrepancies is unclear, but for the major amino acids, blood level measurements are superior. For example, with oral ingestion of tyrosine, only .42 percent is excreted in urine. Urine levels have proven a better measurement than blood levels only in the case of 3-methylhistidine and possibly hydroxyproline, which are relatively unimportant amino acids.

AMINO ACID THERAPY

When taking amino acids for healing purposes, achieving the most clinically effective dose is a challenge, as it is with all nutrient therapy. Niacin, for example, can be effective at 500 mg and also at 4,000 mg. Vitamin C has many benefits at 500 mg. Are the number of benefits that much greater, as some say, at 5,000 mg? Maybe so for one person; maybe not for another. Some people with senility may need 3.5 g of phosphatidylserine. Others, with basic memory problems, may be well served with 200 or 400 mg, a fraction of the amount that generated memory benefits for laboratory animals.

Even if the effect of a given nutrient is known, and even if blood levels and other biochemical markers are considered, the physiological individuality of a person often dictates trying different strengths or different approaches in order to achieve the best result. There is a wide dosing range with many of the amino acids. Continued research and application of amino acids in therapy will help us eventually sort this out.

In general, if taking individual amino acids for healing purposes, it is wise to also take a full amino acid complex. If taking amino acids for general health purposes, we recommend taking a complex that includes all of the essential amino acids. This is the best way to assure that you have adequate amounts of the critical amino acids from which your body can then synthesize whatever nonessential amino acids it may need.

Amino Acid Formulas

Many dietary uses for amino acid are accepted therapy in medical conditions. For instance, an amino acid solution called nephromine, used for kidney failure patients, contains eight essential amino acids as the only source of nitrogen and protein. Electrolytes do not need to be added to the solution, and it prevents any excess nitrogen from adversely affecting the individual.

Liver or hepatic failure patients also require special amino acid formulas. These individuals usually have an abnormal plasma amino acid pattern with high concentrations of the aromatic amino acids phenylalanine, tyrosine, and tryptophan, which reduce the concentration of the branched-chain amino acids leucine, isoleucine, and valine. That is, they do not have the typical proportions usually found among amino acids. A solution of amino acids called hepatamine is used in liver disease. Generally, these amino acid solutions do not cause too many side effects. Infusion of crystalline amino acids may lead to alkalosis. Elevated serum ammonia levels can occur in children, as well as in adults with liver disease, from ordinary amino acid solutions.

Unique Pharmacological Properties of Chronic Supplementation

Interest in long-term therapeutic usage of high doses of amino acids in the treatment of many common health problems is growing. Tryptophan has been used in the treatment of insomnia, depression, pain, and mania. Methionine has been used in the treatment of depression, gallbladder disease, and other medical conditions. Taurine is commonly used therapeutically in Japan, where it is used as an inotrope and anticonvulsant. The effects of long-term chronic loading of amino acids on other plasma amino acids are not well understood.

We retrospectively analyzed plasma amino acids in three patients loaded with methionine alone (1,400 mg per 150 pounds for eleven weeks); four patients loaded with methionine and taurine (1,800 mg methionine per 150 pounds for thirteen weeks, 600 mg taurine per 150 pounds for fourteen weeks); four patients loaded with tryptophan alone (2,500 mg per 150 pounds for six weeks); and four loaded with methionine and tryptophan (800 mg methionine per 150 pounds for nine weeks, 900 mg tryptophan per 150 pounds for ten weeks). We compared these groups with two control groups.

Methionine alone increased plasma methionine and other sulfur amino acids (taurine and cysteine), as well as aminobutyric acid, glycine, and asparagine. Methionine and taurine combined increased the above amino acids plus ornithine and hydroxyproline.

Tryptophan given alone elevated tryptophan, threonine, and arginine. Methionine and tryptophan together elevated methionine, threonine, arginine, taurine, leucine, isoleucine, valine, phenylalanine, tyrosine, serine, hydroxyproline, and lysine.

The addition of a second amino acid again accentuated the increase in other plasma amino acids. All four groups combined (fifteen subjects), compared to twenty-six controls, showed increases in ten amino acids and trends upward in all plasma amino acids. Chronic (long-term, high dose) supplementation of methionine, taurine, or tryptophan lends to an elevation of many other plasma amino acids.

This remarkable elevation probably occurs with all chronic supplementation of amino acids. Carrier or transport systems are probably stimulated. We believe this is a positive effect, because of the previously mentioned decrease in plasma amino acids with advancing age. Chronic supplementation of amino acids, particularly cysteine, is potentially valuable for everyone. The side effect of increased hydroxyproline can probably be corrected by increased vitamin C intake. Further research on this phenomenon is warranted.

We have been particularly impressed by individuals who have been taking one amino acid for years. Recently, we saw a fifty-year-old woman who had been taking 500 mg of L-lysine a day for three years for cold sores. Tests revealed that her lysine levels were one-and-a-half to two times normal, and ten other amino acids were significantly elevated.

A thirty-two-year-old schizophrenic woman on methionine and taurine for several years had methionine levels 50 percent above normal and taurine levels twice normal. Her blood tests also showed eight other amino acids significantly elevated. A twenty-nine-year-old depressed man was taking about 8 g of three different amino acids for several months; he came to us with the highest levels of amino acids in almost every amino acid group.

We have found, therefore, that chronic supplementation of several essential (but not nonessential) amino acids, individually or in combination dosing over time, will lead to gradual buildup, and that plasma levels will continue to increase after several years of taking an amino acid supplement. The generalized increase that occurs from taking one amino acid chronically may be specific toward competing amino acids, yet we have not seen any definite pattern. This fascinating finding, we feel, is significant to overall human nutrition, and I (Dr. Braverman) am continuing my studies.

Adjuncts to Supplementation

At PATH Medical, we find that cranial electrical stimulation (CES), when combined with amino acid therapy, substantially improves results. This technique, which has been referred to throughout this book, generates a gentle, minute low-voltage electrical stimulation of the brain. The medical literature is replete with studies documenting the success of electrotherapy in the treatment of numerous conditions, such as depression, anxiety, alcoholism and substance abuse, withdrawal syndrome, insomnia, schizophrenia, learning disorders, hyperactivity, and even hyperacidity. The CES device is simple to operate. It can be used in a clinic setting or purchased for use at home.

In our clinic, we also regard brain electrical activity mapping (BEAM), which we have discussed frequently throughout this book, as an immensely valuable diagnostic tool for evaluating mental illness, degenerative aging of the brain, and the effectiveness of exciting, restorative nutritional treatments. BEAM is a simple office procedure that provides reliable spectral analysis of alpha and theta waves, evoked potentials, visual evoked response, auditory evoked response, and positive brain wave (P300) voltage. Using BEAM, we can establish a clinically meaningful physiological age and functional status of an individual's brain.

AMINO ACIDS IN CLINICAL CONDITIONS: A SUMMARY

Table 21.4 summarizes the research and literature presented throughout this book. It can be a useful guide to laypeople, nutritionists, and practitioners of integrative medicine.

TABLE 21.4. AMINO ACIDS AND CLINICAL CONDITIONS AND DISEASE

DISEASE	PROBABLE THERAPY	TO BE AVOIDED
Aging	Methionine, tryptophan	
Aggressiveness	Tryptophan	
Alzheimer's disease	All essential amino acids	
Appetite control	Tryptophan, phenylalanine, GABA	
Arthritis	Histidine, cysteine	
Autism	Tryptophan	
Benign prostatic hypertrophy	Glycine	
Cancer	Cysteine, taurine, most essential amino acids	Phenylalanine, tyrosine
Cholesterol (elevated)	Methionine, taurine, glycine, carnitine, arginine	
Chronic pain	Tryptophan, phenylalanine	
Cigarette addiction	Tyrosine	
Cocaine addiction	Tyrosine	
Depression	Tryptophan, phenylalanine, threonine, tyrosine	Arginine
Diabetes	Alanine, cysteine, tryptophan	
Drug addiction	GABA, methionine, tyrosine	
Epilepsy	Glycine, taurine	Glutamic acid, aspartic acid
Gallbladder disease	Methionine, taurine, BCAA, glycine	
Gout	Glycine	
Hair loss	Cysteine, arginine	
Heart failure	Taurine, tyrosine, carnitine	
Herpes	Lysine	Arginine
Hypertension	Tryptophan, GABA, taurine	
Hypoglycemia	Alanine, GABA	

DISEASE	PROBABLE THERAPY	TO BE AVOIDED
Insomnia	Tryptophan	
Kidney failure	All essential amino acids	Nonessential amino acids
Leg ulcer	Topical cysteine, glycine, threonine	
Liver disease	Isoleucine, leucine, valine	
Manic depression	Tryptophan, glycine	
Myasthenia	Glycine	
Osteoporosis	Lysine	
Parkinson's disease	Phenylalanine, tyrosine, tryptophan, methionine, L-dopa	
Radiation toxicity	Cysteine, taurine, methionine, glycine	
Schizophrenia	Isoleucine, tryptophan, methionine	Serine, asparagine, leucine
Stress	Tyrosine, histidine, all essential amino acids	
Suicidal depression	Tryptophan, methionine	
Surgery	BCAAs, all essential amino acids	
Thymus insufficiency	Aspartic acid, threonine	

It is worth noting that deficient or excessive plasma levels of an amino acid do not always provide the basis for therapy. Blood levels are usually excellent guides to therapy, but can be deceptive; for example, short-term stress may elevate plasma tyrosine but long-term stress will deplete it. Time sequence in a disease can make test results ambiguous. Hence, amino acid therapy, like all medical therapies, depends heavily on clinical judgment; therefore, we urge you to work with a healthcare practitioner to assess your body's individual needs for amino acids.

CHAPTER TWENTY-TWO

Continuing Breakthroughs in Amino Acids

Research is moving so fast in discovering the many vital uses and applications of amino acids. Following is a discussion of a few of the latest findings as we go to press.

Research is exploding in the area of amino acids and brain chemistry, where we're finding that if the brain is functioning well, the body will follow suit. The latest scientifically "hot" dramatic studies show that balanced brain chemistry plays a pivotal role in the overall health of the body, particularly in the treatment of substance abuse and weight loss. According to the latest research, brain function is dominated by four core chemical systems: the dopamine group, the acetylcholine group, the GABA group, and the serotonin group. Each system is driven by a particular group of neurotransmitters that promotes specific functions within the brain.

The dopamine, or adrenaline, system of the brain is responsible for promoting energy, power, and metabolism to the brain; the GABA, or calming, system promotes relaxation and mood leveling; the acetylcholine, or cognition, system is responsible for the brain's speed, memory, and ability to think clearly; and lastly, the serotonin, or resting, system allows the body to sleep and controls the brain's on-and-off mechanism. Scientists and clinicians are focusing on how to balance these systems using amino acids, diet, and/or amino acid–based drugs to achieve a wide range of beneficial effects.

The interest in measuring amino acids that has come from measuring plasma homocysteine levels continues. The latest studies show that elevations in this toxic amino acid are implicated in heart disease. Treatment for this problem with pyridoxine (vitamin B_6), cyanocobalamin (vitamin B_{12}), and folic acid has started to turn the ordinary practitioner into a nutritionist. It has spread the concept that measuring plasma amino acids levels can be useful, because it actually gives a rough baseline amount of antioxidants in the blood. Elevations of plasma homocysteine levels essentially reflect a loss of antioxidants, while sufficient levels of cysteine in the blood represent a sufficient amount of antioxidants.

Numerous other studies have shown the benefits of plasma amino acids analyzed in chronic fatigue disorders, which are frequently marked by low tryptophan levels. Measuring aromatic amino acids and branched-chain amino acid levels can help predict how individuals suffering from manic-depressive disorders will respond to antidepressants and anticonvulsants. For example, low aromatic amino acids, such as tyrosine, phenylalanine, and tryptophan, predict response to antidepressants, while increases in branched-chain amino acids predict response to anticonvulsants. Similarly, patients with depression have low blood levels of tyrosine and phenylalanine and respond to such antidepressants as bupropion (Wellbutrin), phentermine hydrochloride (Phentermine), and methylphenidate (Ritalin), or similar medications. Patients with low levels of tryptophan may respond better to Serzone (nefazodone), trazodone (Desyrel), fluoxetine (Prozac) or paroxetine (Paxil).

Low plasma amino acids are found in cases of cirrhosis and renal failure, and the need for supplementing these amino acids can be discerned by measuring the plasma. Elevated levels of aspartate and glutamate can predict deterioration in Parkinson's disease and seizure patients, and blocking these amino acids has important implications in lowering or preventing strokes. Low levels of phosphatidylserine and serine may predict memory problems and disorders associated with aging, while elevation in serine may predict other psychiatric problems. Deficiencies in N-acetyl cysteine have been shown to be associated with bronchitis and lung disease, in addition to many other conditions. N-acetyl cysteine has provoked new interest in the prevention of cancer and toxic drug side effects. Low taurine levels have been associated with eye disorders and can predict possible macular degeneration and other eye diseases.

Arginine has been shown to decrease platelet stickiness and joins garlic, fish oil, aspirin, and vitamin E in preventing stroke and blood clots. It is an excellent alternative for those who cannot tolerate or do not wish to take warfarin (Coumadin). Arginine also raises the endothelial-releasing factor, vasodilates the blood, and helps circulation. Some think arginine may be helpful in reducing cholesterol levels, migraines, and cancer.

Studies on elevation in glutamates and aspartates show that blocking these amino acids and blocking monosodium glutamate (MSG) prevents damage and anesthetizing of the brain. Essentially these are toxic amino acids, but they can be used to stimulate brain activity and memory. High amounts can result in the damaging effects of stroke, migraine headaches, and other toxic conditions. Glutamine supplementation used for gastrointestinal disorders raises tryptophan levels, which in turn may benefit these disorders.

New studies suggest that branched-chain amino acids help cancer patients and the wasting associated with cancer. New studies continue to suggest the benefits of carnitine for heart disease, N-acetyl-carnitine for memory disorders, tyrosine as a natural amphetamine for the brain, and phosphatidylserine for memory. They also suggest that uses of amino acids in clinical therapy continue to be refined. Amino acids do have many useful benefits in medicine. Therefore, plasma amino acids should be measured along with trace elements, vitamins, and fatty acids for complete biochemical evaluation. Amino acids are the building blocks of protein and neurotransmitter systems throughout the body and help the entire health of the body metabolically and hormonally.

Glossary

Acetylcholine. Neurotransmitter made from choline, a substance related to the B vitamins.

Acidosis. Abnormal state of overacidity, or reduced alkalinity, of the blood and body tissues,

Acute. State or condition that comes on quickly and causes relatively severe symptoms, but is of limited duration.

Adenosine triphosphate (ATP). Intermediate compound that supplies energy to cells.

Adrenaline (epinephrine). Hormone secreted by the adrenal gland that produces the "fight or flight" response.

Agonist. Substance that enhances the action of another substance.

Albumin. Principal protein in blood found in tissues and fluid; responsible for osmotic pressure.

Alkaloids. Naturally occurring amines that exhibit pharmacological activity.

Amine. Nitrogen-containing compound.

Amino acid. Group of organic chemical compounds that consists of a basic amino group (nitrogen and hydrogen) and acid from a carboxyl group (carbon, oxygen, and hydrogen) and is used to form the basic structural units of proteins.

Amino acid loading. Experimental process in which one nutrient is given in extremely large doses to overload the system and then to study its effect.

Amino acid pattern. Relative proportions of various amino acids.

Amino aciduria. Excess excretion of amino acids in the urine.

Analgesic. Substance that alleviates the sensation of pain.

Analog. Chemical very similar in structure to an organic compound.

Antagonist. Refers to nutrient interactions that inhibit one another.

Antibody. A protein created by the immune system, in response to a foreign organism or toxin, that is capable of destroying or neutralizing the invader.

ApoE. Protein that transports fat and cholesterol in the bloodstream.

Ataxia. Loss of ability to coordinate muscular movement.

Basal ganglia. Islands of gray matter located in the cerebral hemispheres that are involved in the regulation of voluntary movement.

Beta-alanine. Constituent of of pantothenic acid and coenzyme A derived from of the amino acid alanine.

Blood-brain barrier. Physiological mechanism that alters the permeability of small brain vessels and prevents some substances from entering brain tissue. Many amino acids and substances are blocked from entering into the brain readily without transport system.

Catalepsy. Trancelike state that may occur in schizophrenia or epilepsy in which the muscles are more or less rigid.

Catecholamine. Any of a group of structurally similar compounds, including norepinephrine, epinephrine, and dopamine, that function like adrenaline in the brain, and are made from tyrosine.

Cerebellum. Area of the brain located behind the cerebrum responsible for the regulation and coordination of voluntary muscular movement and for posture and balance.

Chromatography. Technique that physically separates the substances in a liquid.

Chronic. Mild or severe, state or condition that is of long duration.

Chronic fatigue syndrome. Long-term condition characterized by low energy, muscle aches and pain, and depression.

Cirrhosis. A disease in which fibrous tissue replace healthy liver tissue and liver functions are compromised.

Cofactor. Part of an enzyme, which is usually a mineral or trace metal, important for the activity of an enzyme.

Collagen. Protein that is the main component of connective tissue, cartilage, and bone.

Covalent bond. Type of bond between molecules that is neither polarized nor electric.

Cranial electrical stimulation (CES). Safe and gentle low-voltage electrical stimulation of the brain found to promote the neurotransmitter functions of amino acids.

D-, L- and DL- form. Chemical structures in which amino acids occur. Amino acids typically occur in D- and L- forms, and occasionally in DL- form; these terms denote the direction in which the amino acid rotates light. "D" stands for dextro, meaning right; "L" stands for levo, meaning left; and "DL" is a 50/50 mixture of D- and L- forms.

Deamination. Metabolic process whereby the nitrogen portion of an amino acid is removed.

Deoxyribonucleic acid (DNA). Substance in the nuclei of all cells that contains the cell's genetic blueprints and determines the types of life form into which the cells will develop.

Dipeptide. Substance made from the joining of two amino acids.

Dopamine. Stimulatory neurotransmitter commonly associated with mood.

Dopaminergic. Characteristics and activities of dopamine and dopaminelike substances.

Double-blind study. A study in which neither the researcher nor the subject knows when the active agent or a placebo is being used.

Dysthymia. Mild depression.

Electroencephalograpy (EEG). A type of testing used to measure brain-wave activity.

Encephalopathy. Various diseases of the brain that may result in a decline in brain function.

Endorphins. Naturally occurring morphinelike peptide hormones that act as mild mood elevators, control pain perception, and serve as potent analgesics.

Enkephalinase. Enzyme that may act to increase pain levels in the body.

Enkephalins. Naturally occurring morphinelike polypeptides that act as mild mood elevators, control pain perception, and serve as potent analgesics.

Enzyme. Large protein that functions as a catalyst to speed a chemical reaction.

Endogenous amino acids. Amino acids that are recycled from the pool of amino acids within the body.

Eosinophilia myalgia syndrome (EMS). A rare autoimmune disease marked by severe muscle pain, spasms, and weakness; swelling of the arms and legs; numbness; fever and rashes; and in severe cases death.

Exogenous amino acids. Amino acids that are derived from the diet.

Familial amyloidosis. Inherited condition marked by dizziness upon standing, numbness and tingling in the arms and legs, and possibly diarrhea.

Familial spastic paraplegia. Group of disorders characterized by progressive stiffness or spasticity of the legs with varying degress of weakness.

Fatty acid. Acid derived from a series of hydrogen atoms that composes the building blocks of fats. There are three major categories of fatty acids: saturated, polyunsaturated, and monounsaturated.

Fibrillation. Incoordinate contraction of muscle fibers, often involving the heart.

Fibroblasts. Large cell with nuclei found often in newly formed tissue or tissue in the state of being repaired.

Folliculitis. Bacterial infection of the hair follicle.

Friedreich's ataxia. Inherited, progressive nervous system disorder causing loss of balance and corrdination.

Glomerulonephritis. Severe kidney disease.

Glucagon. Hormone produced by pancreatic gland that stimulates an increase in blood glucose levels.

Glucogenic. Glucose-forming.

Gluconeogenesis. Formation of glucose from noncarbohydrate substances such as amino acids.

Glucose. A monosaccharide found in the blood; one of the body's primary energy sources.

Glycogen. Primary storage form of glucose in the body that is converted back into glucose as needed to supply energy.

Glycogenesis. Formation of glycogen from sugar.

Glycogenolysis. Formation of sugar from glycogen in the liver and muscles.

Glycolysis. Conversion of glucose to lactic acid that produces some energy in the form of ATP.

Gram. Unit of measure. One gram is equal to 1,000 milligrams.

Gray matter. Brownish-gray nerve tissue of the brain and spinal cord, composed of nerve cells and fibers, and some supportive tissue.

Hartnup's disease. Inherited disorder of amino acid metabolism characterized by disturbances of gait and coordination; an ataxic disorder.

Helper T cell. Lymphocyte that is under the control of the thymus gland that helps in the immune response.

Hemoglobin. Protein that holds iron in the red blood.

Hepatic encephalopathy. Form of brain damage, resulting from a decline in liver function manifested as speech difficulties, altered sleep, tremors, and other symptoms due to the accumulation of toxins in the brain caused by abnormal functioning of the kidney.

Hippocampus. Important area of the brain that has a central role in memory processes.

Histamine. Substance that plays a central role in allergic reactions and other functions of the immune system.

Homeostasis. Body's ability to keep equilibrium among its parts.

Hydrolysis. Chemical reaction in which breakdown of a substance into new compounds is due to the addition of one or more molecules of water.

Hydroxylase. Primary enzyme in the liver that starts the conversion of aromatic amino acids to neurotransmitters.

Hyperlipoproteinemia. Metabolic disorder characterized by abnormally high cholesterol or triglyceride levels, or both.

Hyperoxalemia. Abnormally high accumulation of oxalates in the blood, associated with the formation of kidney stones.

in vitro. Latin term for studies done in test tubes.

Inborn errors of metabolism. Inability to metabolize or transport an amino acid due to an inherited defect usually in an enzyme.

Inotrope. Drug or nutrient that promotes the pumping action of the heart, for example, calcium or taurine.

Interleukin. Immune system chemicals made by the body that help fight infection.

Ischemia. A decrease in the blood supply to a body organ or tissue.

Keratin. An insoluble protein found in hair, skin, and nails.

Ketone. Substance that is formed as a result of incomplete oxidation of fats.

Ketosis. Process whereby the body burns stored fuel for fat.

Kilogram. Unit of measure in which one kilo is equal to 2.2 pounds.

Krebs cycle. The body's pathway for the metabolism of carbohydrate into energy. Named for British biochemist Hans Krebs, a Nobel prize winner.

Kwashiorkor. A protein deficiency disease seen in malnourished children and characterized by lack of growth, edema, tissue wasting, lowered resistance to disease, and pigment changes in the skin.

Leukocyte. White blood cell

Levodopa (L-dopa). Pharmaceutical drug commonly used in treatment of Parkinson's disease that the body converts into dopamine.

Lymphocyte. A type of white blood cell that is responsible for building immunity in the body.

Macrophage. Substance that has the ability to digest foreign particles, thus protecting the tissues and organs where they are found.

Metabolic pathway. Way in which energy is taken from protein, fat, or carbohydrate.

Metabolite. Substance produced as a result of a metabolic process.

Methylation. Chemical process of adding a methyl group to a compound.

Milligram. Unit of measure; 1,000 milligrams is equal to one gram.

Mitochondria. Microscopic structure found in the cells of almost all living organisms. It contains enzymes responsible for the conversion of food to usable energy.

Molecule. Minute mass of matter; smallest quantity into which a substance can be divided and retain its characteristic properties.

Multiple myeloma. Cancer of the bone marrow.

Myoclonus. Muscle spasms associated with numerous neurological conditions.

Narcolepsy. Condition marked by an uncontrollable desire to sleep or sudden attacks of sleep occurring at intervals.

Necrosis. Death of cells or tissue through injury or disease.

Neonates. Newborns one month or younger.

Net protein utilization (NPU). The way in which protein is utilized. Some foods contain protein that cannot be metabolized adequately.

Neuron. Nerve cell that conducts electrical impulses, causing the release of neurotransmitters.

Neuropathy. Condition resulting from nerve damage.

Neuropeptides. Nerve proteins, or biochemicals, that send chemical messages from the brain to receptor sites in cell membranes.

Neurotransmitter. Chemical typically made from amino acids or peptides involved in the chemical languages by which neurons in the brain communicate; acetylcholine, dopamine, and norepinephrine are considered major neurotransmitters.

Neutrophil. Major constituent of leukocytes, a type of white blood cell important in immune response.

Nucleus raphus magnus. Primary pain-inhibiting center in the brain.

Orotic acid. Intermediate compound in the synthesis of pyrimidines.

Orthostatic hypotension. Sudden fall in blood pressure that occurs when assuming a standing position.

Oxidation. Burning of fuel to supply energy in the body.

Parenteral. Proceeding through the body via channels other than the intestines.

Parkinson's disease. Slowly progressive degenerating nervous system disease characterized by tremors, masklike facial expression, shuffling gait, and muscle rigidity and weakness.

Pellagra. Niacin deficiency disease marked by mental deterioration and disorders of the skin, gastronintestinal tract, and nervous system.

Peptide. Chain of amino acids that serves as an intermediary in protein digestion.

Peptide bond. Substance that links amino acids together.

Phagocyte. Protein that destroys the membranes of invading bacteria, killing the germs.

Phenylketonuria. An inborn error of metabolism of the enzyme necessary for conversion of the amino acid phenylalanine to tyrosine that is characterized by mental retardation.

Phospholipid. Substance consisting primarily of fatty acids and phosphorus, such as lecithin, occurring in all membranes.

Plasma. Liquid portion of blood or lymph devoid of cells.

Polyamine. Amino acid compounds that promote the growth of cells, including possibly cancer cells.

Polypeptides. Protein made up of more than three amino acids.

Porphyrins. Nonprotein nitrogenous tissues constituents.

Precursor. Substance used as a building block for another.

Prolactin. Natural hormone made in the pituitary gland that stimulates milk production.

Protease. Enzyme that catalyzes the breakdown of protein into peptides and amino acids.

Protein. Collection of amino acids; one of the building blocks of the body.

Psychotropic drug. Drug that affects the mind and the psychology of an individual.

Purine. Basic constituent of DNA and RNA and of at least fifty other important compounds.

Pyrimidine. Basic constituent of DNA and RNA and of at least fifty other important compounds.

Pyroluria. Genetically determined chemical imbalance that causes a deficiency of pyridoxine (vitamin B_6) and zinc.

Pyruvate. Common compound in carbohydrate metabolism.

Rate-limiting. Deficiency in one of the compounds that hinders synthesis of a substance.

Reye's syndrome. Rare, serious disease that affects many internal organs, particularly the brain and liver, characterized by fever, vomiting, fatty infiltration of the liver, disorientation, and coma. Most cases occur in children given aspirin or aspirin-containing medications for viral infections, such as the chickenpox or flu.

Ribonucleic acid (RNA). Identical copy of DNA that acts as a messenger, carrying DNA blueprint instructions to the ribosome, a protein-making structure; the RNA messenger then supervises that the blueprint is followed exactly.

Serotonin. Neurotransmitter formed from the amino acid tryptophan that regulates mood, sleep, appetite, and pain.

Serum. Fluid portion of the blood that is left after clotting.

Status epilepticus. Form of epilepsy characterized by long-lasting seizures that can be life-threatening.

Substrate. Substance acted upon by an enzyme.

Synapse. Junction between two neurons where a nerve impulse is transmitted from one neuron to the next.

Telencephalon. Portion of the lower brain that develops into olfactory lobes, cerebral cortex, and corpora striata.

Thymus. Small gland found behind the breastbone that makes some of the hormones that tell the immune system what to do.

Thyroid. Small, butterfly-shaped gland found in the neck that produces hormones that regulate your metabolism.

Transaminases. Important enzymes that metabolize amino acids.

Transamination. Process of transferring amine groups from one amino acid to another.

Transport. Moving one part of the body to another part.

Tripeptide. Combination of three amino acids.

Urea. Major nitrogen-containing product of protein catabolism excreted in urine.

Urea cycle. The body's pathway for ammonia and nitrogen metabolism.

Vasopressin. Hormone, also known as antidiuretic hormone, that may be useful to memory.

White matter. White brain and spinal cord tissue, consisting mostly of myelinated nerve fibers.

Wilson's disease. Genetic disorder characterized by increased intestinal absorption of copper and its accumulation in the brain and other organs.

References

SECTION ONE

Chapter 1: Introduction

Adam, A., and Lederer, E., Muramyl peptides: immunomodulators, sleep factors, and vitamins. *Medicinal Res. Rev.,* 4(2):111–152, 1984.

Adibi, S. A., and Johns, B. A., Partial substitutions of amino acids of a parenteral solution with tripeptides: effects on parameters of protein nutrition in baboons. *Metabolism,* 33(5):420–424, 1984.

Bessman, S. P., The justification theory: the essential nature of the non-essential amino acids. *Nutr. Rev.,* 37(7):209–220, 1979.

Blackburn, G. L., Grant, J. P., and Young, V. R., eds., *Amino Acids: Metabolism and Medical Applications.* Littleton, MA: John Wright, PSG Inc., 1983.

Bralley, A. J., and Lord, R., Treatment of chronic fatigue syndrome with specific essential amino acid supplementation. 2nd International Congress on Amino Acids and Analogues, Vienna, August 5–9, 1991.

Calkins, B. M., Whittaker, D. J., Rider, A. A., and Turjman, N., Diet, nutrition intake, and metabolism in populations at high and low risk for colon cancer. *Amer. J. Clin. Nutr.,* 40:896–905, 1984.

Campbell, T. C., Allison, R. G., and Fisher, K. D., Nutrition toxicity. *Nutr. Rev.,* 39(6):249–256, 1981.

Chalmers, L., *Organic Acids in Man: The Analytical Chemistry, Biochemistry and Diagnosis of the Organic Acidurias.* New York: Chapman and Hall, 1982, p. 221.

Cheraskin, E., Ringsdorf, W. M., and Medford, F. H., The "ideal" daily intake of threonine, valine, phenylalanine, leucine, isoleucine, and methionine. *J. of Orth. Psych.,* 7(3):150–155, 1978.

Darcy, B., Availability of amino acids in monogastric animals. *Diabet. & Metabol.,* 10:121–133, 1984.

Di George, A. M., and Auerbach, V. H., The primary amino-acidopathies: genetic defects in the metabolism of the amino acids. *Ped. Clin. N. Amer.,* 723–744, 1963.

Dravid, A. R., Himwich, W. A., and Davis, J. M., Some free amino acids in dog brain during development. *J. Neurochem.,* 12:901–906, 1965.

Droge, W., Amino acids as immune regulators with special regard to AIDS. 2nd International Congress on Amino Acids and Analogues, Vienna, August 5–9, 1991.

Eagle, H., Amino acid metabolism in mammalian cell cultures. *Science,* 130:432–437, 1959.

Eberle, A. N., New perspective for "natural" therapeutic agents? *Karger Gazette,* No. 52, 1991.

Edvinsson, L., Uddman, R., and Juul, R., Peptidergic innervations of the cerebral circulation: role in subarachnoid hemorrhage in man. *Neurosurg. Rev.,* 13: 265–272, 1990.

Friedman, M., Absorption and utilization of amino acids. *JAMA,* 264(14), October 10, 1990.

Furst, P., Peptides in clinical nutrition. *Clin. Nutr.* 10(Suppl.) 19–24, 1991.

Gage, J. P., Francis, M. J. O., and Smith, R., Abnormal amino acid analyses obtained from *osteogenesis imperfecta* dentin. *J. Dent. Res.* 67(8):1097–1102, August 1988.

Gillies, D. R. N., Hay, A., Sheltway, M. J., and Congdon, P. J., Effect of phototherapy on plasma, 25(OH)-vitamin D in neonates. *Biol. Neonate,* 45(5):228–235, 1984.

Guroff, G., Effects of inborn errors of metabolism on the nutrition of the brain. *Nutrition and the Brain,* Vol. 4. Wurtman, R. J. and Wurtman, J. J., eds. New York: Raven Press, 1979.

Halliday, H. L., Lappin, T. R. J., and McClure, G., Iron status of the preterm infant during the first year of life. *Biol. Neonate,* 45(5):228–235, 1984.

Hanning, R. M., and Zlotkin, S. H., Amino acid and protein needs of the neonate: effects of excess and deficiency. *Seminars in Perinatology,* 13(2):131–141, 1989.

Harris, M., The 100,000-year hunt. *The Sciences* 1:22–33, 1986.

Hellebostad, M., Markestad, T., and Halvorsen, K. S., Vitamin D deficiency rickets and vitamin B-12 deficiency in vegetarian children. *Acta Paediatr. Scand.,* 74:191–195, 1985.

Hesseltine, C. W., The future of fermented foods. *Nutr. Rev.,* 41(10):293–298, 1983.

Hoffer, A., Mega amino acid therapy. *J. Ortho. Psych.,* 9(1):2–5, 1980.

Inglis, M. S., Page, C. M., and Wheatley, D. N., On the essential nature of non-essential amino acids. *Mol. Physiol.,* 5(1–2):115–122, 1984.

Ingram, D. D., et al., U.S.S.R. and U.S. nutrient intake, plasma lipids, and lipoproteins in men ages 40 to 59 sampled from lipid research clinics population. *Preven. Med.,* 14:264–271, 1985.

Inque, Y., Zama, Y., and Suzuki. M., "D-amino acids" as immunosuppressive agents. *Japan. J. Exp. Med.,* 51(6):363–366, 1981.

IRCS Med. Sci.: *Alimentary System: Biochem., Metab. and Nutr.,* 4:393–394, 1976.

Julius, D., Home for an orphan endorphin. *Nature,* Vol. 377, October 12, 1995.

Karkela, J., Marnela, K. M., Odink, J., et al., Amino acids and glucose in human cerebrospinal fluid after acute ischaemic brain damage. *Resuscitation,* 23:145–156, 1992.

Kenakin, T. P., The classification of drugs and drug receptors in isolated tissues. *Pharmacological Rev.,* 165–199, 1984.

Kirschmann, J. D., and Dunne, L. J., *Nutrition Almanac.* New York: McGraw-Hill Book Co., 1984.

Klevay, L. M., Changing patterns of disease: some nutritional remarks. *J. Amer. Coll. Nutr.,* 3:149–158, 1984.

Kolata, G., New neurons form in adulthood. *Science,* 224:1325–1326, June 1984.

Komatsu, T., Kishi, K., Yamamoto, T., and Inque, G., Nitrogen requirement of amino acid mixture with maintenance energy in young men. *J. Nutr. Sci. Vitaminol.,* 29:169–185, 1983.

Kramer, L. B., Osis, D., Coffey, J., and Spencer, H., Mineral and trace element content of vegetarian diets. *J. ACN,* 3:3–11, 1984.

Krnjevic, K., Chemical nature of synaptic transmission in vertebrates. *Physiol. Rev.,* 54:418–540, 1974.

Kurup, P. A., et al., Diet, nutrition intake, and metabolism in populations at high and low risk for colon cancer. *Amer. J. Clin. Nutr.,* 40:942–946, 1984.

Manning, A., TB drug also helps control schizophrenia. *Business Monday,* September 1995.

Matsuo, T., Shimakawa, K., Ikeda, H., and Susuoki, Z., Relation of body energetic status to dietary self-selection in Sprague-Dawley rats. *J. of Nutr. Sci. and Vitaminology,* 30(3):255–264, 1984.

May, M. E., and Hill, J. O., Energy content of diets of variable amino acid composition. *Am. J. Clin. Nutr.,* 52:770–776, 1990.

McBride, J. H., Amino acids and proteins. *Lab. Med.,* table 8, pp. 143–172.

McIntosh, N., Rodeck, C. H., and Heath, R., Plasma amino acids of the mid-trimester human fetus. *Biol. Neonate,* 45(5):218–224, 1984.

Meldrum, B. S., Competitive NMDA antagonists as drugs. In *The NMDA Receptor.* eds. J. C. Watkins and G. L. Gollingridge. IRL Press, Oxford, England: 1989, pp. 207–216.

Monagham, D. T., Bridges, R. J., and Cotman, C. W., The excitatory amino acid receptors: their classes, pharmacology and distinct properties in the function of the central nervous system. *Ann. Rev. Pharm. & Toxicol.,* 69:365–402, 1989.

Nutrition Reviews. Growth of vegetarian children. CRC Handbook of Nutritional Supplements. Boca Raton, FL: CRC Press, Inc., 1983, p. 371.

Oberholzer, V. G., and Briddon, A., A novel use of amino acid ratios as an indicator of nutritional status. London, U.K.

Oldendorf, W. H., Uptake of radio labeled essential amino acids by brain following arterial injection. *Proc. Soc. Exp. Biol. & Med.,* 136:385–386, 1971.

Palombo, J. D., and Blackburn, G. L., Human protein requirements. *N.Y. State J. Med.,* 1762–1763, October 1980.

Pauling, L., Letter to the Editor: Dietary influences on the synthesis of neurotransmitters in the brain. *Nutr. Rev.,* 37(9):302–304, 1979.

Pfeiffer, C., *Mental and Elemental Nutrients.* New Canaan, CT: Keats Publishing, Inc., 1975, 402–408.

Pitkow, H. S., Davis, R. H., and Bitar, M. S., The endocrine mimicking influence of amino acids. 2nd International Congress on Amino Acids and Analogues, Vienna, August 5–9, 1991.

Pitkow, H. S., Davis, R. H., and Bitar, M. S., The anabolic effects of amino acids. 2nd International Congress on Amino Acids and Analogues, Vienna, August 5–9, 1991.

Richardson, M. A., *Amino Acid in Psychiatric Disease.* Washington, D.C.: American Psychiatric Press, 1990, pp. xix and 190.

Rivera, Jr., A., Bell, E. F., Stegink, L. D., et al., Plasma amino acid profiles during the first three days of life in infants with respiratory distress syndrome: effect of parenteral amino acid supplementation. 115(3):465–468, 1989.

Roberts, J. C., Prodrugs of L-cysteine as radioprotective agents. 2nd International Congress on Amino Acids and Analogues, Vienna, August 5–9, 1991.

Robles, R., Gil, A., Faus, M. J., Periago, J. L., Sanchez-Pozo, A., Pita, M. L., and Sanchez-Medina, F., Serum and urine amino acid patterns during the first month of life in small-for-date infants. *Biol. Neonate,* 45(5):209–217, 1984.

Saito, T., Kobatake, K., Ozawa, H., et al., Aromatic and branched-chain amino acid levels in alcoholics. *Alcohol and Alcoholism,* 29(S1):133–135, 1994.

Shaheed, M. M., Plasma amino acid concentration in pre-term babies fed on various milk formulae compared with babies fed breast milk: a pilot study. *Saudi Med.* 10(4), 1990.

Stanbury, Wyndgaarden, Fredrickson, Goldstein, and Brown, eds. *The Metabolic Basis of Inherited Disease.* New York: McGraw-Hill, 1983.

Stegink, L. D., Filer, L. J., and Baker, G. L., Effect of sampling site on plasma amino acid concentration of infants: effect of skin amino acids. *Amer. J. Clin. Nutr.,* 36:917–925, 1982.

Stiegler, H., Wicklmayr, M., Rett, K., et al., The effect of prostaglandin EI on the amino acid metabolism of the human skeletal muscle. *Klin Wochenschr,* 68:380–383, 1990.

Stone, T. W., and Burton, N. R., NMDA receptors and ligands in the vertebrate CNS. *Progr. Neurobiol.,* 30:333–368, 1988.

———, and Perkins, M. N., Quinolinic acid: a potent endogenous excitant at amino acid receptors in the rat CNS. *Aur. J. Pharmacol.,* 72:411–412, 1981.

Stroud, E. D., and Smith, G. G., A search for D-amino acids in tumor tissue. *Biochem. Med.,* 31:254–256, 1984.

Swaiman, K. F., Menkes, J. H., DeVivo, D. C., and Prensky, A. L., Metabolic disorders of the central nervous system. *The Practice of Pediatric Neurology.* New York: C. V. Mosby Co., 1982, 472–513.

Turpeenoja, L., and Lahdesmaki, P., Presynaptic binding of amino acids: characterization of the binding and disassociation properties of taurine, GABA, glutamate, tyrosine and norleucine. *Intern. J. Neuroscience,* 22:99–106, 1983.

Vente, J. P., Von Meyenfeldt, M. F., Van Eijk, H. M. H., et al., Plasma-amino acid profiles in sepsis and stress. *Ann. Surg.* 209(1), January 1989.

Wilson, M. J., and Hatfield, D. L., Incorporation of modified amino acids into proteins *in vivo.* *Biochim. et Biophys. Acta,* 781:205–215, 1984.

Wright, R. A., Nutritional assessment. *JAMA,* 244(6):559–560, 1980.

Zioudrou, C., and Klee, W. A., Possible roles of peptides derived from food proteins in brain function. In: *Nutrition and the Brain, Vol. 4,* Wurtman, R. J., and Wurtman, J. J., eds. New York: Raven Press, 1979.

SECTION TWO

Chapter 2: Phenylalanine

Anderson, A. E., Lowering brain phenylalanine levels by giving other large neutral amino acids. *Arch. Neurol.,* 33(10):684–686, 1976.

Armstrong, M. D., and Tyler, F. H., Studies on phenylketonuria. I. Restricted phenylalanine intake in phenylketonuria. *J. Clin. Invest.,* 34:565–580, 1955.

Aspartame. Dept. of Health and Human Services, Public Health Service, Food and Drug Administration. Summary of Commissioner's Decision. 1983.

Aviation, Space and Environmental Medicine. Amino acid excretion in stress, Vol. 177, February 1975.

Balagot, R., Ehrenpreis, S., Kubota, K., and Greenberg, J., Analgesia in mice and humans by D-phenylalanine: relation to inhibition of enkephalin degradation and enkephalin levels. In: *Advances in Pain Research and Therapy.* Bonica, J. J., et al., eds. New York: Raven Press, 1983, 5:289–93.

Beckmann, H., Strauss, M. A., and Ludolph, E., DL-phenylalanine in depressed patients: an open study. *J. Neural Trans.,* 41:123–24, 1977.

Beckmann, H., Athen, D., Oheanu, M., and Zimmer, R., DL-phenylalanine versus imipramine: a double-blind controlled study. *Arch. Psychiat. Nervenkr.,* 227:49–58, 1979.

Biochemical Pharmo., Dopa and dopamine formation from phenylalanine in human brain. 26:900–902, 1977.

Blomquist, H. K., Gustavson, K. H., and Holmgren, G., Severe mental retardation in five siblings due to maternal phenylketonuria. *Neuropediatrics,* 11(3):256–262, 1980.

Blum, K., et al., Enkephalinase Inhibition: regulation of ethanol intake in genetically predisposed mice, *Alcohol,* 4:449, 1987.

Blum, K., et al., Improvement of inpatient treatment of the alcoholic as a function of neurotransmitter restoration: a pilot study. *International Journal of Addictions,* 23:991, 1988.

Blum, K., et al., Enkephalinase inhibition and precursor amino acid loading improves inpatient treatment of alcohol and polydrug abusers: double-blind placebo-controlled study of the nutritional adjunct SAAVE (a REWARD 1 variant). *Alcohol,* 5: 481, 1989.

Brown, R., et al., Neurodynamics of relapse prevention: a neuronutrient approach to outpatient DUI offenders. *Journal of Psychoactive Drugs,* 22:173, 1990.

Blum, K., et al., Reduction of both drug hunger and withdrawal against advice rate of cocaine abusers in a 30 day inpatient treatment program with the neuronutrient Tropamine. *Current Therapeutic Research,* 43: 1204, 1988.

Blum, K., et al., Neuronutrient effects on weight loss on carbohydrate bingers: an open clinical trail. *Current Therapeutic Research,* 48: 217, 1990.

Blum, K., et al., Enkephalinase inhibition and precursor amino acid loading improves inpatient treatment of alcohol and polydrug abusers: double-blind placebo-controlled study of the nutritional adjunct SAAVE (a REWARD 6 variant). *Alcohol,* 5: 481, 1989.

Borison, R. L., Maple, P. J., Havdala, S., and Diamond, B. I., Metabolism of an amino acid with antidepressant properties. *Res. Commun. Chem. Pathol. Pharmacol.,* 21:363–66, 1978.

Boulton, A. A., Trace amines and the neurosciences: an overview. In: *Neurobiology of the Trace Amines.* Boulton, A. A., Baker, G. B., Dewhurst, W. G., and Sandler, M., eds., Clifton, NJ: The Humana Press, 1984.

Boundry, V. A., et al., Agonist and antagonists differentially regulate the high affinity state of the D2L receptor in human embryonic kidney 293 cells. *Molecular Pharmacology,* 48:956, 1995.

Budd, K., Use of D-phenylalanine, an enkephalinase inhibitor, in the treatment of intractable pain. In: *Advances in Pain Research and Therapy.* Bonica, J. J., Liebeskind, J. C., and Albe-Fessard, D. G., eds. New York: Raven Press, 1983, 5:305–308.

Bruckm, A., et al., Positron emission tomography shows that impaired frontal lobe functioning in Parkinson's disease is related to dopaminergic hypofunction in the caudate nucleus. *Neuroscience Letter,* 311(2). 81–4, September 28, 2001.

Carlsson, A., A paradigm shift in brain chemistry. *Science,* 294(5544), 1021–4, November 2001.

Chemistry. Elements in hair provide diagnostic clues: Phenylketonuria (hereditary error in metabolism). Vol. 29, March 1979.

Cheraskin, E., Ringsdorf, W. M., and Medford, F. H., The "ideal" intake of threonine, valine, phenylalanine, leucine, isoleucine, and methionine. *J. Ortho. Psych.,* 7(3):150–155, 1978.

Cho, S., and McDonald, J. D., Effects of maternal blood phenylalanine level on mouse maternal phenylketonuria offspring. *Mol Genet Mebab,* 74(4), 420–5, December 2001.

Comings, D. E., et al., The dopamine D@ receptor (DRD2) gene. A genetic risk factor in smoking. *Pharmacogenetics,* 6:73, 1996.

Couzin, J., Parkinson's disease. Dopamine may sustain toxic protein. *Science,* 294(5545), 1257–8, November 2001.

Defrance, J. F., et al., Enhancement of attention processing by Kantroll (tm) in healthy humans: a pilot study. Electroencephalography, 28:68, 1997.

Di Chiara, G. D., Imperato, A., Drugs abused by human preferentially increase synaptic dopamine concentrations on the mesolimbic system in freely moving rats. *Proceedings of the National Academy of Science* U.S.A., 85:5274, 1988.

Donzelle, G., et al., Curing trial of complicated oncologic pain by D-phenylalanine. *Anesth. Analg.,* 38:655–58, 1981.

Ehrenpreis, S., Balagot, R. C., Comaty, J. E., and Myles, S. B., Naloxone reversible analgesia in mice produced by D-phenylalanine and hydrocinnamic acid, inhibitors of carboxypeptidase. In: *Advances in Pain Research and Therapy.* Bonica, J. J., Liebeskind, J. C., and Albe-Fessard, D. G., eds. New York: Raven Press, 1979, 3:479–488.

Fait, G., et al., High levels of catecholamines in human semen. *Andrologia,* 33(6), 347–50, November 2001.

Fox, A., Phenylalanine: resistance to disease through nutrition. *Let's LIVE,* November 1983, 16–26.

———, and Fox, B., *DLPA: To End Chronic Pain and Depression.* New York: Long Shadow Books, 1985.

Friedman, M., and Gumbmann, M. R., The nutritive value and safety of D-phenylalanine and D-tyrosine in mice. *J. Nutr.,* 114:2089–2096, 1984.

Guroff, G., Effects of inborn errors of metabolism on the nutrition of the brain. In: *Nutrition and the Brain.* Wurtman, R. J., and Wurtman, J. J., eds. New York: Raven Press, 1979, 29–68.

Halbriech, U., et al., Increased imidazoline and alpha2 adrenergic binding in platelets of women with dysphoric premenstrual syndromes. *Biological Psychiatry,* 34:676, 1993.

Halbriech, U., et al., Low plasma gamma-aminobutyric acid levels during the late luteal phase of women with PMDD. *American Journal Psychiatry,* 153:718, 1996.

Harper, B. L., and Morris, D. L., Implications of multiple mechanisms of carcinogenesis for short-term testing. *Teratogenesis, Carcinogenesis, & Mutagenesis,* 4(6):505, 1984.

Harrison, R. E. W., and Christian, S. T., Individual housing stress elevates brain and adrenal tryptamine content. *Neurobiol. Trace Amines,* 249–256, 1984.

Heiblim, D. I., Evans, H. E., Glass, L., and Agbayani, M. M., Amino acid concentrations in cerebrospinal fluid. *Arch. Neurol.*, 35:765–768, 1978.

Heller, B., Pharmacological and clinical effects of DL-phenylalanine in depression and Parkinson's disease. In: *Modern Pharmacology-toxicology, Noncatecholic Phenylethylamines,* Part 1. Mosnaim, A. D., and Wolfe, M. E., eds. New York: Marcel Dekker, 1978, 397–417.

Huxley Institute, *CSF Newsletter.* News Briefs, 11(4), October 1984.

Hyodo, M., Kitade, T., and Hosoka, E., Study on the enhanced analgesic effect induced by phenylalanine during acupuncture analgesia in humans: *Adv. Pain Res. Ther.*, 5:577–582, 1983.

Iwasaki, Y., Sato, H., Ohkubo, A., Sanjo, T., and Tutagawa, S., Effect of spontaneous portal-systemic shunting on plasma insulin and amino acid concentrations. *Gastroenterology*, 78:677–683, 1980.

Jakubovic, A., Psychoactive agents and enkephalin degradation. In: *Endorphins and Opiate Antagonists in Psychiatric Research.* Shah, N.S., and Donald, A.G., eds. New York: Plenum Publishing Corp., 1982, 89–99.

Jones, R. S. G., Trace biogenic amines: a possible functional role in the CNS. *Trends in Pharmacological Sciences,* 4:426–429, 1983.

Juorio, A. V., A possible role for tyramines in brain function and some mental disorders. *Gen. Pharma.,* 13:181–183, 1982.

Lancet. Eat your way to a headache. pp. 1–4, December 1980.

Kaats, G. R., et al., Evidence of chromium picolinate supplementation on body-composition: a randomized double-masked, placebo-controlled study. Current Therapeutic Research, 57:747, 1996.

Lawson, D. H., Stockton, L. H., Bleier, J. C., Acosta, P.B., Heymsfield, S. B., and Nixon, D. W., The effect of a phenylalanine and tyrosine restricted diet on elemental balance studies and plasma aminograms of patients with disseminated malignant melanoma. *Amer. J. Clin. Nutr.,* 41(1):73–84, 1985.

Lofft, J. G., and Bridenbaugh, R. H., The availability of D-phenylalanine and DL-phenylalanine. Letters to the editor, *Am. J. Psychiatr.,* 142(2):269–270, 1985.

Louis, E. D., et al, Clinical correlates of action tremor in Parkinson's disease. *Arch Neurology,* 58(10), 1630–4, October 2001.

Mann, J., Peselow, E. D., Snyderman, S., and Gershon, S., D-Phenyl-alanine in endogenous depression. *Am. J. Psychiatr.,* 137(12):12, 1980.

Marco, C., Alejandre, M. J., Zafra, M. F., Segovia, J. L., and Garcia-Peregrin, E., Induction of experimental phenylketonuria-like conditions in chick embryo. Effect on amino acid concentration in brain, liver and plasma. *Neurochem. Int.,* 6(4):485–489, 1984.

Milner, J. A., Garton, R. L., and Burns, R. A., Phenylalanine and tyrosine requirements of immature beagle dogs. *J. Nutr.,* 114:2212–2216, 1984.

Morgan, M. Y., Milsom, J. P., and Sherlock, S., Plasma ratio of valine, leucine and isoleucine to phenylalanine and tyrosine in liver disease. *Gut* 19:1068–1073, 1978.

Noble, E. P., et al., D2 dopamine receptor gene and cigarette smoking: a reward gene? *Medical Hypotheses,* 42:257, 1994.

Nutrition Action. The aspartame debate. May 1984.

Nutrition Reviews. The dietary treatment of phenylketonuria. 41(1):11–14, 1983.

————, Phenylalanine-tyrosine conversion in 1 hour in 18 families with one or more non-specific retarded children. 37(7):217, 1979.

Nutrition Week. Food industry funds aspartame studies. April 12, 1984.

Nutzenadel, W., Fahr. K., and Lutz, P., Absorption of free and peptide-linked glycine and phenylalanine in children with active celiac disease. *Pediatr. Res.,* 15:309–312, 1981.

Portoles, M., Minana, M. D., Jorda, A., and Grisolia, S., Caffeine intake lowers the level of phenylalanine, tyrosine and thyroid hormones in rat plasma. *IRCS Med. Sci.,* 12:1002–1003, 1984.

Rapkin, A., et al., Trytophan loading test in premenstrual syndrome. *Journal Obstetrics & Gynecology,* 10:140, 1989.

Ratzmann, G. W., Grimm, U., Jahrig, K., and Knapp, A., On the brain barrier system function and changes of cerebrospinal fluid concentrations of phenylalanine and tyrosine in human phenylketonuria. *Biomed. Biochim. Acta,* 43(2):197–204, 1984.

Robinson, N., and Williams, C. B., Amino acids in human brain. *Clin. Chim. Acta,* 12:311–317, 1965.

Sabelli, H. C., Gut flora and urinary phenylacetic acid. *Science,* 226(11):996, 1984.

Satou, T., et al., The prevention of pneumonia in the elderly by dopamine agonists. *Nippon Ronen Igakkai Zasshi,* 38(6), 778–9, November 2001.

Schuett, V. E., and Brown, E. S., Diet policies of PKU clinics in the United States. *Amer. J. Public Health,* 74(5):501–502, 1984.

Searle Food Resources, Inc. Safety studies bibliography for aspartame, September 1983.

Seppala, T., Linnoila, M., Sondergaard, I., Elonen, E., and Mattila, M. J., Tyramine pressor test and cardiovascular effects of chlorimipramine and nortriptyline in healthy volunteers. *Bio. Psych.,* 16(1):71, 1981.

Shen, R. S., and Abell, C. W., Phenylketonuria: a new method for the simultaneous determination of plasma phenylalanine and tyrosine. *Science,* 197(8):665–667, 1977.

Smith, R. J., Aspartame approved despite risks. *Science,* 213:986–987, August 1981.

Spitz M. R., et al., Case-control study of the dopamine receptor gene and smoking status on lung cancer patients. *Journal of the National Cancer Institute,* 90:358, 1998.

Swaiman, K. F., Menkes, J. H., DeVivo, D. C., and Prensky, A. L., Metabolic disorders of the central nervous system. In: *The Practice of Pediatric Neurology.* New York: C.V. Mosby Co., 1982, 472–513.

Tews, J. K., Carter, S. H., Roa, P. D., and Stone, W. E., Free amino acids and related compounds in dog brain: post-mortem and anoxic changes, effects of ammonium chloride infusion, and levels during seizures induced by picrotoxin and by pentylenetetrazol. *J. Neurochem.,* 10:641–653, 1963.

Thanos, P. K., et al., Over expression of the D2 receptors reduces alcohol self-administration. *Journal of Neurochemistry,* 78:1094, 2001.

Walsh, D. A., and Christian, Z. H., The effects of phenylalanine on cultured rat embryos. *Teratogenesis, Carcinogenesis, & Mutagenesis,* 4:505–513, 1984.

Wannemacher, R. W., Klainer, A. S., Dinterman, R. E., and Beisel, W. R., The significance and mechanism of an increased serum phenylalanine-tyrosine ratio during infection. *Amer. J. Clin. Nutr.,* 29:997–1006, 1976.

Williams, C. M., Couch, M. W., and Midgley, J. M., Natural occurrence and metabolism of the isomeric octapamines and synephrines. In: *Neurobiology of the Trace Amines.* Boulton, A. A., Baker, G. B., Dewhurst, W. G., and Sandler, M., eds. Clifton, NJ: Humana Press, 1984, 97–106.

Wood, D. R., et al., Treatment of attention deficit disorder with DL-phenylalanine. *Psychiatric Research,* 16:21, 1985.

Yaryura-Tobias, J. A., Heller, B., Spatz, H., and Fischer, E., Phenylalanine for endogenous depression. *J. Ortho. Psych.,* 3(2):80–81, 1974.

Yokogoshi, H., Roberts, C. H., Caballero, B., and Wurtman, R. J., Effects of aspartame and glucose administration on brain and plasma levels of large neutral amino acids and brain 5-hydroxyindoles. *Amer. J. Clin. Nutr.,* 40:1–7, 1984.

Yonkers, K. A., et al., Sertraline as a treatment for premenstrual dysphoric syndrome. *Psychopharmacology Bulletin,* 32:411996.

Yonkers, K. A., The association between premenstrual dysphoric disorder and other mood disorders. *Journal of Clinical Psychiatry,* 58(supplement 15):19, 1997.

Zioudrou, C., and Klee, W. A., Possible roles of peptides derived from food proteins in brain function. In: *Nutrition and the Brain.* Wurtman, R. J., and Wurtman, J. J., eds. New York: Raven Press, 1979.

Chapter 3: Tyrosine

Ablett, R. F., MacMillan, M., Sole, M. J., Toal, C. B., and Anderson, G. H., Free tyrosine levels of rat brain and tissues with sympathetic innervations following administration of L-tyrosine in the presence and absence of large neutral amino acids. *J. Nutr.,* 114:835–839, 1984.

Agharanya, J. C., Alonso, R., and Wurtman, R. J., Changes in catecholamine excretion after short-term tyrosine ingestion in normally fed human subjects. *Amer. J. Clin. Nutr.,* 34:82–87, 1981.

All-Ericsson, C., et al., Insulin-like growth factor-1 receptor in uveal melanoma: a predictor for metastatic disease and a potential therapeutic target. *Invest Ophthalmology Visual Science,* 43(1), 1–8, January 2002.

Alonso, R., Agharanya, J. C., and Wurtman, R. J., Tyrosine loading enhances catecholamine excretion. *J. Neural Transmis.,* 49:31–43, 1980.

Amer. J. Clin. Nutr. The case for and against regulating the protein quality of meat, poultry, and their products. 40:675–684, 1984.

Anderson, G. M., Gerner, R. H., Cohen, D. J., and Fairbanks, L., Central tryptamine turnover in depression, schizophrenia, and anorexia: measurement of indoleacetic acid in cerebrospinal fluid. *Biol. Psych.,* 19(10):1427, 1984.

Anton, A. H., Crumrine, R. S., Stern, R. C., and Izant, R. J., Inhibition of catecholamine biosynthesis by carbidopa and metyrosine in neuroblastoma. *Ped. Pharmac.,* 3:107–117, 1983.

Bennet, W. M., Connacher, A. A., Jung, R. T., et al., Effects of insulin and amino acids on leg protein turnover in IDDM patients. *Diabetes,* 40(4), April 1991.

Benoit, R. M., Eiseman, J., Jacobs, S. C., et al., Reversion of human prostate tumorigenic growth by azatyrosine. *Current Contents,* Comment, 23(40), October 2, 1995.

Bere, A., and Helene, C., Binding of copper and zinc ions to polypeptides containing glutamic acid and tyrosine residues. *Int. J. Biolog. Macromolecules,* Vol. 1, 227–232, 1979.

Boyd, A. E., Leibovitz, B. E., and Pfeiffer, J. B., Stimulation of human-growth hormone secretion by L-dopa. *New Engl. J. Med.,* 283:1425–1429, 1970.

Cahill, A. L., and Ehret, C. F., Circadian variations in the activity of tyrosine hydroxylase, tyrosine aminotransferase, and tryptophan hydroxylase: relationship to catecholamine metabolism. *J. Neurochem.*, 37(5): 1109–1115, 1981.

Carranza, D., Coto, F., Quirce, C. H., Odio, M., and Maickel, R. P., Differential effects of L-tyrosine and L-tryptophan on stress induced alterations in adrenocortical function in rats. *Pharmacologist*, 22:3, 1980.

Clark, J. T., Smith, E. R., and Davidson, J. M., Enhancement of sexual motivation in male rats by yohimbine. *Science*, 225:847–848, 1984.

Clinical Psychiatry News. Biochemical tests may become basic in diagnosing depression. Vol. 6. No. 6, 1, 58, 1976.

Conlay, L. A., Tyrosine administration decreases vulnerability to ventricular fibrillation in the normal canine heart. *Science*, 211:727, February 1981.

———, Tyrosine increases blood pressure in hypotensive rats. *Science*, 212:559–560, May 1981.

———, Maher, T. J., and Wurtman, R. J., Tyrosine's pressor effect in hypotensive rats is not mediated by tyramine. *Life Sci.*, 35:1207–1212, 1984.

Cotzias, G. C., Miller, S. T., Nicholson, A. R., Maston, W. H., and Tang, L. C., Prolongation of the life-span in mice adapted to large amounts of L-dopa. *Proc. Nat. Acad. Sci.*, 71(6):2466–2469, June 1974.

———, Papavasiliou, P. S., and Gellene, R., Modification of Parkinsonism—chronic treatment with L-dopa. *New Engl. J. Med.*, 280(7):337–345, February 1969.

———, Miller, S. T., Tang, L. C., and Papavasiliou, P. S., Levodopa, fertility, and longevity. *Science*, 196:549–550, April 29, 1977.

Dasgupta, J. D., Swarup, G., and Garbers, D. L., Tyrosine protein kinase activity in normal rat tissues: brain. *Advances in Cyclic Nucleotide & Protein Phosphorylation Res.*, 17:461–470, 1984.

Della-Fera, M. A., Experimental phenylketonuria: replacement of carboxyl terminal tyrosine by phenylalanine in infant rat brain tubulin. *Science*, 206:463–464, 1979.

Denis, L., et al., Diet and its preventive role in prostatic disease. *European Urology*, 35(5–6), 377–87, 1999.

Druml, W., Hubl, W., Roth, E., et al., Utilization of tyrosine-containing dipeptides and N-acetyl-tyrosine in hepatic failure. *Current Contents*, 21(4), April 1995.

Fitzgerald, M., McIntosh, N., and Rieder, M. J., Plasma amino acids in adolescents and adults with phenylketonuria on three different levels of protein intake. Pain and analgesia in the newborn. *Arch. Dis. Child.*, 64:441–443, 1989, *N. Engl. J. Med.*, 1990, Letter to the Editor, 323:1205, 1990.

Friedman, M., and Gumbmann, M. R., The nutritive value and safety of D-phenylalanine and D-tyrosine in mice. *J. Nutr.*, 114:2089–2096, 1984.

Furst, P., Conditionally indispensable amino acids (glutamine, cysteine, tyrosine, arginine, ornithine, taurine) in enteral feeding and dipeptide concept. *Nestle Nutritional Workshop Ser Clinical Performance Program*, 3, 199–217, 2000.

Gadisseux, P., Ward, J. D., Young, H. F., and Becker, D. P., Nutrition and the neurosurgical patient. *J. Neurosurg.*, 60:219–232, 1984.

Gelenberg, A. J., and Wurtman, R. J., L-tyrosine in depression. *Lancet*, October, 1980.

——, Wojcik, J. D., Gibson, C. J., and Wurtman, R. J., Tyrosine for depression. *J. Psychiat. Res.,* 17(2):175–180, 1982–83.

Gerdes, A. M., Nielsen, J. B., Lou, H., et al., Plasma amino acids in term neonates and infants with phenylketonuria before and after institution of the diet. *Acta. Paediatr. Scand.,* 79:64–68, 1990.

Goldberg, I. K., L-tyrosine in depression. *Lancet,* August, 1980.

Goodnick, P. J., Evans, H. E., Dunner, D. L., and Fieve, R. R., Amino acid concentrations in cerebrospinal fluid: effects of aging, depression and probenecid. *Biol. Psych.,* 15(4):557–563, 1980.

Guidosti, A., Gale, K., Toffano, G., and Vargas, F. M., Tolerance to tyrosine hydroxylase activation in N. accumbens and C. striatum after repeated injections of "classical" and "atypical" antischizophrenic drugs. *Life Sci.,* 23:501–506, 1978.

Guroff, G., Effects of inborn errors of metabolism on the nutrition of the brain. In: *Nutrition and the Brain,* Vol. 4, Wurtman, R. J., and Wurtman, J. J., eds. New York: Raven Press, 1979.

Harris, A., and Pathe, G., Effect of L-tyrosine and exercise on eating behavior. *J. Amer. Col. Nutr.,* 1983.

Harrison, R. E. W., and Christian, S. T., Individual housing stress elevates brain and adrenal tryptamine content. *Neurobiology of the Trace Amines,* Boulton, A.A., et al., eds. Clifton, NJ: Humana Press, 1984, 249–255.

Heiblim, D. I., Evans, H. E., Glass, L., and Agbayani, M. M., Amino acid concentrations in cerebrospinal fluid. *Arch. Neurol.,* 35:765–768, 1978.

Heird, W. C., Dell, R. B., Driscoll, J. H., Grebin, B., and Winters, R. W., Metabolic acidosis resulting from the intravenous alimentation mixtures containing synthetic amino acids. *New Engl. J. Med.,* 287(19):943–948, 1972.

Hermann, M. E., Monch, E., Reinbacher, M., et al., Phenylalaninfreie aminosaurenmischung: Stoffwechselwirkung in abhangigkeit von der einzeldosis. *Monatsschr. Kinderheilkd,* 139: 670–675, 1991.

Horne, M. K., Cheng, C. H., and Wooten, G. F., The cerebral metabolism of L-dihydroxyphenylalanine. *Pharmacol.,* 28:12–26, 1984.

Hughes, E. C., Weinstein, R. C., Gott, P., and Pingelli, R., *Hyposensitivity Diets for the Diagnosis and Management of Sensitivity to Foods.* Los Angeles, CA: Depts. of Otolaryngology and Neurology, LAC-USC Med. Ctr. and School of Med., U. of Southern California, 1984.

Kaneyuki, T., Morimasa, T., and Shohmori, T., Relationship of tyrosine concentration to catecholamine levels in rat brain. *Acta Med. Okayama,* 38(4):403–407, 1984.

King, R. A., and Olds, D. P., Tyrosine uptake in normal and albino hair bulbs. *Arch. Dermatol. Res.,* 276:313–316, 1984.

Krieger, D. T., and Martin, J. B., Brain peptides. *New Engl. J. Med.,* pp. 876–885, April, 1981.

Lefebure, B., Castot, A., Danan, G., Elmalem, J., Jean-Pastor, M. J., and Efthymiou, M. L., Antidepressant-induced hepatitis: a report of 91 cases. *Therapie,* 39(5):509–516, 1984.

Mackey, S. A., and Berlin, Jr., C. M., Effect of dietary aspartame on plasma concentrations of phenylalanine and tyrosine in normal and homozygous phenylketonuric patients. Department of Pediatrics, Milton S. Hershey Medical Center, Pennsylvania State University, Hershey, PA.

Maes, M., Jacobs, M. P., Suy, E., et al., Suppressant effects of dexamethasone on the availability of plasma L-tryptophan and tyrosine in healthy controls and in depressed patients. *Acta. Psychiatr. Scand.,* 81:199–223, 1990.

Mandell, A. J., Redundant mechanisms regulating brain tyrosine and tryptophan hydroxylases. *Ann. Rev. Pharmacol. Toxicol.,* 18:461–493, 1978.

Markianos, M., and Tripodianakis, J., Low plasma dopamine-B-hydroxylase in demented schizophrenics. *Biol. Psychiatry,* 20:94–119, 1985.

Markovitz, D. C., and Fernstrom, J. D., Diet and uptake of aldomet by the brain: competition with natural large neutral amino acids. *Science,* 197:1013–1015, 1977.

Masse, P.G., et al., Testing the tyrosine/ catecholamine hypothesis of oral contraceptive-induced psychological side-effect. *Ann Nutrition Metabolism,* 45(3), 102–9, 2001.

McCabe, E. R. B., and McCabe, L., Issues in the dietary management of phenylketonuria: breast-feeding and trace-metal nutriture. B. F. Stolinsky Research Laboratories Department of Pediatrics, University of Colorado Health Sciences Center, Denver, CO.

Miranda, M., Botti, D., and Di Cola, M., Possible genotoxity of melanin synthesis intermediates: tyrosinase reaction products interact with DNA *in vitro. Mol. Gen. Genet.,* 193:395–399, 1984.

Morre, M. C., Hefti, F., and Wurtman, R. J., Regional tyrosine levels in rat brain after tyrosine administration. *J. Neural Transmis.,* 49:45–50, 1980.

Nutrition Reviews. Amniotic fluid protein: a nutritional function. 11:341–344, 1976.

Neurogenesis, Inc. Neurotransmitter precursor amino acids and vitamins.

Papkoff, H., Murthy, H. M. S., and Roser, J. F., Effect of tyrosine modification on the biological and immunological properties of equine chorionic gonadotropin. *Proc. Soc. Exper. Bio. Med.,* 177:42–46, 1984.

Pardridge, R., Regulation of amino acid availability to the brain. In: *Nutrition and the Brain,* Wurtman, R. J., and Wurtman, J. J., eds. New York: Raven Press, 1977, 141–204.

Pfeiffer, C. C., and Braverman, E. R., Folic acid and vitamin B12 therapy for the low-histamine high-copper biotype of schizophrenia. In: *Folic Acid in Neurology, Psychiatry, and Internal Medicine,* Botez, M. I., and Reynolds, E. H., eds. New York: Raven Press, 1979, 483–488.

Portoles, M., Minana, M.-D., Jorda, A., and Grisolia, S., Caffeine intake lowers the level of phenylalanine, tyrosine and thyroid hormones in rat plasma. *IRCS Med. Sci.,* 12:1002–1003, 1984.

Potocnik, U., and Widhalm, K., Long-term follow-up of children with classical phenylketonuria after diet discontinuation: A review. *Am. Col. Nutr.* 13(3): 232–236, 1994.

Quirce, C. M., and Odio, M., L-tyrosine alters chronic restraint-induced elevations in rat biogenic amines and peripheral stress markers. *Pharmacologist,* 22:3, 1980.

Rajfer, S. I., Anton, A. H., Rossen, J. C., and Goldberg, L.I., Beneficial hemodynamic effects of oral levodopa in heart failure. *New Eng. J. Med.,* 310:1357–1362, 1984.

Reeves, P. G., and O'Dell, B. L., The effect of dietary tyrosine levels on food intake in zinc-deficient rats. *J. Nutr.,* 114:761–767, 1984.

Reinstein, D. K., Lehnert, H., and Wurtman, R. J., Neurochemical and behavioral consequences of stress: effects of dietary tyrosine. *J. Amer. Col. Nutr.,* 3(3), 1984.

Robinson, R., and Williams, C. B., Amino acids in human brain. *Clin. Chim. Acta,* 12:311–317, 1965.

Seshia, S. S., Perry, T. L., Dakshinamurti, K., and Snodgrass, P. J., Tyrosinemia and intractable seizures. *Epilepsia,* 25(4):457–463, 1984.

Shetty, P. S., Jung, R. T., and James, W. P. T., Effect of catecholamine replacement with levodopa on the metabolic response to semi starvation. *Lancet,* pp. 77–79, January 1979.

Stoerner, J. W., Butler, I. J., Morriss, F. H., Howell, R., Seifert, W. E., Caprioli, R. M., Adcock, E. W., and Denson, S. E., CSF neurotransmitter studies. *Am. J. Dis. Child,* 134:492–494, 1980.

Takahashi, Y., Kipnis, D. M., and Daughaday, W. H., Growth hormone secretion during sleep. *J. Clin. Invest.,* 47:2079–2090, 1968.

Tews, J. K., Carter, S. H., Roa, P. D., and Stone, W. E., Free amino acids and related compounds in dog brain: post-mortem and anoxic changes, effects of ammonium chloride infusion, and levels during seizures induced by picrotoxin and by pentylenetetrazol. *J. Neurochem.,* 10:641–653, 1963.

Thurmond, J. B., and Brown, J. W., Effect of brain monoamine precursors on stress-induced behavioral and neurochemical changes in aged mice. *Brain Res.,* 93–102, 1984.

Undenfriend, S., Factors in amino acid metabolism which can influence the central nervous system. *Amer. J. Clin. Nutr.,* 12:287–290, April 1963.

van der Kolk, B., Greenberg, M., Boyd, H., and Krystal, J., Inescapable shock, neurotransmitters, and addiction to trauma: toward a psychobiology of post traumatic stress. *Biol. Psych.,* 20:314–325, 1985.

Wagernmakers, A.J., Amino acids supplements to improve athletic performance. *Current Opinion and Clinical Nutrition Metabolism Care,* 2(6), 539–44, November 1999.

Weisburd, S., Food for mind and mood. *Science News,* 125:216–218, April 7, 1984.

Weldon, V. V., Gupta, S. K., Klingensmith, G., Clarke, W. L., Duck, S. C., and Haymond, M. W., Evaluation of growth hormone release in children using arginine and L-dopa in combination. *J. Ped.,* 87(4):540–544, 1975.

Wilcox, M., and Franceshini, N., Illumination induces dye incorporation in photoreceptor cells. *Science,* 225:851–853, August, 1984.

Yu, S., Effects of low levels of dietary tyrosine on the hair color of cats. *Journal Small Animal Practice,* 42(4), 447–63, April 2001.

Chapter 4: Tryptophan

Abbar, M., et al., Suicide attempts and the tryptophan hydroxylase gene. *Molecular Psychiatry,* 6(3), 268–73, May 2001.

Agarwal, D. P., Ziemsen, B., Goedde, H. W., Philippu, G., Milech, U., and Schrappe, O., Free and bound plasma tryptophan levels in psychiatric disorders. In: *Progress in Tryptophan and Serotonin Research,* Schlossberger, H. G., Kochen, W., Linzen, B., and Steinhart, H., eds. Berlin: Walter de Gruyter,1984, 391–396.

Allegri, G., Angi, M. R., Costa, C., and Bettero, A., Tryptophan and kynurenine in senile cataract. In: *Progress in Tryptophan and Serotonin Research,* 469–472.

Anderson, G. M., Feibel, F. C., Wetlaufer, L. A., et al., Effect of a meal on human whole blood serotonin. *Gastroenterology,* 88:86–89, 1985.

Anderson, L. E., Morris, J. E., Sasser, L. B., Loscher, W., Effects of 50- or 60-hertz, 100 micro T magnetic field exposure in the DMBA mammary cancer model in Sprague-Dawley rats: possible explanations for different results from two laboratories. *Environ Health Perspect.,* 108(9):797–802, September 2000.

Anderson, R. A., Lincoln, G. A., and Wu, F. C. W., Melatonin potentiates testosterone-induced suppression of luteinizing hormone secretion in normal men. *Current Contents, Comment,* 22(1), January 3, 1994.

Anderson, S. A., and Raiten, D. J., Safety of amino acids used as dietary supplements. Bethesda, MD, July 1992.

Asberg, M., Bertilsson, L., Tuck, D., Cronholm, B., and Sjoqvist, F., Indoleamine metabolites in the cerebrospinal fluid of depressed patients before and during treatment with nortriptyline. *Clin. Pharm. Ther.*, 14(2), 277–286, 1973.

Ashley, D. V., Fleury, M., Hardwick, S., Leathwood, P. D., and Moennoz, D., Effects of large neutral amino acids on tryptophan transport into the brain during development. In: *Progress in Tryptophan and Serotonin Research*, pp. 583–586.

——, Finot, P. A., and Liardon, R., Contribution of exogenous N-15-tryptophan to plasma and red blood cell tryptophan and kynurenine in healthy humans. In: *Progress in Tryptophan and Serotonin Research*, pp. 587–590.

Aviram, A., and Gulyassay, P. F., Impaired absorption of tryptophan in uremia. *Harefuah*, 79:114–117, 1970.

Axford, S., Mutton, O., and Adams, A., Beyond pumpkin seeds. St. Andrew's Hospital, Thorpe, Norwich, UK, NR7 OSS.

Azad, K. A., et al., Vegetarian diet in the treatment of fibromyalgia. *Bangladesh Medical Res. Counc. Bull.*, 26(2), 41–7, August 2000.

Bachmann, C., and Colombo, J., Increased tryptophan uptake into the brain in hyperammonemia. *Life Sci.*, 33:2417–2424, 1983.

Bagiella, E., Cairella, M., Del Ben, M., et al., Changes in attitude toward food by obese patients treated with placebo and serotoninergic agents. *Cur. Ther. Res.*, 50(2), August 1991.

Barr, L. C., Goodman, W. K., McDougle, C. J., et al., Tryptophan depletion in patients with obsessive-compulsive disorder who respond to serotonin reuptake inhibitors. *Arch. Gen. Psychiatry* (U.S.), 51(4):309–317, April 1994.

Bassant, M. H., Fage, D., Dedek, J., Cathala, F., Court, L., and Scatton, B., Monoamine abnormalities in the brain of scrapie-infected rats. *Brain Res.*, 308:182–185, 1984.

Baumann, P., and Gaillard, M., Insulin coma therapy: decrease of plasma tryptophan in man. *J. Neural. Transmis.*, 39:309–313, 1976.

Baumgarten, H. G., and Schlossberger, H. G., Anatomy and function of central serotonergic neurons. In: *Progress in Tryptophan and Serotonin Research*, pp. 173–188.

Beasley, B. L., Nutt, J. G., Davenport, R. W., and Chase, T. N., Treatment with tryptophan of levodopa-associated psychiatric disturbances. *Arch. Neurol.*, 37(3):155–156, 1980.

Bender, D. A., Effects of oestrogens on the metabolism of tryptophan—implications for the interpretation of the tryptophan load test for vitamin B6 nutritional status. In: *Progress in Tryptophan and Serotonin Research*, pp. 637–640.

Benkelfat, C., Ellenbogen, M. A., Dean, P., et al., Mood-lowering effect of tryptophan depletion. *Arch. Gen. Psychiatry*, 51:687–697, 1994.

Bhagavan, H., An interview. *Am. J. Psychiatry*, 6(4):317–326, 1977.

Bhajan, Y., Solving sleep problems with melatonin. *Nutrition News*, 1973.

Biesalski, H. K., Free radical theory of aging. *Curr. Opin. Clin. Nutr. Metab. Care*, 5(1), 5–10, January 2002.

Biology., *Science News*, Vol. 144, 1993.

Blazejova, K., Nevsimalova, S., Illnerova, H., Hajek, I., Sonka, K., Sleep disorders and the 24-hour profile of melatonin and cortisol. *Sb. Lek.*, 101(4), 347–51, Czech., 2000.

Braverman, E. R., and Pfeiffer, C. C., Suicide and biochemistry. *Biol. Psych.,* 20:123–124, 1985.

Broderick, P. A., and Bridger, W. M., A comparative study of the effect of L-tryptophan and its acetylated derivative N-acetyl-L-tryptophan on rat muricidal behavior. *Biol. Psych.,* 19(1):89–94, 1984.

Brotto, L. A., Gorzalka, B. B., LaMarre, A. K., Melatonin protects against the effects of chronic stress on sexual behavior in male rats. *Neuroreport,* 12(16), 3465–9, November 16, 2001.

Brown, G. M., Melatonin in psychiatric and sleep disorders. *CNS Drugs,* 3(3):209–226, 1995.

Brugger, P., Marktl, W., and Herold, M., Impaired nocturnal secretion of melatonin in coronary heart disease. *Lancet,* 345:1408, 1995.

Bunce, G. E., Hess, J. L., and Davis, D., Cataract formation following limited amino acid intake during gestation and lactation. *Society Exper. Biol. Med.,* 176:485–489, 1984.

Burrors, M., As L-tryptophan illustrates, taking dietary supplements is chancy. *The New York Times,* December 20, 1989.

Byerley, W. F., Judd, L. L., Reimherr, F. W., et al., 5-Hydroxytryptophan: a review of its antidepressant efficacy and adverse effects. *J. Clin. Psychopharmacology,* 7(3), 1987.

———, and Risch, S. C., Depression and serotonin metabolism: rationale for neurotransmitter precursor treatment. *J. Clin. Psychopharmacology,* 5(4), 1985.

Caroleo, M.C., Frasca, D., Nistico, G., et al., Melatonin as immunomodulator in immunodeficient mice. *Immunopharmacology,* 23(2):81–89, March–April 1992. ISSN 0162–3109, Journal Code: GY3.

Chadwick, C., Phipps, D. A., and Powell, C., Serum tryptophan and cataract. *Lancet,* 1981.

Charney, D. S., Henninger, G. R., Reinhard, J. F., Sternberg, D.-E., and Hafstead, K. M., The effect of IV L-tryptophan on prolactin, growth hormones and mood in healthy subjects. *Psychopharmacology,* 78:38–45, 1982.

Chiancone, F. M., Il metabolismo triptofano-acido icotinico nelle malattie psichiatriche. *Acta Vitam. et Enzym.,* XXII (3–4): 111–134.

Childs, P. A., Rodin, I., Martin, N. J., et al., Effect of fluoxetine on melatonin in patients with seasonal affective disorder and matched controls. *Brit. J. Psychiatry,* 166:196–198, 1995.

Chouinard, G., Young, S. N., Annabelle, L., Sourkes, T. L., and Kiriakos, R. Z., Tryptophan-nicotinamide combination in the treatment of newly admitted depressed patients. *Commun. in Psych.,* 2:311–318, 1978.

———, Lawrence, A., Young, S. N., and Sourkes, T. L., A controlled study of tryptophan-benserazide in schizophrenia. *Commun. in Psych.,* 2:21–31, 1978.

Christensen, H. N., Implications of the cellular transport step for amino acid metabolism. *Nutrition Reviews,* 35(6):129–133, 1977.

Christian and Pegram, DMT: Clue to insomnia. *Med. World News.* October 17, 1977, p. 93.

Cleare, A. J., and Bond, A. J., Effects of alterations in plasma tryptophan levels on aggressive feelings. *Arch. Gen. Psychiatry* (U.S.), 51(12):1004–1005, 1994.

Cooper, A. J., Tryptophan antidepressant "physiological sedative": fact or fancy? *Psychopharmacology,* 61:97–102, 1979.

Coppen, A., Eccleston, E. G., and Peet, M., Plasma tryptophan binding and depression. *Advances in Bioch. Psychopharm.,* 11:325–333, 1974.

Coppen, A. J., Gupta, R. K., Eccleston, E. G., Wood, K. M., Wakeling, A., and De Sousa, V. F. A., Plasma-tryptophan in anorexia nervosa. *The Lancet,* May 1, 1976.

————, and Wood, K., Total and non-bound plasma-tryptophan in depressive illness. *Lancet,* 1977.

Cos, S., and Blask, D. E., Melatonin modulates growth factor activity in MCD-7 human breast cancer cells. *USA J. Pineal Research,* 17:1, 25–32, August 1994.

Coscina, D. V., and Stancer, H. C., Selective blockade of hypothalamic hyperphagia and obesity in rats by serotonin-depleting midbrain lesions. *Science,* 195:415–417, 1977.

Cowley, G., Melatonin. *Newsweek,* August 7, 1995.

Curzon, G., Ettlinger, G., Cole, M., and Walsh, J., The biochemical, behavioral, and neurologic effects of high L-tryptophan intake in the rhesus monkey. *Neurology,* 13(5), 431–438, 1963.

————, Kantamaneni, B. D., Lader, M. H.. and Greenwood, M.-H., Tryptophan disposition in psychiatric patients before and after stress. *Psych. Med.,* 9:457–463, 1979.

Dam, H., Mellerup, E. T., and Rafaelsen, O. J., Diurnal variation of total plasma tryptophan in depressive patients. *Acta Psychiat. Scand.,* 69:190–196, 1984.

D'Elia, G., Lehmann, J., and Raotma, H., Evaluation of the combination of tryptophan and ECT in the treatment of depression. *Acta Psychiat. Scand.,* 56:303–318, 1977.

————, Lehmann, J., and Raotma, H., Evaluation of the combination of tryptophan and ECT in the treatment of depression. *Biochem. Anal. Acta Psychiat. Scand.,* 56:319–334, 1977.

de Montis, M. G., Olianas, M. C., Mulas, G., and Tagliamonte, A., Evidence that only free serum tryptophan exchanges with the brain. *Pharm. Res. Commun.,* 9, 2, 1977.

Dennery, P. A., Melatonin: the next panacea? *Pediatr Res.,* 50(6), 680, December 2001.

Donald, E. A., and Bosse, The vitamin B6 requirement in oral contraceptive users. Assessment by tryptophan metabolites, vitamin B6, and pyridoxic acid levels in urine. *Amer. J. Clin. Nutr.,* 32:1024–1032, 1979.

Donaldson, T., Klatz, R., Denckla, W. D., et al., Melatonin and breast cancer. *Life Extension Report,* 13(5), April, 1993.

Effect of drugs on melatonin. *CNS Drugs,* 3(3):213, 1995.

Evans, G. W., Normal and abnormal zinc absorption in man and animals: the tryptophan connection. *Nut. Reviews,* 38:137–141, 1980.

Evers, B. M., Hurlbut, S. C., Tyring, S. K., et al., Novel therapy for the treatment of human carcinoid. *Ann. Surg.,* 213(5):411–416, May 1991.

Eynard, N., Flachaire, E., Lestra, C., et al., Platelet serotonin and free and total plasma tryptophan in healthy volunteers during 24 hours. *Clin. Chem.* (U.S.), 39 (11, pt. 1): 2337–2340, 1993.

Farkas, T., Dunner, D. L., and Fieve, R. R., L-tryptophan in depression. *Biol. Psych.,* 11(3), 1976.

FDA widens its recall of L-tryptophan. *The New York Times,* March 23, 1990.

Feltkamp, H., Meurer, K. A., and Godehardt, E., Tryptophan-induced lowering of blood pressure and changes in serotonin uptake by platelets in patients with essential hypertension. *Klinische Wochenschrift,* 62(23): 1115–1119, 1984.

Fernstrom, J. D., Tryptophan availability and serotonin synthesis in rat brain—effects of experimental diabetes. In: *Progress in Tryptophan and Serotonin Research,* pp. 161–172.

————, and Wurtman, R. J., Brain serotonin content: physiological dependence on plasma tryptophan levels. *Science,* 173:149–151, 1971.

————, and Lytle, L. D., Corn malnutrition, brain serotonin and behavior. *Nutr. Reviews,* 34(9), 1976.

Fishlock, D., Glaucoma: a treatment without tears. *Financial Times,* 17(1):19, 1979.

Flannery, M. T., Wallach, P. M., Espinoza, L. R., et al., A case of the eosinophilia-myalgia syndrome associated with use of an L-tryptophan product. *Ann. Int. Med.,* 112:300–301, 1990.

Fontenot, J. M., and Levine, S. A., Melatonin deficiency: its role in oncogenesis and age-related pathology. *J. Orthomol. Med.,* 5(1), 1990.

Friedman, M., Nielsen, H. K., Steinhart, H., Bechandersen, S., Geeraerts, F., Schimpfessel, L., and Crokaert, R., The *in vivo* effect of sodium fluoride on the key enzymes of tryptophan metabolism. In: *Progress in Tryptophan and Serotonin Research,* pp. 677–680.

Fujii, E., Nomoto, T., and Muraki, T., Effects of two 5-hydroxytryptamine agonists on head-weaving behavior in streptozotocin-diabetic mice. *Diabetologia,* 34:537–541, 1991.

Fujiki, H., Suganuma, M., Tahira, T., Esumi, M., Nagao, M., Wakabayashi, K., and Sugimura, T., New biological significance of indole-containing compounds as initiators or tumor promoters in chemical carcinogenesis. In: *Progress in Tryptophan and Serotonin Research.*

Furst, P., Guarnieri, G., and Hultman, E., The effect of the administration of L-tryptophan on synthesis of urea and gluconeogenesis in man. *Scandi. J. Clin. Lab. Investigation,* 127(2), 183–191, 1971.

Gagnier, J.J., The therapeutic potential of melatonin in migraines and other headache types. *Altern. Med. Rev.,* 6:383–389, 2001.

Gal, E. M., Hydroxylation of tryptophan and its control in brain. *Pav. J. Biol. Sci.,* 10(3):145–160, 1975.

Garcia, J. J., Reiter, R. J., Karbownik, M., Calvo, J. R., Ortiz, G. G., Tan, D. X., Martinez-Ballarin, E., Acuna-Castroviejo, D., N-acetylserotonin suppresses hepatic microsomal membrane rigidity associated with lipid peroxidation. *Eur. J. Pharmacol.,* 428(2), 403–12, October 5, 2001.

Geeraerts, F., Schimpfessel, L., and Crokaert, R., The *in vivo* effect of sodium fluoride on the key enzymes of tryptophan metabolism. In: *Progress in Tryptophan and Serotonin Research.*

Gibbons, J. L., Barr, G. A., Bridger, W. H., and Leibowitz, S. F., Manipulations of dietary tryptophan: effects on mouse killing and brain serotonin in the rat. *Brain Res.,* 169:139–153, 1979.

Gilka, L., Schizophrenia: a disorder of tryptophan metabolism. *Acta Psychiat. Scand.,* Suppl. 258, 16–82, 1975.

Gillman, P. K., Bartlett, J. R., Bridges, P. K., Kantamaneni, B.-D., and Curzon, G., Relationships between tryptophan concentrations in human plasma, cerebrospinal fluid and cerebral cortex following tryptophan infusion. *Neuropharmacology,* 19:1241–1242, 1980.

Giraldi, T., Perissin, L., Zorzet, S., et al., Stress, melatonin, and tumor progression in mice. *Ann. NY Acad. Sci.,* 719:526–536, 1994.

Giron-Caro, F., Munoz-Hoyos, A., Ruiz-Cosano, C., Bonillo-Perales, A., Molina-Carballo, A., Escames, G., Macias, M., and Acuna-Castroviejo, D., Melatonin and beta-endorphin changes in children sensitive to olive and grass pollen after treatment with specific immunotherapy. *Int, Arch. Allergy Immunology.* 281:R1647–1664, 2001.

Glazer, W. M., Woods, S. W., Goff, D., Should Sisyphus have taken melatoniun? *Arch. Gen. Psychiatry,* 58(11), 1049–52, November 2001.

Godefroy, F., Weifugazza, J., and Besson, J. M., Effects of antirheumatic drugs and tricyclic antidepressants on total and free serum tryptophan levels in arthritic rats. In: *Progress in Tryptophan and Serotonin Research,* pp. 409–412.

Gordon, M. L., et al., Eosinophilic fasciitis associated with tryptophan ingestion: a manifestation of eosinophilia-myalgia syndrome. *JAMA,* 265(17), May 1, 1991.

Grant, A., Melatonin. *Health Gazette,* 18(2), February 1995.

Gratz, R., Induction of tyrosine aminotransferase by tryptophan in rat liver. In: *Progress in Tryptophan and Serotonin Research,* pp. 689–696.

Haimov, I., Laudon, M., Zisapel, N., et al., Sleep disorders and melatonin rhythms in elderly people. *Brit. Med. J.,* 309:167, July 16 1994.

Hankes, L. V., Jansen, C. R., Debruin, E. P., and Schmaeler, M., Effect of a B-vitamin on tryptophan metabolism in South African Bantu with pellagra. In: *Progress in Tryptophan and Serotonin Research,* pp. 339–346.

Hankes, L.V., et al., Vitamin effects on tryptophan-niacin metabolism in primary hepatoma patients. *Advanced Exp. Medical Biology,* 467, 283–7, 1999.

Hartmann, E., Cravens, J., and List, S., Hypnotic effects of L-tryptophan. *Arch. Gen. Psychiatry,* 31, September 1974.

———, L-Tryptophan: a rational hypnotic with clinical potential. *Am. J. Psychiatry,* 134:4, April 1977.

———, L-tryptophan as an hypnotic agent: a review. *Waking and Sleeping,* 1:155–161, 1977.

———, and Spinweber, C. L., Sleep induced by L-tryptophan: effect of dosages within the normal dietary intake. *J. Nervous & Ment. Dis.,* 167(8), 1979.

Hayakawa, T., and Iwai, K., Effect of tryptophan and/or casein supplementation on NAD levels in livers of the rats fed on niacin and protein-free diet. *J. Nutr. Sci. Vitaminol.,* 30:303–306, 1984.

Heeley, A. F., Piesowicz, A. T., and McCubbing, D. G., The biochemical and clinical effect of pyridoxine in children with brain disorders. *Clin. Sci.,* 35:381–389, 1968.

Heindel, J. J., and Riggs, T. R., Amino acid transport in vitamin B6-deficient rats: dependence on growth hormone supply. *American Physiological Society,* 235(3): E316–E323, 1978.

Heine, W.E., The significance of tryptophan in infant nutrition. *Advanced Exp. Medical Biology,* 467, 833–40, 1999.

Hernandez-Rodriguez, J., and Manjarrez-Gutierrez, G., Macronutrients and neurotransmitter formation during brain development. *Nutritional Review,* 59(8 pt 2), S49–57, August 2001.

Hijikata, Y., Katsuko, H., Shiozaki, Y., Murata, K., and Sameshima, Y., Determination of free tryptophan in plasma and its clinical applications. *J. Clin. Chem. Clin. Biochem.,* 22(4), 1984.

Hirata, H., Asanuma, M., Cadet, J. L., Melatonin attenuates methamphetamine-induced toxic effects on dopamine and serotonin terminals in mouse brain. *Synapse,* 30(2):150–5, October 1998.

Hoes, M. J., Xanthurenic acid excretion in urine after oral intake of 5 grams L-tryptophan by healthy volunteers: standardization of the reference values. *J. Clin. Chem. Clin. Biochem.,* 19:259–264, 1981.

Hoffer, A., Mega-amino acid therapy. *J. Ortho. Psych.* 9 (1): 2–5, 1980.

Hortin, G. L., Landt, M., and Powderly, W. G., Changes in plasma amino acid concentrations in response to HIV-1 infection. *Clin. Chem.* (U.S.), 40(5):785–789, May 1994.

Hudson, J. I., Pope, Jr., H. G., Daniels, S. R., et al., Eosinophilia-myalgia syndrome or fibromyalgia with eosinophilia? *JAMA,* 269(24), June 23/30, 1993.

Huffer, V., Levin, L., and Aronson, H., Oral contraceptives: depression & frigidity. *J. Nerv. Ment. Dis.,* 151:35–41, 1970.

Hussan, I., Mesples, B., Bac, P., Vamecq, J., Evrard, P., Gressens, P., Melatoninergic neuroprotection of the murine periventricular white matter against neonatal excitotoxic challenge. *Ann. Neurol.* 51(1):82–92, January 2002.

Ikeda, S., and Kotake, Y., Urinary excretion of xanthurenic acid and zinc in diabetes. In: *Progress in Tryptophan and Serotonin Research,* pp. 355–358.

Internal Medicine News. Carbidopa with L-5-HTP held effective for intention myoclonous. 9(15), 1976.

Iuvone, M. P., Catecholamines and indoleamines in retina. *Federation Proceedings,* 43(12), 1984.

Jaffe, I., Kopelman, R., Baird, R., et al., Eosinophilic fasciitis associated with the eosinophilia-myalgia syndrome. *Am. J. Med.,* 88, May 1990.

Jan, J. E., and Espezel, H., Melatonin treatment of chronic sleep disorders. *Devel. Med. of Child Neur.,* 37:279–281, 1995.

———, ———, and Appleton, R. E., The treatment of sleep disorders with melatonin. *Devel. Med. of Child Neur.,* 36:97–207, 1994.

Jones, M. R., Cheek, J. M., Tamaki, J., et al., Plasma amino acid concentrations in premature infants: effect of sampling site. *Am. J. Clin. Nutr.,* 50:1389–1394, 1989.

Joseph, M. H., Johnson, L. A., and Kennett, G. A., Increased availability of tryptophan to the brain in stress is not mediated via changes in competing amino acids. In: *Progress in Tryptophan and Serotonin Research,* pp. 387–390.

Joseph, M. S., Brewerton, D., Reus, V. I., and Stebbins, G. T., Plasma L-tryptophan/neutral amino acid ratio and dexamethasone suppression in depression. *Psychiatry Res.,* 11:185–192, 1984.

Kalyanasundraram, S., and Ramanamurthy, P. S. V., Tryptophan metabolism in undernourished developing rat brain. In: *Progress in Tryptophan and Serotonin Research,* pp. 567–570.

Kamb, M. L., Murphy, J. J., Jones, J. L., et al., Eosinophilia-myalgia syndrome in L-tryptophan-exposed patients. *JAMA,* 267(1), January 1, 1992.

Kantak, K. M., Hegstrand, L. R., Whitman, J., and Eichelman, B., Effects of dietary supplements and tryptophan-free diet on aggressive behavior in rats. *Pharmacol. Biochem. Behav.,* 12:173–179, 1980.

Karadotti, R., Axelsson, J., Melatonin secretion in sad patients and healthy subjects matched with respect to age and sex. *Int. J. Circumpolar Health,* 60(4), 548–51, November 2001.

Kaufman, L. D., and Philen, R. M., Tryptophan: current status and future trends for oral administration. *Drug Safety,* 8(2), 1993.

Kaysen, G. A., and Kropp, J., Dietary tryptophan supplementation prevents proteinuria in the seven-eighths nephrectomized rat. *Kidney Int.,* 23:473–479, 1983.

Kennedy, S. H., Melatonin disturbances in anorexia nervose and bulimia nervosa. *Int. J. Eating Disorders,* 16(3):257–265, 1994.

Kent, S., *Life Extension Magazine,* 7(11), Suppl., November 1994.

Khan, R., Burton, S., Morley, S., et al., The effect of melatonin on the formation of gastric stress lesions in rats. *Experientia,* 46:88–89, 1990.

Kimura, M., Yagi, N., and Itokawa, Y., Effect of subacute manganese feeding on serotonin metabolism in the rat. *J. Toxicol. Environ. Health,* 4:701–707, 1978.

Kirchlechner, V., Hoffman-Ehrhart, B., Kovacs, J., Waldhauser, F., Melatonin production is similar in children with monosymptomatic nocturnal enuresis or other forms of enuresis/incontinence and in controls. J. Urol., 166(6), 2407–10, December 2001.

Koskiniemi, M. L., Deficient intestinal absorption of L-tryptophan in progressive myoclonus epilepsy without lafora bodies. J. Neuro. Sci., 47:1–6, 1980.

Koyama, T., Lowy, M. T., Jackman, H. L., and Meltzer, H. Y., Plasma indoles and hormones following a 5-hydroxytryptophan (5-HTP) or tryptophan (TRP) load in affective disorders. Abstracts of panels and posters presented at the annual meeting of the American College of Neuropsychopharmacology, Nashville, TN, December 10–14, 1984.

Krieger, I., and Statter, M., Picolinic acid/tryptophan increase zinc uptake. Am. J. Clin. Nutr., 46:511–517, 1987.

Krieger, I., Picolinic acid in the treatment of disorders requiring zinc supplementation. Nutr. Rev., 38(4), 1980.

Krizova, L., and et al., Effect of nonessential amino acids on nitrogen retention in growing pigs fed on a protein-free diet supplemented with sulphur amino acids, threonine and tryptophan. Journal of Animal Physiology and Animal Nutrition, 85(9–10), 325–32, October 2001.

Kroger, H., and Gratz, R., Induction of tyrosine aminotransferase under the influence of D-galactosamine. Int. J. Biochem., 16(6):703–705, 1984.

Krstulovic, A. M., Brown, P. R., Rosie, D. M., and Champlin, P. B., High-performance liquid-chromatographic analysis for tryptophan in serum. Clin. Chem., 23(11), 1984–1988, 1977.

L-tryptophan: An amino acid that enhances gain by easing exercise pain. Men's Health, p. 7.

Lacoste, V., Wirz-Justice, A., Graw, P., Puhringer, W., and Gastpar, M., Intravenous L-5-hydroxytryptophan in normal subjects: an interdisciplinary precursor loading study. Pharmakopsychiat., 9:289–294, 1976.

Lancet. Uptake of dopamine and 5-hydroxytryptamine by platelets from patients with Huntington's chorea. January 1977.

Latham, C. J., and Blundell, J. E., Evidence for the effect of tryptophan on the pattern of food consumption in free feeding and food deprived rats. Life Sci., 24:1971–1978, 1979.

Laurichesse, H., and et al., Threonine and Methionine are limiting amino acids for protein synthesis in patients with AIDS. Journal of Nutrition, 128(8), 1342–8, August 1998.

Leary, W. E., Levels of a hormone are lower in those with the condition. The New York Times, January 8, 1991.

Leclercq, C., Christiaens, F., Maes, M., et al., Suppressive effects of dexamethasone on the availability of L-tryptophan and tyrosine to the brain of healthy controls. Amino Acids: Chemistry, Biology and Medicine, eds. Lubec and Rosenthal. ESCOM, pp. 694–695.

Lehmann, J., Mental and neuromuscular symptoms in tryptophan deficiency. Acta Psychiat. Scand. Suppl., 237, 1972.

———, Tryptophan deficiency stupor—a new psychiatric syndrome. Acta Psychia. Scand. Suppl., 300: 1982.

———, Persson, S., Walinder, J., and Wallin, L., Tryptophan malabsorption in dementia. Improvement in certain cases after tryptophan therapy as indicated by mental behavior and blood analysis. Acta Psychiat. Scand., 64:123–131, 1981.

Lehnert, H., Beyer, J., Hellhammer, D. H., Effects of L-tyrosine and L-tryptophan on the cardiovascular and endocrine system in humans. Amino Acids: Chemistry, Biology and Medicine, eds. Lubec and Rosenthal. ESCOM, pp. 618–619.

Leone, A. M., and Skene, D., Melatonin concentrations in pineal organ culture are suppressed by sera from tumor-bearing mice. *J. Pineal Res.,* 17:1, 17–19, August 1994.

Levitt, A. J., Brown, G. M., Kennedy, S. H., et al., Tryptophan treatment and melatonin response in a patient with seasonal affective disorder. *J. Clin. Psychopharmacol,* 11(1), February 1991.

Lewis, A. E., Actions and uses of melatonin & melatonin with accessory factors. *Townsend Letter for Doctors,* December 1994.

Lewis, P. D., Perry, G. C., Morris, T. R., English, J., Supplementary dim light differently influences sexual maturity, oviposition time, and melatonin rhythms in pullets. *Poult. Sci.,* 80(12): 1723–8, December 2001.

Lieberman, H. R., Corkin, S., Spring, B. J., Growdon, J. H., and Wurtman, R. J., Mood, performance, and pain sensitivity: changes induced by food constituents. *J. Psychiat. Res.,* 17(2):135–145, 1982–83.

Life Extension Update. Tryptophan: a clarification of our position. 1(7), November 1984.

Lopez-Ibor, J. J., The involvement of serotonin in psychiatric disorders and behavior. *Brit. J. Psychiatry,* and 153, Suppl. 3, 26–39, 1988.

Loscher, W., Pagliusi, S. R., and Muller, F., L-5-hydroxytryptophan correlation between anticonvulsant effect and increases in levels of 5-hydroxyindoles in plasma and brain. *Neuropharmacology,* 23(9):1041–1048, 1984.

Lovell, R.A., and Freedman, D. X., Stereospecific receptor sites for d-lysergic acid diethylamide in rat brain: Effects of neurotransmitters, amine antagonists, and other psychotropic drugs. *Mol. Pharmac.,* 12:620–630, 1976.

Lunenfeld, B., Aging men—challenges ahead. *Asian J. Androl.* (3), 161–8, September 3, 2001.

Manowitz, P., Menna-Perper, M. M., Mueller, P. S., Rochford, J., and Swartzburg, M., Effect of insulin on human plasma tryptophan and nonesterified fatty acids. *Proc. Soc. Exp. Biol. Med.,* 156:402–405, 1977.

———, Gilmour, D. G., and Racevskis, J., Low plasma tryptophan levels in recently hospitalized schizophrenics. *Biol. Psych.,* 6(2):109–118, 1973.

Martin, J. R., Mellor, C. S., and Fraser, F. C., Familial hyperstryptophanemia in two siblings. *Clin. Genet.,* 47:180–183, 1995.

Martin, R. W., and Duffy, J., Eosinophilic fasciitis associated with use of L-tryptophan: a case-control study and comparison of clinical and histopathologic features. *Mayo Clin. Proc.,* 66:892–898, 1991.

Martins, Jr., E., Ligeiro de Oliverira, A. P., Fialho de Araujo, A. M., Tavares de Lima, W., Cipolla-Neto, J., Costa Rosa, L. F., Melatonin modulates allergic lung inflammation. *J. Pineal Res.,* 31(4), 363–9, November 2001.

McConnell, H. M., Another way EMFs might harm tissues. *Health Physics,* February 19, 1994.

Matthies, D. L., and Jacobs, F. A., Rat liver is not damaged by high dose tryptophan treatment. *J. Nutr.* (U.S.), 123(5):852–859, May 1993.

Mawson, A. R., Corn, tryptophan and homicide. *J. Ortho. Psych.,* 7(4):227–30, 1978.

Melatonin update. *Life Extension Update,* 8(6), June 1, 1995.

Melatonin again proves effective for cancer patients. *Life Extension Update,* 6(9), September 1993.

Menna-Perper, M., Swartzburg, M., Mueller, P. S., Rochford, J., and Manowitz, P., Free trypto-phan response to intravenous insulin in depressed patients. *Biol. Psych.,* 18(7):771–780, 1983.

Miller, L. T., Johnson, A., Benson, E. M., and Woodring, M. J., Effect of oral contraceptives and pyridoxine on the metabolism of vitamin B6 and on plasma tryptophan and amino nitrogen. *Amer. J. Clin. Nutr.,* 28:846–853, 1975.

Miller, M. W., Drug companies and health-food stores fight to peddle melatonin to insomni-acs. *The Wall Street Journal,* August 31, 1994.

Millward, J., Can we define indispensable amino acid requirements and assess protein quality in adults? *J. Nutr.* (U.S.), 124, 8, Suppl. 1509s–1516s, August 1994.

Minami, M., Yu, P. H., Davis, B. A., et al., Inhibition of tryptophan hydroxylase by 6, 7-dihy-droxy-N-cyanomethyl-1, 2, 3, 4-tetrahydroisoquinoline, a cyanomethyl derivative of dopamine formed from cigarette smoke. *Neurosic. Lett.* (Ireland), 160 (2):217–220, October 1, 1993.

Modlinger, R. S., Schonmuller, J. M., and Arora, S. P., Stimulation of adolesterone, renin, and cortisol by tryptophan. *J. Clin. Endocrin. Metab.,* 48(4):599–603, 1979.

Moller, S. E., and Amdisen, A., Plasma neutral amino acids in mania and depression: variation during acute and prolonged treatment with L-tryptophan. *Biol. Psychiat.,* 14(1):131–139, 1979.

Montenero, A. S., Sullo tossicita e tollerabilita del triptofano e di suoi metaboliti. *Acta Vitamin. Enzymol.,* 32:188, 1978.

Montgomery, G. W., Flux, D. S., and Greenway, R. M., Tryptophan deficiency in pigs: changes in food intake and plasma levels of glucose, amino acids, insulin and growth hormone. *Hor-mone & Metabolic Res.,* 12(7):304–309, 1980.

Montilla, P., Cruz, A., Padillo, F. J., Tunez, I., Gascon, F., Munoz, M. C., Gomez, M., Pera, C., Melatonin versus vitamin E as protective treatment against oxidative stress after extra-hepatic bile duct ligation in rats. 31:138–144.

Moore, P., et al., Rapid tryptophan depletion plus a serotonin 1A agonist: competing effects on sleep in healthy men. *Neuropsychopharmacology,* 25(5 Suppl.), S40–4, November 2001.

Munoz-Clares, R. A., Lloyd, P., Lomax, M. A., Smith, S. A., and Pogson, C. I., Tryptophan metabolism and its interaction with gluconeogenesis in mammals: studies with the guinea pig, Mongolian gerbil and sheep. *Arch. Biochem. Biophys.* 209(2):713–717, 1981.

Munsat, T. L., Hudgson, and Johnson, M., Serotonin myopathy. *Neurology,* 384, April 1976.

Murialdo, G., Fonzi, S., Costelli, P., et al., Urinary melatonin excretion throughout the ovarian cycle in menstrually related migraine. *Cephalalgia* (*Oslo*), 14:205–209, 1994.

Murphy, D. G. M., Murphy, D. M., Abbas, M., et al., Seasonal affective disorder: response to light as measured by electroencephalogram, melatonin suppression, and cerebral blood flow. *Brit. J. Psychiatry,* 163:327–331, 1993.

Mustonen, A. M., Nieminen, P., Hyvarinen, H., Asikainen, J., Exogenous melatonin elevates the plasma leptin and thyroxine concentrations of the mink (Mustela vison). *Z Natorforsch* [C]. 55(9–10):806–13, September–October 2000.

Narasimhachari, and Himwich, H. E., Gas chromatographic-mass spectrometric identification of N:N-dimethyltryptamine in urine samples from drug-free chronic schizophrenic patients and its quantitation by the technique of single (selective) ion monitoring. *Biochem. Biophys. Res. Commun.,* 55(4):1064–1071, 1973.

Nasrallah, H. A., Dunner, F. J., and McCalley-Whitters, M. A., Placebo-controlled trial of valpo-rate in tardive dyskinesia. *Biol. Psych.,* 20:199–228, 1985.

Nedopil, N., Einhaupl, K., Ruther, E., and Steinburg, R., L-tryptophan in chronic insomnia. In: *Progress in Tryptophan and Serotonin Research,* pp. 305–309.

Nielsen, D. A., Goldman, D., Virkkunen, M., et al., Suicidality and 5-hydroxyindoleacetic acid concentration associated with a tryptophan hydroxylase polymorphism. *Arch. Gen. Psychiatry.* (U.S.), 51 (1):34–38, January 1994.

Nielson, H. K., and Hurrell, R. F., Content and stability of tryptophan in foods. In: *Progress in Tryptophan and Serotonin Research,* pp. 527–534.

Niskamen, P., Huttunen, M., Tamminen, T., and Jaaskelainen, J., The daily rhythm of plasma tryptophan and tyrosine in depression. *Brit. J. Psychiat.,* 128:67–73, 1976.

Norden, M., The risk associated with not taking tryptophan. *The Nutrition Reporter,* 5(4).

———, Risk of tryptophan depletion following amino acid supplementation. *Arch. Gen. Psychiatry.* (U.S.), 50(12):1000–1001, December 1993.

NYU Medical Center. Five ways to relieve temporary insomnia. *Health Letter,* No. 5.

Ogren, S. O., Holm, A. C., Hall, H., and Lindberg, U. H., Alaproclate, a new selective 5-HT uptake inhibitor with therapeutic potential in depression and senile dementia. *J. Neural. Transmission,* 59:265–288, 1984.

Ormsbee, H. S., Silber, D. A., and Hardy, F. E., Serotonin regulation of the canine migrating motor complex. *J. Pharmacol. Experiment. Therapeut.,* 231(2):436, 1984.

Palfreyman, M. G., Mcdonald, I. A., Zreika, M., et al., Tyrosine and tryptophan analogues as MAO-inhibiting prodrugs. *Amino Acids: Chemistry, Biology and Medicine,* eds. Lubec and Rosenthal. ESCOM, pp. 370–371.

Pardridge, W. M., Tryptophan and hepatic encephalopathy. *The Lancet,* May 1975.

Pariza, M. W., and Leighton, T. J., Food components help prevent cancer. *C&EN,* April 24, 1989.

Park, S., et al., Increased binding at 5-HT(1A), 5-HT(1b), and 5-HT(2A) receptors and 5-HT transporters in diet-induced obese rat. *Brain Res,* 847(1), 90–7, November 1999.

Penz, A. M., Clifford, A. J., Rogers, Q. R., and Kratzer, F. H., Failure of dietary leucine to influence the tryptophan-niacin pathway in the chicken. *J. Nutr.,* 114:33–41, 1984.

Peters, J. C., Bellissimo, D. B., and Harper, A. E., L-tryptophan injection fails to alter nutrient selection by rats. *Physiol. Behav.,* 32:253–259, 1983.

Peuschel, S. M., Yeatman, S., and Hum, C., Discontinuing the phenylalanine-restricted diet in young children with PKU. *J. Amer. Diet. Assoc.,* 70(5):838–844, 1977.

———, Reed, R. B., Cronk. C. E., and Goldstein, B. I., 5-hydroxytryptophan and pyridoxine. *Am. J. Dis. Child.,* 134, September 1980.

Pfeiffer, C. C., and Bacchi, D., Copper, zinc, manganese, niacin and pyridoxine in the schizophrenias. *J. Applied Nutr.,* 27 (2,3): 9–39, 1975.

Pharmacological effects of melatonin administration. *CNS Drugs,* 3(3): 212, 1995.

Picone, T. A., Daniels, T. A., Ponto, K. H., et al., Cord blood tryptophan concentrations and total cysteine concentrations. *Current Contents,* Comment, 17(8), February 20, 1989.

Pierpaoli, W., and Mastroni, G. J. M., Melatonin: a principal neuroimmunoregulatory and anti-stress hormone: its anti-aging effects. *Immunology Letters,* 16: 355–362, 1987.

———, and Regelson, W., Pineal control of aging: effect of melatonin and pineal grafting on aging mice. *Proc. Natl. Acad. Sci. USA,* 91:787–791, January 1994.

———, ———, and Colman, C., *The Melatonin Miracle.* New York: Simon & Schuster, 1995.

Pires, M. L., Benedito-Silva, A. A., Pinto, L., Souza, L., Vismari, L., Calil, H. M., Acute effects of low doses of melatonin on the sleep of young healthy subjects. *J. Pineal Res.*, 31(4), 326–32, November 2001.

Poldinger, W., Calanchini, B., and Schwarz, W., A functional-dimensional approach to depression: serotonin deficiency as a target syndrome in a comparison of 5-hydroxytryptophan and fluvoxamine. *Psychopathology*, 24:53–81, 1991.

Ponter, A. A., Seve, B., and Morgan, L. M., Intragastric tryptophan reduces glycemia after glucose, possible via glucose-mediated insulinotropic polypeptide, in early-weaned piglets. *J. Nutr.* (U.S.), 124(2):259–267, February 1994.

Pratt, J. A., Jenner, P., Johnson, A. L., Shorvon, S. D., and Reynolds. E. H., Anticonvulsant drugs alter plasma tryptophan concentrations in epileptic patients: implications for antiepileptic action and mental function. *J. Neurol. Neurosurg. Psych.*, 47:1131–1133, 1984.

Prevention Magazine. New hope for victims of Parkinson's disease, 42–44, September 1976.

Price, L. H., Charney, D. S., Pedro, M. D., et al., Clinical data on the role of serotonin in the mechanism(s) of action of antidepressant drugs. *J. Clin. Psychiatry*, 51, Suppl. 4, 44–50, 1990.

———, L. H., Ricaurte, G. A., Krystal, J. H., et al., Neuroendocrine and mood responses to intravenous L-tryptophan in 3, 4-methylenedioxymethamphetamine (MDMA) Users. *Arch. Gen. Psychiatry*, 46, January 1989.

Puhringer, W., Wirz-Justice, A., Graw, P., Lacoste, V., and Gastpar, M., Intravenous L-5-hydroxytryptophan in normal subjects: an interdisciplinary precursor loading study. *Pharmakopsychatrie Neuro-Psychopharmakologie*, 9:259–266, 1976.

Puig-Domingo, M., Webb, S. M., Serrano, J., et al., Brief report: melatonin-related hypogonadotropic hypogonadism. *New Eng. J. Med.*, 327(19), November 5, 1992.

Quadbeck, H., Lehmann, E., and Tegeler, J., Comparison of the antidepressant action of tryptophan, tryptophan/5-hydroxytryptophan combination and nomifensine. *Neuropsychobiology*, 11(2):111–115, 1984.

Raba, M., Reiderer, P., Danielcyk, W., and Seemano, D., The influence of L5-hydroxytryptophan (L5-HTP) on clinical and biochemical parameters in depressive patients. In: *Progress in Tryptophan and Serotonin Research*, pp. 401–404.

Raghuram, T. C., and Krishnaswamy, K., Serotonin metabolism in pellagra. *Arch. Neurol.*, 32:708–710, 1975.

Rao, G. N., Ney, E., Herbert, R. A., Effect of melatonin and linolenic acid on mammary cancer in transgenic mice with c-neu breast cancer oncogene. *Breast Cancer Res. Treat.* 64(3):287–96, December 2000.

Rapkin, A., Chung, L. C., and Reading, A., Tryptophan loading test in premenstrual syndrome. *J. Obst. Gyn.*, 10:140–144, 1989.

Reddi, E., Rodgers, M. A. J., Spikes, J. D., and Jori, G., The effect of medium polarity on the hematoporphyrin-sensitized photooxidation of L-tryptophan. *Photochem. Photobiol.*, 40(4): 415–421, 1984.

Reeves, J. E., and Lahmeyer, H. W., Tryptophan for insomnia. *JAMA*, 262(19), November 17, 1989.

Reich, T., and Winokur, G., Postpartum psychoses in patients with manic depressive disease. *J. Nerv. Ment. Dis.*, 151:60–68, 1970.

Reiter, R. J., Tryptophan metabolism in the pineal gland. In: *Progress of Tryptophan and Serotonin Research*, pp. 251–258.

Reiter, R. J., Tan, D. X., Poeggeler, B., et al., Melatonin as a free radical scavenger: implications for aging and age-related diseases. *Ann. N.Y. Acad. of Sci.*

Reynolds, R. D., Serotonergic drugs and the serotonin syndrome. *Am. Fam. Physician* (U.S.), 49(5):1083, 1086, April 1994.

Rimler, A., Clig, Z., Levy-Rimler, P. M., Lupowitz, K., Klocker H., Matzkin, H., Bartsch, G., Zisapel, N., Melatonin elicits nuclear exclusion of the human androgen receptor and attenuates its activity. *Prostate*, 49:145–164, 2001.

Rimon, R., Latvala, M., Hyyppa, M., and Kampman, R., Cerebrospinal fluid tryptophan and brain atrophy in patients with chronic schizophrenia. *Ann. Clin. Res.,* 14:133–136, 1982.

Richardson, M. A., Amino acids in psychiatric disease. *J. App. Nutr.,* 44(1), 1992.

Root-Bernstein, R. S., and Westall, F. C., Serotonin binding sites I. structures of sites on myelin basic protein, LHRH, MSH, ACTH, interferon, serum albumin, ovalbumin and red pigment concentrating hormone. *Brain Research Bulletin,* 12:425–436, 1984.

Rudorfer, M. V., Scheinin, M., Karoum, F., Ross, R. J., Potter, W.-Z., and Linnoila, M., Reduction of norepinephrine turnover by serotonergic drug in man. *Biol. Psych.,* 19(2):179–193, 1984.

Russ, M. J., Ackerman, S. H., Banay-Schwartz, M., et al., L-tryptophan does not affect food intake during recovery from depression. *Int. J. Eating Disorders,* 10(5):539–546, 1991.

Ryoo, Y. W., Suh, S. I., Mun, K. C., Kim, B. C., and Lee, K. S., The effects of the melatonin on ultraviolet-B irradiated cultural dermal fibroblasts. *J. Dermatol. Sci.,* 27:162–169, 2001.

Saavedra, J. M., and Axelrod, J., Psychotomimetic N-methylated tryptamines: formation in brain in vivo and *in vitro. Science,* 175(3):1365–1366, 1972.

Sadovsky, E., et al., Prevention of hypothalamic habitual abortion by periactin. *Harefuah,* 78:332–333, 1970.

Satel, S. L., Krystal, J. H., Delgado, P. L., et al., Tryptophan depletion and attenuation of cue-induced craving for cocaine. *Am. J. Psychiatry,* 152:5, May 1995.

Schenker, J. G., and Jungereis, E., Serum copper levels in normal pregnancy. *Harefuah,* 78:330–331, 1970.

Schneider-Helmert, D., and Spinweber, C. L., Evaluation of L-tryptophan for treatment of insomnia: a review. *Psychopharmacology,* 89:1–7, 1986.

Schweigert, B. S., Urinary excretion of amino acids by the rat, *Science,* 315–318, November 1977.

Science, Lithium increases serotonin release and decreases metabolism: implications for theories of schizophrenia. 205(9), 1979.

Segura, R., and Ventura, J. L., Effect of L-tryptophan supplementation on exercise performance. *Int. J. Sports Med.* 9: 301–305, 1988.

Selman, J., Rissenberg, M., and Melius, J., Eosinophilia-myalgia syndrome: follow-up survey of patients, New York, 1990–1991. *MMWR,* 40(24), June 21, 1991.

Seltzer, S., Dewart, D., Pollack, R. L., and Jackson, E., The effects of dietary tryptophan on chronic maxillofacial pain and experimental pain tolerance. *J. Psychiat. Res.,* 17(2):181–186, 1982–83.

Sepping, P., Wood, W., Bellamy, C., Bridges, P. K., O'Gorman, P., Bartlett, J. R., and Patel, V. K., Studies of endocrine activity, plasma tryptophan and catecholamine excretion on psychosurgical patients. *Acta Psychiat. Scand.,* 56:1–14, 1977.

Shansis, F. M., and et al., Behavioral effects of acute tryptophan depletion in healthy male volunteers. *Journal of Psychopharmacology,* 14(2), 157–63, June 2000.

Shamir, E., Barak, Y., Shalman, I., Laudon, M., Zisapel, N., Tarrasch, R., Elizur, A., Weizman, R., Melatonin treatment for tardive dyskinesia: a double -blind, placebo-controlled, crossover study. *Arch. Gen. Psychiatry,* 58(11), 1049–52, November 2001.

Sharma, M., Gupta, Y, K., Effect of chronic treatment of melatonin on learning, memory and oxidative deficiencies induced by intracerebroventricular streptozotocin in rats. *Pharmacol. Biochem. Behav.,* 70(2–3), 325–31, October–November 2001.

Shaw, D. M., Tidmarsh, S. F., and Karajgi, B., Trytophan, affective disorder and stress. *J. Affective Disorders,* 321–325, 1980.

Shen, Y. X., Wei, W., Yang, J., Liu, C., Dong, C., Xu, S. Y., Improvement of melatonin and memory impairment induced by amyloid bgr;-peptide 25-35 in elder rats. *Acta Pharmacol. Sin.,* 22(9), 797–803, September 2001.

Shibata, K., et al., Efficiency of D-Tryptophan as niacin in rats. *Bioscience Biotechnology Biochemistry,* 64(1), 206–9, January 2000

Short, R. V., Hormone of darkness. *Brit. Med. J.,* 307:952–953, October 16, 1993.

Silver, R. M., The eosinophilia-myalgia syndrome. *Pfizer Labs Mediguide to Inflammatory Diseases,* Vol. 10, issue 3.

Slutsker, L., Hoesly, F. C., Miller, L., et al., Eosinophilia-myalgia syndrome associated with exposure to tryptophan from a single manufacturer. *JAMA,* 264(2), July 11, 1990.

Smith, Q. R., Fukui, S., Robinson, P., et al., Influence of cerebral blood flow on tryptophan uptake into brain. *Amino Acids: Chemistry, Biology and Medicine,* eds. Lubec and Rosenthal. ESCOM, p. 364.

Spillmann, M. K., and et al., Tryptophan depletion in SSRI-recovered depressed outpatients. *Psychopharmacology,* 155(2), 123–7, May 2001.

Studies documenting the safety and effectiveness of melatonin have been reported in leading magazines and newspapers. *Harvard Health Letter,* 18(8), June 1993.

Sulman, F. G., and Pfeiffer, Y., The role of serotonin in gynecology and obstetrics. *Israel Pharmaceut. J.,* 16:83–85, 1973.

Suzuki, T., Yuyama, S., Sasaki, A., Yamada, M., and Kumagai, R., Influence of excess leucine intake on the conversion of tryptophan to NAD in rats fed low protein diet. In: *Progress in Tryptophan and Serotonin Research,* pp. 599–602.

Tagaya, H., Matsuno, Y., and Atsumi, Y., Psychiatric treatment for the disorder of sleep-wake schedule: 2 cases of non-24-hour sleep-wake syndrome. *Jap. J. Psych. of Neur.,* 48(2), 1994.

Tahmoush, A. J., Alpers, D. H., and Feigin, R. D., Hartnup disease: clinical, pathological, and biochemical observations. *Arch. Neurol.,* 33:797–806, 1976.

Terron, M. P., Cubero, J., Marchena, J. M., Barriga, C., Rodriguez, A. B., Melatonin and aging: *in vitro* effect of young and mature ring dove physiological concentrations of melatonin on the phagocytic function of heterophils from old ring dove. *Exp. Gerontol.,* 37(2–3):421–6, January 3, 2002.

Toglia, J. U., Melatonin: a significant contributor to the pathogenesis of migraine. *Med Hypotheses,* 57:432–434, 2001.

Trichopoulous, D., Are electric or magnetic fields affecting mortality from breast cancer in women? *J. Nat. Cancer Inst.,* 86(12), June 15, 1994.

Traber, J., Davies, M. A., Dompert, W. U., Glaser, T., Schuurman, T., and Seidel, P.-R., Brain serotonin receptors as a target for the putative anxiolytic TVX Q 7821. *Brain Res. Bulletin,* 12:741–744, 1984.

Traskman-Bendz, L., Asberg, M., Bertilsson, L., and Thoren, P., CSF monoamine metabolites of depressed patients during illness and after recovery. *Acta Psychiatr. Scand.,* 69:333–342, 1984.

Treneer, C. M., and Bernstein, I. L., Learned aversions in rats fed a tryptophan-free diet. *Physio. & Behav.,* 27:757–760, 1981.

Tricoire, H., Locatelli, A.,Chemineau, P., Malpaux, B., Melatonin enters the cerebrospinal fluid through the pineal recess. *Endocrinolog,* 143(1), 84–90, January 2002.

Triebwasser, K. C., Swan, P. B., Henderson, L. M., and Budny, J. A., Metabolism of D-and L-tryptophan in dogs. *J. Nutr.,* 106(5):797–806, 1976.

Tzischinsky, O., and Lavie, P., Melatonin and sleep. *Sleep* (Israel), 17(7):638–645, October 1994.

Utiger, R. D., Melatonin: the hormone of darkness. *New Eng. J. Med.,* 327(19), November 5, 1992.

Valcavi, R., Zini, M., Maestroni, G. J., et al., Melatonin stimulates growth hormone secretion through pathways other than the growth hormone-releasing hormone. Switzerland, February 18, 1993.

Valzelli, L., Bernasconi, S., and Garattini, S., *Brain Tryptophan and Foods.* Milan, Italy: Instituto di Ricerche Farmacologiche "Mario Negri," 1981.

van Hiele, L. J., 1-5-Hydroxytryptophan in depression: the first substitution therapy in psychiatry? *Neuropsychobiology,* 6:230–240, 1980.

van Praag, H. M., Precursors of serotonin, dopamine, and norepinephrine in the treatment of depression. *Advan. Biol. Psych.,* 14:54–68, 1984.

———, H., and de Haan, S., Depression vulnerability and 5-hydroxytryptophan prophylaxis. *Psychiatry Res.,* 3:75–83, 1980.

Vannucchi, H., Mello, J. A., and Dutra, J. E., Tryptophan metabolism in alcoholic pellagra patients: measurements of urinary metabolites and histochemical studies of related muscle enzymes. *Amer. J. Clin. Nutr.,* 35:1368–1374, 1982.

Vannucchi, H., Moreno, F. S., Amarante, A. R., et al., Plasma amino acid patterns in alcoholic pellagra patients. *Alcohol & Alcoholism,* 26(4): 431–436, 1991.

Wannamaker, S. S., and Maxted, W. R. Characterization of bacteriophages from nephritogenic group A *streptococci. J. Infec. Dis.,* 121:407–418, 1970.

Wassmer, E., Carter, P. F., Quinn, E., McLean, N., Welsh, G., Seri, S., Whitehouse, W. P., Melatonin is useful for recording sleep EEGs: a prospective audit of outcome. *Dev. Med. Child. Neurol.,* 43(11), 735–8, November 2001.

Webb, M., and Kirker, J. G., Severe post-traumatic insomnia treated with L-5-hydroxytryptophan. *Lancet,* June 1981.

Webb, S. M., and Puig-Domingo, M., Role of melatonin in health and disease. *Clin. Endocr.,* 42:221–234, 1995.

Weifugazza, J., Godefroy, F., Bineauthurotte, M., and Besson, J. M., Plasma tryptophan levels and 5-hydroxytryptamine synthesis in the brain and the spinal chord in arthritic rats, In: *Progress in Tryptophan and Serotonin Research,* pp. 405–408.

Weil-Fugazza, J., Godefroy, F., Bineau-Thurotte, M., et al., Plasma tryptophan levels and 5-hydroxytryptamine synthesis in the brain and the spinal cord in arthritic rats. Walter de Gruyler & Co., pp. 405–408, 1984.

Weinberger, S. B., Knapp, S., and Mandell, A. J., Failure of tryptophan load-induced increases in brain serotonin to alter food intake in the rat. *Life Sci.,* 22:1595–1602, 1978.

Wilcock, G. K., et al., Tryptophan/trazodone for aggressive behavior. *Lancet,* 1:930, 1987.

Williams, W.A., et al., Effects of acute tryptophan depletion on plasma and cerebrospinal fluid tryptophan and 6 hyroxyindoleacetic acid in normal volunteers. *Journal of Neurochemistry,* 72(4), 1641–7, April 1999.

Wolden-Hanson, T., Mitton, D. R., McCants, R. L., Yellon, S. M., Wiolkinson, C. W., Matsumoto, A. M., Rasmussen, D. D., Daily melatonin administration to middle-aged male rats suppresses body weight, intra abdominal adiposity, and plasma leptin and insulin independent of food intake and total body fat. *Endocrinology,* 141(2):487–97, February 2000.

Wolf, W. A., and Kuhn, D. M., Effects of L-tryptophan on blood pressure in normotensive and hypertensive rats. *J. Pharmacol. Exper. Therapeut.,* 230(2):324–329.

Wong, K. L., and Tyce, G. M., Effect of administration of 5-hydroxytryptophan and an inhibitor of L-aromatic amino acid decarboxylase on glucose metabolism in rat brain. *Neurochem. Res.,* 4:277–287, 1979.

Wong, P. W. K., Forman, P., Tabahoff, B., and Justice P., A defect in tryptophan metabolism. *Pediat. Res.,* 10:725–730, 1976.

Wood, K., Swade, C., Harwood, J., Eccleston, E., Bishop. M., and Coppen, A., Comparison of methods for the determination of total and free tryptophan in plasma. *Clin. Chim. Acta,* 80:229–303, 1977.

Wurtman, J. J., Carbohydrate craving, mood changes, and obesity. *J. Clin. Psychiatry,* 49:8 (Suppl.), August 1988.

Wurtman, R. J., Behavioral effects of nutrition. *Lancet,* May 1983.

———, Hefti, F., and Melamed, E., Precursor control of neurotransmitter synthesis. *Pharmaco. Rev.,* 32(4):315–330, 1981.

Wurtman, et al., Composition and method for suppressing appetite for calories as carbohydrates. *United States Patent,* 4,210,637. July 1, 1980.

Yap, S. H., Hafkenscheid, J. C. M., and van Tongeren, J. H. M., Important role of tryptophan on albumin synthesis in patients suffering from anorexia nervosa and hypoalbuminemia. *Amer. J. Clin. Nutr.,* 289(12): 1356–1363, 1975.

Zarcone, V., Kales, A., Scharf, M., Tan, T. L., Simmons, J. Q., and Dement, W. C., Repeated oral ingestion of 5-hydroxytryptophan: the effect on behavior and sleep processes in two schizophrenic children. *Arch. Gen. Psychiat.,* 15(28), 1973.

Zhdanova, I. V., Wurtman, R. J., Lynch, H. J., et al., Sleep-inducing effects of low doses of melatonin ingested in the evening. *Clin. Pharmacol. & Thera.,* 57(5):552–558, May 1995.

Zigman, S., The role of tryptophan oxidation in ocular tissue damage. *Progress in Tryptophan and Serotonin Research,* pp. 449–468.

Zimmerman, M., Keep your internal clock from "tocking" when it should be "ticking!" *Swanson's Health Shopper,* November 1993.

Zimmerman, R. C., McDougle, C. J., Schumacher, M., et al., Effects of acute tryptophan depletion on nocturnal melatonin secretion in humans. *J. Clin. Endocrinol. Metab.* (U.S.), 76(5):11600–11604, May 1994.

SECTION THREE

Chapter 5: Methionine

Agnoli, A., Andreoli, V., Casacchia, M., and Cerbo, R., Effect of S-adenosyl-L-methionine (SAMe) upon depression symptoms. *J. Psychiat. Res.,* 13:43–54, 1976.

Aksnes, A., Methionine sulphoxide: formation, occurrence and biological availability. *Fisk. Dir., Ser. Ernaering,* II(5):125–153, 1984.

———, Studies on the *in vivo* utilization and the *in vitro* enzymatic reduction of methionine sulphoxide in rats and rat tissues. *Ann. Nutr. Metab.,* 28:288–296, 1984.

Anagnostou, A., Schade, S. G., and Fried, W., Stimulation of erythropoietin secretion by single amino acids. *Proceed. Soc. Exper. Biol. Med.,* 159:139–141, 1978.

Benesh, F. C., and Carl, G. F., Methyl biogenesis. *Bio. Psychiat.,* 13(4):465–480, 1978.

Bidard, J. N., Darmenton, P., Cronenberger, L., and Pacheco, H., Effect de la S-adenosyl-L-methionine sur le catabolisme de la dopamine. *J. Pharmacol. (Paris),* 8, I:83–93, 1977.

Biochemical Pharmacology. Effect of exogenous S-adenosyl-L-methionine on phosphatidyl-choline synthesis by isolated rat hepatocytes. 33(9):1562–1564, 1984.

Bouchard, R., and Conrad, H. R., Sulfur metabolism and nutrition changes in lactating cows associated with supplemental sulfate and methionine hydroxy analog. *Can. J. Anim. Sci.,* 54(12):587–593, 1974.

Brune, G. G., and Himwich, H. E., Effects of methionine loading on the behavior of schizophrenic patients. *J. Nervous & Mental Dis.,* 134, 5:447–450, 1962.

Campbell, R. A., Polyamines and atherosclerosis. *Lancet,* March 1979.

Caruso, I., Fumagelli, M., Boccassini, L., Puttini, P. S., Cliniselli, G., and Cavallari, G., Antidepressant activity of S-adenysylmethionine. *Lancet,* July 1984, p. 904.

Catto, E., Algeri, S., Brunnello, N., and Stramentinoli, G., Brain monomine changes following the administration of S-adenosyl methionine (SAMe). *Neuropharmacol.,* 2:1978.

Chance, W.T., et al., Methionine sulfoximine intensifies cancer anorexia. *Pharmacological Biochemistry and Behavior,* 39(1), 115–8, May 1991.

Cheraskin, E., Ringsdorf, W. M., and Medford, F. H., The "ideal" intake of threonine, valine, phenylalanine, leucine, isoleucine, and methionine. *J. Ortho. Psychiat.,* 7, 3:15–155, 1978.

Colin, M., Effect of adding methionine to drinking water on growth of rabbits. *Nutr. Rep. Inter.,* 17(3):397–402, 1978.

Crome, P., et al., Oral methionine in treatment of severe paracetamol (acetaminophen) overdose. *Lancet,* 2:829–830, 1976.

Darby, W. J., Broquist, H. P., and Olson, R. E., eds. *Annual Review of Nutrition,* Vol. 4. Palo Alto, CA: Annual Reviews, Inc. 170–181, 1984.

Davis, A., *Let's Eat Right to Keep Fit.* New York: Harcourt Brace Jovanovich, Inc., 1970.

De Gandarias, J. M., et al, Brain met-enkephalin immonostaining after subacute and sub-chronic exposure to benzene. *Bull Environmental Contam. Toxicology,* 52(1), 163–70, January 1994.

De Maio, et al., *Clinical and Biochemical Trial of Adenosyl Methionine in Heroin Addicts.* Milan, Italy: Psychiatr. Emerg. Service "R. Bozzi."

Di Buono, M. and et al, Dietary cysteine reduces the methionine requirement in men. *American Journal of Clinical Nutrition,* 74(6), 761–6, December 2001.

Di George, A. M., and Auerbach, V. H., The primary amino-acidopathies: genetic defects in the metabolism of the amino acids. *Ped. Clin. N. Amer.,* August 1963.

Eichholzer, M., et al., Folate and the risk of colorectal, breast and cervix cancer: the epidemiological evidence. *Swiss Medical Weekly,* 131(37–38), 539–49, September 22, 2001.

Ekperigin, H. E., Histopathological and biochemical effects of feeding excess dietary methionine to broiler chicks. *Avian Dis.,* 25:1, January/March, 1981.

Eloranta, T. O., and Raina, A. M., S-adenosylmethionine metabolism and its relation to polyamine synthesis in rat liver: effect of nutritional state, adrenal function, some drugs and partial hepatectomy. *Biochem. J.,* 168:179–185, 1977.

Epner, D. E., Can dietary methionine restriction increase the effectiveness of chemotherapy in treatment of advanced cancer. *Journal of American Coll. Nutrition,* 20(5 Suppl.), 443S–449S, October 2000.

Fau, D., Chanez, M., Bois-Joyeux, B., Delhomme, B., and Peret, J., Phosphate, pyrophosphate and adenine nucleotides equilibrium in rat liver after ethionine ingestion and during ischaemia. *Nut. Rep. Inter.,* 24(9):531–541, 1981.

Feer, H., Biochemistry of depression. *Schweiz. Med. Wschr.,* 107:1177–1180, 1977.

Fetrow, C. W., Efficacy of the dietary supplement S-adenosyl-L-methionine. *Ann Pharmacother,* 35(11), 1414–25, November 2001.

Finkelstein, J. D., Martin J. J., Kyle, W. E., and Harris, B. J., Methionine metabolism in mammals: regulation of methylenetetrahydrofolate reductase content of rat tissues. *Arch. Biochem. Biophys.,* 191(1):153–160, 1978.

———, Harris, B. J., Grossman, M. R., and Morris, H. P., S-adenosylhomocysteine metabolism in rat hepatomas. *Proceed. Soc. Exper. Bio. Med.,* 159:313–316, 1978.

———, Kyle, W. E., Harris, B. J., and Martin, J. J., Methionine metabolism in mammals: concentration of metabolites in rat tissues. *J. Nutr.,* 112(5):1011–1018, 1982.

Flora, G. J., Beneficial effects of S-adenosyl-L-methionine on aminolevulinic acid, dehydratase, glutathione, and lipid peroxidation during acute lead-ethanol administration in mice. *Alcohol,* 18(2–3), 103–8, June–July 1999.

Fomon, S. J., Ziegler, E. E., Filer, L. J., Nelson, S. E., and Edwards, B. B., Methionine fortification of a soy protein formula fed to infants. *Amer. J. Clin. Nutr.,* 32:2460–2471, 1979.

Forman, H. J., Rotman, E. I., and Fisher, A. B., Roles of selenium and sulfur-containing amino acids in protection against oxygen toxicity. *Lab. Invest.,* 49(2):148–153, 1983.

Freier, S., Faber, J., Goldstein, R., and Mayer, M., Treatment of acrodermatitis enteropathica by intravenous amino acid hydrolysate. *J. Ped.,* 82 (1):109–112, 1973.

Frezza, M., Pozzato, G., Chiesa, L., Stramentinoli, G., and Di Padova, C., Reversal of intrahepatic cholestasis of pregnancy in women after high dose S-adenosyl-L-methionine administration. *Hepatol.,* 4(2):274–278, 1984.

Gallistl, S., Determinants of homocysteine during weight reduction in obese children and adolescents. *Metabolism,* 50(10), 1220–3, October 2001.

Gambino, R., Improved rubella antibody test. *Metpath,* 1984.

Gaull, G. E., and Tallan, H. H., Methionine adenosyltransferase deficiency: new enzymatic defect associated with hypermethioninemia. *Science,* 186:59–60, 1974.

Ginefri-Gayet, M., and Gayet, J., Possible link between brain serotonin metabolism and methionine sulfoximine-induced hypothermia and associated behavior in the rat. 43(1), 173–9, September 1992.

Glanville, N. T., and Anderson, G. H., Altered methionine metabolism in streptozotocin-diabetic rats. *Diabetologia,* 27(10):468–471, 1984.

Goldstein, L., Beck, R. A., and Phillips, R., The cortical egg stimulant effect in rabbits of DL-methionine exceeds that of L-methionine. *Fed. Proc.,* 31:250, 1972.

Graham, G. G., MacLean, W. C., and Placko, R., Plasma amino acids of infants consuming soybean proteins with and without added methionine. *J. Nutr.,* 106 (9)1307–1313, 1976.

Grillo, M. A., and Bedino, S., S-adenosylmethionine decarboxylase in liver, heart and pancreas of pyridoxine-deficient chickens. *Italian J. Biochem.,* 26(5):342–346, 1977.

Guroff, G., Effects of inborn errors of metabolism on the nutrition of the brain. *Nutr. Brain,* 4:29, 1979.

Harper, et al., Recommended dietary allowances. *Rev. Physiol. Chem.,* 17:37, 1979.

Harter, J. M., and Baker, D. H., Factors affecting methionine toxicity and its alleviation in the chick. *J. Nutr.,* 108(7):1061–1070, 1978.

Heiblim, D. I., Evans, H. E., Glass, L., and Agbayani, M. M., Amino acid concentrations in cerebrospinal fluid. *Arch. Neurol.,* 35:765–767, 1978.

Hidiroglou, M., and Jenkins, K. J., Influence de la defaunation sur l'utilisation de la selenomethionine chez le mouton. *Ann. Biol. Anim. Bioch. Biophys.,* 14, I:157–165, 1974.

Hladovec, J., Methionine, pyridoxine and endothelial lesion in rats. *Blood Vessels,* 17:104–109, 1980.

Hyafil, F., and Blanquet, S., Methionyl-tRNA synthetase from escherichia coli: substituting magnesium by manganese in the L-methionine activating reaction. *Eur. J. Biochem.,* 74:481–493, 1977.

Jaenicke L., and Gross, R., Zur bestimmung der methionin-synthetase in menschlichen geweben und ihrer biologischen bedeutung. *Klin. Wachr.,* 50:985, 1972.

Joint FAO/WHO Ad Hoc Committee on Energy and Protein Requirements 1973 Report. *FAO Nutrition Meetings Report Series No. 52.* World Health Org. Tech. Rep. Ser. No. 522, 1973.

Kies, C., Fox, H., and Aprahamian, S., Comparative value of L-, DL-, and D-methionine supplementation of an oat-based diet for humans. *J. Nutr.,* 105(7):809–814, 1975.

Kinderlehrer, J., B-6—may be the answer to heart disease. *Prevention,* September 1979.

Kobayashi, K., et al., S-adenosyl-Lmethionine ameliorates reduces local cerebral glucose utilization following brain ischemia in the rat. *Japanese Journal of Pharmacology,* 52(1), 141–8, January 1990.

Kremzner, L. T., and Starr, R. M., Effect of methionine on histamine and spermidine tissue levels. *Fed. Proc.,* Vol. 25, 1966.

Kroger, H., Gratz, R., Museteanu, C., and Haase, J., Influence of nicotinic acid amide, tryptophan, and methionine upon galactosamine-induced hepatitis. *Naturwissenschaften,* 66:476, 1979.

Leeming, T. K., and Donaldson, W. E., Effect of dietary methionine and lysine on the toxicity of ingested lead acetate in the chick. *J. Nutr.,* 114:2155–2159, 1984.

Marcolongo, R., Giordano, N., Colombo, B., Cherie-Ligniere, G., Todesco, S., Mazzi, A., Mattara, L., Leardini, G., Passeri, M., and Cucinotta, D., Double-blind multicentre study of the activity of S-adenosyl-methionine in hip and knee osteoarthritis. *Curr. Ther. Res.,* 37, 1985.

Matsuo, T., Seri, K., and Kato, T., Comparative effects of S-methylmethionine (vitamin U) and methionine on choline-deficient fatty liver in rats. *Arzneim.-Forsch./Drug Res.,* 30 (1):68–69, 1980.

Mijatovic, V., and et al., Homocysteine in postmenopausal women and the importance of hormone replacement therapy. *Clinical Chemistry and Lab Medicine,* 39(8), 754–7, August 2001.

Miller, J., and Landes, D. R., Hematological response of rats to diets containing either marginal or adequate levels of methionine, iron and zinc. *Nutr. Reports Int.,* 11(2):103–112, 1975.

Mitchell, A. D., and Benevenga, N. J., The role of transamination in methionine oxidation in the rat. *J. Nutr.,* 108(1):67–78, 1978.

Miyachi, Y., et al., Rapid decrease in brain enkephalin content after low-dose whole-body X-irradiation of the rat. *Journal Radiat. Res.,* 33(1), 11–5, March 1992.

Morrison, L. D., Brain S-adenosylmethionine levels are severely decreased in Alzheimer's disease. *Journal of Neurochemistry,* 67(3), 1328–31, September 1996.

Muccioli, G., and et al., Effect of S-adenosyl-L-methionine on brain muscarinic receptors of aged rats. *European Journal of Pharmacology,* 227(3), 293–9, November 1992.

Mudd, S. H., and Levy, H. L., Disorders of transsulfuration. In: *The Metabolic Basis of Inherited Disease,* eds. Stanbury, J. B., et al., New York: McGraw-Hill Book Co., pp. 458–503, 1978.

Murphy, D. R., et al., Methionine intolerance: a possible risk factor for coronary artery disease. *JACC,* 6(4):725–730, 1985.

Muscettola, G., Galzenati, M., and Balbi, A., SAM versus placebo: a double-blind comparison in major depressive disorders. *Lancet,* 198, July 1984.

Nat. Acad. Sci., Recommended dietary allowances. 8:44, 1974.

Nutrition Reviews., High protein diets and bone homeostasis. 39(1): 11–12, 1981.

———, Methionine and the "methyl folate trap." 36(8): 255–258, 1978.

Peng, Y. S., and Evenson, J. K., Alleviation of methionine toxicity in young male rats fed high levels of retinol. *J. Nutr.,* 109(2):281–290, 1979.

Peters, W. H., Lubs, H., Knoke, M., and Zschiesche, M., Ergebnisse oraler methioninbelastungen bei normalpersonen and leberkranken unter anwendung eines analysen-kurzprogramms. *Acta Biol. Med. Germ.,* 36:1435–1443, 1977.

Pfeiffer, C. C., and Iliev, V., Blood histamine decreasing and CNS effect in man of DL-methionine exceeds that of L-methionine. *Fed. Proc.,* 31:250, 1972.

Podgornaia, E. K., Changes in the levels of met-enkephalin in various brain structures during formation of immune response. *Biull. Eksp. Biol. Medicine,* 123(2), 170–2, February 1997.

Poulton, J. E., and Butt, V. S., Purification and properties of S-adenosyl-L-methionine: caffeic acid O-methyltransferase from leaves of spinach beet (*beta vulgaris L.*). *Biochim. Biophys. Acta,* 403:301–314, 1976.

Prebluda, H. J., and Lubowe, I. I., Methionine in cosmetics and pharmaceuticals. *Proc. Scientific Section Toilet Goods Assoc.,* 32, December 1959.

Printen, K. J., Brummel, M. C., Cho, E. S., and Stegink, L. D., Utilization of D-methionine during total parenteral nutrition in post surgical patients. *Amer. J. Clin. Nutr.,* 32:1200–1205, 1979.

Reynolds, E. H., Carney, M. W. P., and Toone, B. K., Methylation and mood. *Lancet,* pp. 196–197, July 1984.

Robinson, N., and Williams, C. B., Amino acids in human brain. *Clin. Chim. Acta,* 12:311–317, 1964.

Roesel, R. A., Coryell, M. E., Blankenship, P. R., Thevaos, T. G., and Hall, W. K., Interference by methenamine mandelate in screening for organic and amino acid disorders. *Clin. Chim. Acta,* 100:55–58, 1980.

Rotruck, J. T., and Boggs, R. W., Effects of excess dietary L-methionine and N-acetyl-L-methionine on growing rats. *J. Nutr.,* 107, 3:357–362, 1977.

Rubin, R. A., Ordonez, L. A., and Wurtman, R. J., Physiological dependence of brain methionine and S-adenosylmethionine concentrations on serum amino acid pattern. *J. Neurochem.,* 23:237–231, 1974.

Sarwar, G., and Beare-Rogers, J. L., Methionine and arginine supplementation of casein-based high fat diets: effects on rat growth. *Nutr. Res.,* 4:347–351, 1984.

Science. Natural amino acids. 97(5)2526:493, 1943.

Selhub, J., Folate, vitamin B12, and vitamin B6 and one carbon metabolism. *Journal of Health Nutrition and Aging,* 6(1), 39–42, 2002.

Seri, K., Matsuo, T., Asano, M., and Kato, T., Mode of hypocholesterolemic action of S-methyl-methionine (vitamin U) in mice. *Arzneim.-Forsch.,* 11(12):1857–1858, 1979.

Shoob, H. D., Dietary methionine is involved in the etiology of neutral tube defect-affected pregnancy in humans. *Journal of Nutrition,* 131(10), 2653–8, October 2001.

Soper, H. A., ed., *Handbook of Biochemistry,* Cleveland, OH: The Chemical Rubber Co., 1968.

Spector, R., Coakley, G., and Blakely, R., Methionine recycling in brain: a role for folates and vitamin B-12. *J. Neurochem.,* 34(1):132–137, 1980.

Steadman, T. R., and van Peppen, J. F., A methionine substitute: 4-methylthiobutane-1, 2-diol. *Agricult. Food Chem.,* 23(6): 1137, 1975.

Stegink, L. D., Moss, J., Printen, K. J., and Cho, E. S., D-methionine utilization in adult monkeys fed diets containing DL-methionine. *J. Nutr.,* 110(6):1240–1246, 1980.

———, Filer, L. J., and Baker, G. L., Plasma methionine levels in normal adult subjects after oral loading with L-methionine and N-acetyl-L-methionine. *J. Nutr.,* 110(1):42–49, 1980.

———, Plasma and urinary methionine levels in one-year-old infants after oral loading with L-methionine and N-acetyl-L-methionine. *J. Nutr.,* 112(4):597–603, 1982.

Taylor, M., Dietary modification of amphetamine stereotyped behavior: the action of tryptophan, methionine, and lysine. *Psychopharma.,* 61:81–83, 1979.

Teeter, R. G., Baker, D. H., and Corbin, J. E., Methionine essentiality for the cat. *J. Anim. Sci.,* 46(5): 1287–1292, 1978.

Tews, J. K., Carter, S. H., Roa, P. D., and Stone, W. E., Free amino acids and related compounds in dog brain: post-mortem and anoxic changes, effects of ammonium chloride infusion, and levels during seizures induced by pictrotosin and by pentylenetetrazol. *J. Neurochem.,* 10:641–653, 1963.

Toader, C., Acalovschi, I., and Szantay, I., Protein metabolism following surgical stress. Pre- and postoperative methionine incorporated in serum albumin. *Clin. Chim. Acta,* 37:189–192, 1972.

Van Trump, J., and Miller, S. L., Prebiotic synthesis of methionine. *Science,* 178:859, 1972.

Ward, M., et al,, Effect of supplemental methionine on plasma homocysteine concentrations in healthy men. *International Journal of Vitamin Nutrition Res.,* 71(1), 82–6, January 2001.

Wilson, M. J., and Hatfield, D. L., Incorporation of modified amino acids into proteins *in vivo*. *Biochim. et Biophys. Acta,* 781:205–215, 1984.

Woodham, A. A., Cereals as protein sources. *Proc. Nutr. Soc.,* 36:137–142, 1977.

Yamamoto, Y., Katayama, H., and Muramatsu, K., Beneficial effect of methionine and threonine supplements on tyrosine toxicity in rats. *J. Nutr. Sci. Vitaminol.,* 22:467–475, 1976.

Yanagita, T., Enomoto, N., and Sugano, M., Hepatic triglyceride accumulation as an index of the bioavailability of oxidized methionine to the growing rat. *Agricult. Biol. Chem.,* 48(3):815–816, 1984.

Yokota, F., Matsuno, N., and Suzue, R., Developmental and convalescent changes of the anemia caused by excess methionine in the rat. *J. Nutr. Sci. Vitaminol.,* 25:411–417, 1979.

Yoo, J.-S., and Hsueh, A. M., Amino acid(s) fortification of defatted glandless cottonseed flour. *Nutr. Rep. Inter.,* 31(1):157, 1985.

Zappia, V., Zydek-Cwick, C. R., and Schlenk, F., The specificity of S-adenosylmethionine derivatives in methyl transfer reactions. *J. Biolog. Chem.,* 244 (16):4499–4509, 1969.

Zeisel, S.H., Choline: needed for normal development of memory. *Journal American Coll. Nutrition,* 19(5 Suppl.), 528S–531S, October 2000.

Zezulka, A. Y., and Calloway, D. H., Nitrogen retention in men fed varying levels of amino acids from soy protein with or without added L-methionine. *J. Nutr.,* 106(2):212–221, 1976.

Zioudrou, C., and Klee, W. A., Possible roles of peptides derived from food proteins in brain function. *Nutr. & Brain,* 4:125, 1979.

Chapter 6: Homocysteine

Aleman, G., Homocysteine metabolism and risk of cardiovascular diseases: importance of the nutritional status on folic acid, vitamins B6 and B12. *Rev. Invest. Clinical,* Vol. 53(2), p. 141–51, March–April 2001.

Andreotti, F., Homocysteine and arterial occlusive disease: a concise review. *Cardiologia,* Vol. 44(4), p. 341–5, July 1999.

Badawy, A.A., Moderate alcohol consumption as a cardiovascular risk factor: the role of homocysteine and the need to re-explain the "French Paradox." *Alcohol,* Vol.36 (3), p. 185–8, May 2001.

Barber, J. R., and Clarke, S., Inhibition of protein caroxyl methylation by S-adenosyl-L-homocysteine in intact erythrocytes. *J. Biol. Chem.,* 259(11):7115–7122, 1984.

Brenton, D. P., Cusworth, D. C., Dent, C. E., and Jones, E. E., Homocystinuria: clinical and dietary studies. *Quart. J. Med.,* 35:325, 1966.

Broekmans, W. M., Fruits and vegetables increase plasma carotenoids and vitamins and decrease homocysteine in humans. Vol. 130(6), p. 1115–23, June 2000.

Calabrese, E. J., Environmental validation of the homocystine theory of arteriosclerosis, *Med. Hypoth.,* 15:361–367, 1984.

Cohn, J. E., Homocysteine, HIV, and heart disease. *AIDS Treatment News,* Vol. 370, p. 5–6, August 24, 2001.

Crooks, P. A., Tribe, M. J., and Pinney, R. J., Inhibition of bacterial DNA cytosine-5-methyltransferase by S-adenosyl-L-homocysteine and some related compounds. *J. Pharm. Pharmacol.,* 36:85–89, 1984.

De la Vega, M. J., High prevalence of hyperhomocystinemia in chronic alcoholism: the importance of the thermolabile form of the enzyme methylenetetrahydrofolate reductase. *Alcohol*, Vol. 25(2), p. 59–67, October 2001.

Dekou, V., Gene-environment and gene-gene interaction in the determination of plasma homocysteine levels in healthy middle-aged men. *Thromb Haemost*, Vol. 85(1), p. 67–74, January 2001.

Fettman, M. J., Effects of dietary cysteine on blood sulfur amino acid, glutathione, and malondialdehyde concentration in cats. *American Journal Vet. Res.*, Vol. 60(3), p. 328–33, March 1999.

Fonseca, V., Effects of a high-fat-sucrose diet on enzymes in homocysteine metabolism in the rat. *Metabolism*, Vol. 49(6), p. 736–41, June 2000.

Freeman, J. M., Finkelstein, J. D., and Mudd, S. H., Folate-responsive homocystinuria and "schizophrenia": a defect in methylation due to deficient 5, 10-methylenetetrahydrofolate reductase activity. *New Eng. J. Med.*, 292(10):491–496.

Gariballa, S. E., Nutritional factors in stroke. *British Journal of Nutrition*, Vol. 84(1), p. 5–17, July 2000.

Gerritsen, T., and Waisman, H. A., Homocystinura: cystathionine synthase deficiency. In: *Metabolic Errors of Nutrients*, Hommes, F. A., and Vandenberg, C. J., eds. New York: Academic Press, 1973, 403–407.

Gibson, J. B., Carson, N. A. J., and Neill, D. W., Pathological findings in homocystinuria. *J. Clin. Path.*, 17:427, 1964.

Glen, R. H., and et al., Cardiovascular disease risk factors and diet of Fulani pastoralists of northern Nigeria. *American Journal of Clinical Nutrition*, Vol. 74(6), p. 730–6, December 2001.

Gonzalez-Gross, M., Nutrition and cognitive impairment in the elderly. *Br. Journal of Nutrition*, Vol. 86(3), p.313–21, September 2001.

Harker, et al., Homocystine-induced arteriosclerosis. *J. Clin. Invest.*, 58:731–41, 1976.

Hermann, W., Total homocysteine, vitamin B12, and total antioxidant status in vegetarians. *Clinical Chemistry*, Vol. 47(6), p. 1094–101, June 2001.

Hollowell, J. G., Coryell, M. E., Hall, W. K., Findley, W. K., and Thevaos, T. G., Homocystinuria as affected by pyridoxine, folic acid and vitamin B12. *Proc. Soc. Exp. Biol. Med.*, 129:327, 1968.

Ishizaka, T., and Ishizaka, K., Activation of mast cells for mediator release through IgE receptors. *Prog. in Allergy*, 34:188–235, 1984.

Jacob, R. A., Folate nutriture alters choline status of women and men fed low choline diets. *Journal Nutrition*, Vol. 129(3), p. 712–7, March 1999.

Jacques, P. F., Determinants of plasma total homocysteine concentration in the Framingham Offspring cohort. *American Journal Clinical Nutrition*, Vol. 73(3), p. 613–21, March 2001.

Kaletha, K., Homocysteine as a risk factor for atherosclerosis. *Prezegl Lek*, Vol. 57(10), p. 591–5, 2000.

Kass-Annese, B., Alternative between total homocysteine and the likelihood for a history of acute myocardial infarction by race and ethnicity: results from the Third National Health and Nutrition Examination Survey. *American Heart Journal*, Vol. 139(3), p. 446–53, March 2000.

Krishnaswamy, K., Importance of folate in human nutrition. *Br. Journal of Nutrition*, 85 Suppl. 2, p. s115–24, May 2001.

Kurowska, E.M., HDL-cholesterol-raising effect of orange juice in subjects with hypercholesterolemia. *American Journal of Clinical Nutrition*, Vol. 72(5), p. 1095–100, November 2000.

Leuenberger, S., Faulborn, J., Sturrock, G., Gloor, B., Rehorek, R., and Baumgartner, R., Vaskulare und okulare Kompikationen bei cinem Kind mit Homocystinurie. *Schweiz. Med. Wschr.*, 114:793–798, 1984.

Litwin, M., Folate, vitamin B12, and sulfur acid levels in patients with renal failure. *Pediatric Nephrology*, Vol. 16(2), p. 127–32, February 2001.

Louis-Coindet, J., Sarda, N., Pacheco, H., and Jouvet, M., Effect of S-adenosyl-L-homocysteine upon sleep in p-chlorophenylalanine pretreated rats. *Brain Res.*, 294:239–245, 1984.

Lowenthal, E. A., Homocysteine elevation in sickle cell disease. *Journal American Coll. Nutrition*, Vol. 19(5), p. 608–12, October 2000.

Macy, P. A., Homocysteine: predictor of thrombotic disease. *Clinical Lab Science*, Vol. 14(4), p. 272–5, Fall 2001.

McCarron, D. A., Reducing cardiovascular disease risk with diet. *Obesity Res.*, 9 Suppl. 4, p. 335s–340s, November 2001.

McKusick, V. A., Hall, J. G., and Char, F., The clinical and genetic characteristics of homocystinuria in inherited disorders of sulphur metabolism. *Proc. 8th Symposium of the Soc. for the Study of Inborn Errors of Metab.*, Belfast, 1970. eds. Carson, N. A. J., and Raine, D. N., London: Livingstone, 1971.

Molloy, A. M., Homocysteine, folate enzymes and neural tube defects. *Haematologica*, Suppl. EHA-4, p. 53–6, June 1999.

Morris, M. S., Total homocysteine and estrogen status indicators in the Third National Health and Nutrition Examination Survey. *American Journal Epidermiol*, Vol. 152(2), p. 140–8, July 2000.

Mudd, H., Schneider, J. A., Spielberg, S. P., Boxer, L., Oliver, J., Corash, L., and Sheetz, M., Genetic disorders of glutathione and sulfur amino-acid metabolism. *Ann. Inter. Med.*, 93:330–346, 1980.

Nutrition Reviews. Inhibition of platelet aggregation and clotting by pyridoxal-5′-phosphate. 40(2):55–56, 1982.

Papaioannou, R., Beyond homocysteine: a thesis for defective cross-linking as a fundamental cause in arteriosclerosis. *Med. Hypothesis*, 1985.

Perna, A. F., Homocysteine and chronic renal failure. *Miner Electrolyte Metabolism*, Vol. 25(4–6), p. 279–85, July–December 1999.

Pfeiffer, C. C., *Mental and Elemental Nutrients*, New Canaan, CT: Keats Publishing, Inc., 1975.

Price, J., Vickers, C. F. H., and Brooker, B. K., A case of homocystinuria with noteworthy dermatological features. *J. Ment. Defic. Res.*, 12:111, 1968.

Ribes, A., Vilaseca, M. A., Briones, P., Maya, A., Sabater, J., Pascual, P., Alvarez, L., Ros, J., and Pascual, E. G., Methylmalonic aciduria with homocystinuria. *J. Inher. Metab. Dis.*, 7(2): 129–130, 1984.

Rosenberg, I. H., B vitamins, homocysteine, and neurocognitive function. *Nutrition Review*, Vol. 8, p. s69–74, August 2001.

Schatz, R. A., Wilens, T. E., and Sellinger, O. Z., Decreased transmethylation of biogenic amines after *in vivo* elevation of brain S-adenosyl-L-homocysteine. *J. Neurochem.*, 36(5):1739–1748, 1981.

⸻, Decreased *in vivo* protein and phospholipid methylation after *in vivo* elevation of brain S-adenosyl-homocysteine. *Biochem. & Biophys. Res. Comm.*, 98(4): 1097–1107, 1981.

Scherer, C. S., Excess dietary methionine markedly increases the vitamin B6 requirement of young chicks. *Journal of Nutrition,* Vol. 130(12), p. 3055–8, December 2000.

Seman, L. J., Lipoprotein, homocysteine, and remnantlike, particles: emerging risk factors. *Current Opinion Cardiol.,* Vol. 14(2), p. 189–91, March 1999.

Sesmilo, G., and et al., Effects of growth hormone administration on homocysteine levels in men with GH deficiency: a randomized controlled trial. *J Clinical Endocrinology Metab.* Vol. 86(4), p. 1518–24, April 2001.

Shih, V. E., and Efron, M. L., Pyridoxine-unresponsive homocystinuria. *New Eng. J. Med.,* 283(11):1206–1208, 1970.

Shinnar, S., and Singer, H. S., Cobalamin C mutation (methylmalonic aciduria and homocystinuria) in adolescence. *Mass. Med. Soc.,* 1984.

Smolin, L. A., Benevenda, N. J., and Berlow, S., The use of betaine for the treatment of homocystinuria. *J. Ped.,* 99(3):467–472, 1981.

Spaeth, G. L., The usefulness of pyridoxine in the treatment of homocystinuria: a review of postulated mechanisms of action and a new hypothesis. *Birth Defects: Original Article Series,* XII(3):347–354, 1976.

Stanbury, J. B., Wyngaarden, J. B., and Frederickson, D. S., eds., *The Metabolic Basis of Inherited Disease.*

Stolzenberg-Solomon, R., Pancreatic cancer risk and nutrition-related methyl-group availability indicators in male smokers. *Journal National Cancer Institute,* Vol. 91(6), p. 535–41, March 1999.

Strittmatter, W. J., Hirata, F., and Axelrod, J., Phospholipid methylation unmasks cryptic B-adenergic receptors in rat reticulocytes. *Science,* June 1979.

Thomson, S. W., Correlates of total plasma homocysteine: folic acid, copper, and cervical dysplasia. *Nutrition,* Vol. 16(6), p. 411–6, June 2000.

Ulvik, A., and et al., Smoking, folate and methylenetetrahydrofolate reductase status as interactive determinants of adenomatous and hyperplastic polyps of colorectum. *American Journal Genet,* Vol. 101(3), p. 246–254, July 1, 2001.

Ventura, P., Hyperhomocystinemia and related factors in 600 hospitalized elderly subjects. *Metabolism,* Vol. 50(12), p. 1466–71, December 2001.

Vina, J. R., Blood sulfur-amino acid concentration reflects an impairment of liver transsulfuration pathway in patients with acute abdominal inflamer processes. *Br. Journal of Nutrition,* Vol. 85(2), p. 173–8, February 2001.

Ward, M., et al., Effect of supplemental methionine on plasma homocysteine concentrations in healthy men: a preliminary study. *International Vitamin Nutrition Res.,* Vol.71 (1), p. 82–6, January 2001.

Wendel, U., and Bremer, H. J., Betaine in the treatment of homocystinuria due to 5,10-methylenetetrahydrofolate reductase deficiency. *Eur. J. Pediatr.,* 142:147–150, 1984.

Wilcken, D. E. L., and Gupta, V. J., Cysteine-homocysteine mixed disulphide: differing plasma concentrations in normal men and women. *Clin. Sci.,* 57:211–215, 1979.

Winston, M., Diet controversies in lipid therapy. *Journal of Cardiovascular Nursing,* Vol. 14(2), p. 29–38, January 2000.

Witte, K. K., Chronic heart failure and micronutrients. *Journal Am. Coll. Cardiol.,* Vol. 37(7), p. 1765–74, June 1, 2001.

Chapter 7: Cysteine

Allan, C.B., Lacourciere, G.M., and Stadtman, T.C., Responsiveness of selenoproteins to dietary selenium. *Annu. Rev. Nutr.,* 19:1–16, 1999.

Altschule, M. D., Siegel, E. P., and Henneman, D. F., Blood glutathione level in mental disease before and after treatment. *Arch. Psych.,* 71:69, 1955.

————, Goncz, R. M., and Murname, J. P., Effect of pineal extracts on blood glutathione level in psychotic patients. *AMA Arch. of Neuro. & Psych.,* 67:615, 1952.

Ames, B. N., Dietary carcinogens and anticarcinogens: oxygen radicals and degenerative diseases. *Science,* 221:1256–1260, 1983.

Ampola, M. G., Efron, M. L., Bixby, E. M., and Meshover, E., Mental deficiency and a new aminoaciduria. *Amer. J. Dis. Child.,* 117:66–70, 1969.

Anderson, G. H., Sulfur balances in intravenously fed infants: effects of cysteine supplementation. *Amer. J. Clin. Nutr.,* 36:862–867, 1982.

Arrick, B. A., and Nathan, C. F., Glutathione metabolism as a determinant of therapeutic efficacy: a review. *Cancer Res.,* 44(10):4224–4233, 1984.

Ashoub, A., and Hussein, L., The vitamin B2 status among Egyptian school students suffering from various afflictions as evaluated by the erythrocyte glutathione reductase assay. *Nutr. Reports Int.,* 29(2): 291–302, 1984.

Atroshi, F., and Sandholm, M., Red blood cell glutathione as a marker of milk production in Finn sheep. *Res. Vet. Sci.,* 33(2):256–259, 1982.

Baas, P., van Mansom, I., van Tinteren, H., et al., Effect of N-acetylcysteine on photofrin-induced skin photosensitivity in patients. *Lasers in Surg. & Med.,* 16:359–367, 1995.

Bakker, J., Zhang, H., Depierreux, M., et al., Effects of N-acetylcysteine in endotoxic shock. *J. Crit. Care,* 9(4):236–243, December 1994.

Baldetorp, L., and Martensson, J., Urinary excretion of inorganic sulfate, ester sulfate, total sulfur and taurine in cancer patients. *Acta Med. Scand.,* 208:293–295, 1980.

Ballatori, N., and Clarkson, T. W., Dependence of biliary excretion of inorganic mercury on the biliary transport of glutathione. *Biochem. Pharmacol.,* 33:(7):1093–1098, 1984.

————, and Clarkson, T. W., Developmental changes in the biliary excretion of methylmercury and glutathione. *Science,* 216(2):61–62, 1982.

Balli, R., Controlled trial on the use of oral acetylcysteine in the treatment of glue-ear following drainage. *Eur. J. Resp. Dis.,* 61:158, Suppl. 111, 1980.

Beloqui, O., Prieto, J., Suarez, M., et al., N-acetyl cysteine enhances the response to interferon-alpha in chronic hepatitis C: a pilot study. *J. Interferon Res.,* 13:279–282, 1993.

Birwe, H., Schneeberger, W., and Hesse, A., Investigations of the efficacy of ascorbic acid in cystinuria. *Urol. Res.,* 19:199–201, 1991.

Blume, K.-G., Paniker, N. V., and Beutler, E., Enzymes of glutathione synthesis in patients with myeloproliferative disorders. *Clin. Chim. Acta,* 45:281–285, 1973.

Boers, G. H. J., Smals, A. G. H., Trijbels, F. J. M., et al., Heterozygosity for homocystinuria in premature peripheral and cerebral occlusive arterial disease. *New Eng. J. Med.,* 313(12), September 19, 1995.

Boesby, S., Man, W. K., Mendez-Diaz, R., and Spencer, J., Effect of cysteamine on gastroduodenal mucosal histamine in rat. *Gut,* 242:935–939, 1983.

Boesgaard, S., Iversen, H. K., Wroblewski, H., et al., Alteres peripheral vasodilator profile of nitroglycerin during long-term infusion of N-acetylcysteine. *J. Am. Coll. Cardiol.,* 23:163–169, 1994.

Bongers, V., de Jong, J., Steen, I., et al., Antioxidant-related parameters in patients treated for cancer chemoprevention with N-acetylcysteine. *Eur. J. Cancer,* 31A(6):921–923, 1995.

Boushey, C. J., Beresford, S. A. A., Omenn, G. S., et al., A quantitative assessment of plasma homocoysteine as a risk factor for vascular disease. *JAMA,* 274(13):1049–1057, October 4, 1995.

Boyd, S. C., Sasame, H. A., and Boyd, M. R., Gastric glutathione depletion and acute ulcerogenesis by diethylmaleate given subcutaneously to rats. *Life Sci.,* 28:2987–2992, 1981.

Breslow, J. L., Azrolan, N., and Bostom, A., N-acetylcysteine and lipoprotein(a). *Lancet,* 339:126, January 11, 1992.

British Med. Bulletin. Iron absorption and supplementation. 37:25, 1981.

Buchanan, J. H., and Otterburn, M. S., Some structural comparisons between cysteine-deficient and normal hair-keratin. *IRCS Med. Sci.,* 12:691–692, 1984.

Bunce, G. E., Nutrition and cataract. *Nutr. Rev.,* 37(11):337, 1979.

Capel, I. D., Jenner, M., Williams, D. C., Donaldson, D., and Nath, A., The effect of prolonged oral contraceptive steroid use on erythrocyte glutathione peroxidase activity. *J. Steroid Biochem.,* 14:729–732, 1981.

Chasseaud, L. F., The role of glutathione and glutathione S-transferases in the metabolism of chemical carcinogens and other electrophilic agents. *Adv. Cancer Res.,* 29:176–244, 1975.

Chaudhari, A., and Dutta, S., Alterations in tissue glutathione and angiotensin converting enzyme due to inhalation of diesel engine exhaust. *J. Toxicol. Environ. Health,* 9(2):327–337, 1982.

Clemencon, G. H., Fehr, H. F., and Finger, J., Diversion of bile and pancreatic secretion in the rat and its effect on cysteamine-induced duodenal and peptic ulcer development under maximal acid secretion. *Scand. J. Gastroenterol.,* 19(92):112–115, 1984.

Craan, A. G., Mini review: cystinuria: the disease and its models. *Life Sci.,* 28:5–22, 1981.

Deneke, S. M., and Fanburg, B. L., Normobaric oxygen toxicity of the lung. *New Eng. J. Med.,* 7:76–86, 1980.

DeVries, N., and DeFlora, S., N-acetyl-l-cysteine. *J. Cell Biochem. Suppl.,* 17F:270–277, 1993.

Di Buono, M., Dietary cysteine reduces the methionine requirement in men. *American Journal of Clinical Nutrition,* Vol. 74(6), p. 761–6, December 2001.

Domingo, J. L., and Liobet, J. M., The action of L-cystine in acute cobalt chloride intoxication. *Revista Espanola de Fisiologia,* 40:231–236, 1984.

Doni, M. G., Avventi, G. L., Bonadiman, L., and Bonaccorso, G., Glutathione peroxidase, selenium, and prostaglandin synthesis in platelets. *Amer. Physio. Soc.,* 800–803, 1981.

Droge, W., Cysteine and glutathione deficiency in AIDS patients: a rationale for the treatment with N-acetylcysteine. *Pharmacology,* 46:61–65, 1993.

Dubick, M. A., Heng, H. S. N., and Rucker, R. B., Metabolism of ascorbic acid and glutathione in response to ozone and protein deficiency. *Fed. Proc.,* 41:4, 1982.

Edgren, M., Larsson, A., Nilsson, K., Revesz, L., and Scott, O.-C. A., Lack of oxygen effect in glutathione-deficient human cells in culture. *Int. J. Radiat. Bio.,* 37(3):299–306, 1980.

Ehrich, M., Biochemical and pathological effects of clostridium difficile toxins in mice. *Toxicon.,* 20(6):983–989, 1982.

Emerson Ecologics, Inc. NAC (N-Acetyl-L-Cysteine). NAC 91-09b.

Estensen, R. D., N-acetylcysteine suppression of the proliferative index in the colon of patients with previous adenomatous colonic polyps. *Center Letter,* Vol. 147(1–2), p. 109–14, December 1,1999.

Evered, D. F., and Wass, M., Transport of glutathione across the small intestine of the rat *in vitro. Proc. Physio. Soc.,* April 1970.

Factor, P., Ridge, K., Alverdy, J., and Sznajder, J.I., Continuous enternal nutrition attenuates pulmonary edema in rats exposed to 100% oxygen. *J Appl Physiol,* 89:1759–1765.

Fan, J., and Shen, S. J., The role of Tamm-Horsfall mucoprotein in calcium oxalate crystallization. N-acetylcysteine: a new therapy for calcium oxalate urolithiasis. *Br. J. Urol.,* 74:288–293, 1994.

Fernandez, M. A., and O'Dell, B. L., Effect of zinc deficiency on plasma glutathione in the rat. *Proc. Soc. Exper. Biol. & Med.,* 173:564–567, 1983.

Folkers, K., Dahmen, J., Ohta, M., Stepien, H., Leban, J., Sakura, N., Lundanes, E., Rampold, G., Patt, Y., and Goldman, R., Isolation of glutathione from bovine thymus and its significance to research relevant to immune systems. *Biochem. Biophys. Res. Commun.,* 97(2):590–594, 1980.

Forman, H. J., Rotman, E. I., and Fisher, A. B., Roles of selenium and sulfur-containing amino acids in protection against oxygen toxicity. *Lab. Invest.,* 49(2):148, 1983.

Frank, H., Thiel, D., and Langer, K., Determination of N-acetyl-L-cysteine in biological fluids. *Biomed. App.,* 309(2):261–268, 1984.

Frank, T., Kuhl, M., Makowski, B., Bitsch, R., Jahreis, G., and Hubscher, J., Does a 100-km walking affect indicators of vitamin status? *Int. J. Vitam. Nutr. Res.,* 70:238–250, 2000.

Friedman, M., and Gumbmann, M. R., The utilization and safety of isomeric sulfur-containing amino acids in mice. *J. Nutr.,* 114:2301–2310, 1984.

Fritz, G., Ronquist, G., and Hugosson, R., Perspectives of adenylate kinase activity and glutathione concentration in cerebrospinal fluid of patients with ischemic and neoplastic brain lesions. *Euro. Neuro.,* 21:41–47, 1982.

Fujii, S., Dale, G. L., and Beutler, E., Glutathione-dependent protection against oxidative damage of the human red cell membrane. *Blood,* 63(5):1096–1101, 1984.

Fujinami, S., Hijikata, Y., Shiozaki, Y., et al., Profiles of plasma amino acids in fasted patients with various liver diseases. *Hepato-Gastroenterol.,* 37: (Suppl. II) 81–84, 1990.

Gatton-Umphress, T. L., Weber, K. A., and Seidler, N. W., Methionine metabolism: A window on carcinogenesis? *Brief Review Hospital Practice* (Kansas City, MO). September 30, 1993.

Geerling, B. J., Badart-Smook, A., van Deursen, C., van Houwelingen, A.C., Russel, M.G., Stockbrugger, R. W., Brummer, R. J., Nutritional supplementation with N-3 fatty-acids and anti-oxidants in patients with Crohn's disease in remission: effects on antioxidant status and fatty acid profile. *Inflamm. Bowel Dis.,* 6:77–84, 2000.

Girardi, G., and Elias, M. M., Effectiveness of N-acetylcysteine in protecting against mercuric chloride-induced nephrotoxicity. *Toxicology,* 67:155–164, 1991.

Glatt, H., Protic-Sabljic, M., and Oesch, F., Mutagenicity of glutathione and cysteine in the Ames test. *Science,* 220:961–962, 1983.

Glatzle, D., Vuilleumier, J. P., Weber, F., and Decker, K., Glutathione reductase test with whole blood, a convenient procedure for the assessment of the riboflavin status in humans. *Separatum Experientia,* 30:665–667, 1974.

Glazenburg, E. J., Jekel-Halsema, M. C., Baranczyk-Kuzma, A., Krugsheld, K. R., and Mulder, G. J., D-Cysteine as a selective precursor for inorganic sulfate in the rat *in vivo. Biochem. Pharm.,* 33(4):625–628, 1984.

Green, G. M., Cigarette smoke: protection of alveolar macrophages by glutathione and cystine. *Science,* 162:810–811, 1968.

Grundfest, W. S., Homocysteine and marginal vitamin deficiency. *JAMA,* 270(22), December 8, 1993.

Habior, A., and Danowski, S. T., Effect of D-penicillamine on liver glutathione. *Res. Commun. Chem. Pathol. Pharmacol.,* 34(1):153–156, 1981.

Hamilton, M. L., Van Remmen, H., Drake, J. A., Yang, H., Guo, Z. M., Kewitt, K., Walter, C.A., Richardson, A., Does oxidative damage to DNA increase with age? *Proc. Natl. Acad. Aci. U.S.A.,* 28:10469

Hazelton, G. A., and Lang, C. A., Glutathione contents of tissues in the aging mouse. *Biochem. Soc.,* 188:25–30, 1980.

Helms, R. A., Cysteine supplements results in normalization of plasma taurine concentrations in children receiving home parental nutrition. *J. Periatrics,* Vol. 134(3), p. 358–61, March 1999.

Hesse, A., High-performance liquid chromatographic determination of urinary cysteine and cystine. *Clin. Chim. Acta,* 199:33–42, 1991.

Hoffer, A., Editorial: mega amino acid therapy. *Ortho. Psych.,* 9(1):2–5, 1980.

Holoye, P. Y., Duelge, J., Hansen, R. M., Ritch, P. S., and Anderson, T., Prophylaxis of ifosfamide toxicity with oral acetylcysteine. *Sem. Oncol.,* 10(1):66–71, 1983.

Hospital Practice. Toxic effects of OTC analgesics, "health food" supplements reported. 29–30, June 1984.

Hsu, J. M., Lead toxicity as related to glutathione metabolism. *J. Nutr.,* III:26–33, 1981.

———, Rubenstein, B., and Paleker, A. G., Role of magnesium in glutathione metabolism of rat erythrocytes. *Amer. Inst. Nutr.,* 488–496, July 1981.

———, Zinc deficiency and glutathione linked enzymes in rat liver. *Nutr. Rep. Int.,* 25(3):573–582, 1982.

Husain, S., and Dunlevy, D., Possible role of glutathione (GSH) in phencyclidine (PCP) toxicity and its protection by N-acetylcysteine (NAC). *Pharmacologist,* 243(3):1982.

Igarashi, T., Satoh, T., Ueno, K., and Kitagawa, H., Species difference in glutathione level and glutathione related enzyme activities in rats, mice, guinea pigs and hamsters. *J. Pharm. Dyn.,* 6:941–949, 1983.

Itinose, A. M., Doi-Sakuno, M. L., and Bracht, A., N-acetylcysteine stimulates hepatic glycogen deposition in the rat. *Res. Commun. Chem. Pathol. Pharmacol.,* 83:87–92, 1994.

James, M. B., Hair growth benefits from dietary cysteine-gelatin supplementation. *J. Appl. Cosmetol.,* 2:15–27, 1983.

Janssen, M. J. F. M., van den Berg, M., Stehouwer, C. D. A., et al., Hyperhomocysteinaemia: a role in the accelerated atherogenesis of chronic renal failure? *Netherlands J. Med.,* 46:244–251 1995.

Jensen, G. E., and Clausen, J., Glutathione peroxidase activity in vitamin E and essential fatty acid-deficient rats. *Ann. Nutr. Metab.,* 25:27–37, 1981.

Jensen, L. S., and Maurice, D. V., Influence of sulfur amino acids on copper toxicity in chicks. *J. Nutr.,* 109:91–97, 1979.

Johnson, M. V., Novel treatments after experimental brain injury. *Semin Neonatol.,* Vol. 5(1), p. 75–89, February 2000.

Johnston, R. E., Hawkins, H. C., and Weikel, J. H., The toxicity of N-acetylcysteine in laboratory animals. *Sem. Oncol.,* 10(1):17–24, 1983.

Joseph, J. A., Denisova, N. A., Bielinki, D., Fisher, D. R., Shukitt-Hale, B., Oxidative stress protection and vulnerability in aging: putative nutritional implications for intervention. *Mech. Aging Dev.,* 31:116(2–3):141–53, 2000.

Kaplowitz, N., The importance and regulation of hepatic glutathione. *Yale J. Bio. Med.,* 54:497–502, 1981.

Karlsen, R. L., Grofova, I., Malthe-Sorensson, D., Fonnum, F., and Jayaraj, A. P., Dissecting aneurysm of aorta in rats fed with cysteamine. *Brit. J. Exp. Path.,* 64:158, 1983.

Kawata, M., and Suzuki, K. T., The effect of cadmium, zinc or copper loading on the metabolism of amino acids in mouse liver. *Toxicology Letters,* 20:149–154, 1984.

Kerai, M. D., Taurine: protective properties against ethanol-induced hepatic steatosis and lipid peroxidation during chronic ethanol consumption in rats. *Amino Acid,* Vol. 15(1–2), p. 53–76, 1998.

Kim, J. A., Baker, D. G., Hahn, S. S., Goodchild, N. T., and Constable, W. C., Topical use of N-acetylcysteine for reduction of skin reaction to radiation therapy. *Sem. Oncol.,* 10(1):86–88, 1983.

Kinscherf, R., Fischbach, T., Mihm, S., et al., Effect of glutathione depletion and oral N-acetylcysteine treatment on CD4+ and CD8+ cells. *FASEB J.,* 8:448–451, 1994.

Kowluru, R. A., Engerman, R. L., and Kern, T. S., Abnormalities of retinal metabolism in diabetes or experimental galactosemia VIII. Prevention by aminoguanidine. *Curr. Eye Res.* 21:814–819, 2000.

Kraemer, R., and Geubelle, F., Evaluation of mucolytic drugs by lung function studies in children. *Eur. J. Resp. Dis.,* 61:122–126, 1980.

Kuna, P., Petyrek, P., and Dostal, M., Modification of toxic and radioprotective effects of cystamine by glutathione in mice. *Radiobio. Radiother.,* 599–601, May 1978.

Lafleur, M. V. M., Woldhuis, J., and Loman, H., Effects of sulphydryl compounds on the radiation damage in biologically active DNA. *J. Radiat. Biol.,* 37(5):493–498, 1980.

Lands, L., NAC, glutamine, and alpha lipoic acid. *AIDS Treat. News,* Vol. 268, p. 2–7, April 4, 1997.

Larsson, A., Orrenius, S., Holmgren. A., and Mannervik, B., Functions of glutathione, biochemical, physiological, toxicological and clinical aspects. *Annal. Biochem.,* 139(1):126, 1984.

Le, B., and Steel, R. D., Effect of portacaval shunt on sulfur amino acid metabolism in rats. *Amer. J. Physiol.,* 241(6):503–508, 1981.

Leibach, F. H., Pillion, D. J., Mendicino, J., and Pashley, D., The role of glutathione in transport activity in kidney. In: *Functions of Glutathione in Liver and Kidney,* eds. Sies and Wendel. New York: Springer-Verlag, 1978, 170–180.

Lemy-Debois, N., Frigerio, G., and Lualdi, P., Oral acetylcysteine in bronchopulmonary disease. Comparative clinical trial with bromhexine. *Eur. J. Resp. Dis.,* 61:78–80, 1980.

Leuchtenberger, C., and Leuchtenberger, R., The effects of naturally occurring metabolites (L-cysteine, vitamin C) on cultured human cells exposed to smoke of tobacco or marijuana cigarettes. *Cytometry,* 5:396–402, 1984.

Levey, H. L., Phenylketonuria: old disease, new approach to treatment. *National Academy of Science U.S.A.,* Vol. 96(5), p.1811–3, March 2, 1999.

Levy, L., and Vredevoe, D. L., The effect of N-acetylcysteine on cyclophosphamide immunoregulation and antitumor activity. *Sem. Oncol.,* 10(1):7–16, 1983.

Livardjani, F., Lediga, M., Koppa, P., et al., Lung and blood superoxide dismutase activity in mercury vapor exposed rats: effect of N-acetylcysteine treatment. *Toxicology,* 66:289–295, 1991.

Loehrer, P. J., Williams, S. D., and Einhorn, L. H., N-acetylcysteine and ifosfamide in the treatment of unresectable pancreatic adenocarcinoma and refractory testicular cancer. *Sem. Oncol.,* 10(1):72–75, 1983.

Luder, E., Kattan, M., Thornton, J. C., et al., Efficacy of a nonrestricted fat diet in patients with cystic fibrosis. *AJDC,* 143, April 1989.

Macara, I. G., Kustin, K., and Cantley, L. C., Glutathione reduces cytoplasmic vanadate mechanism and physiological implications. *Biochim. et Biophys. Acta,* 629:95–106, 1980.

Maldonado, J., Gil, A., Faus, M. J., et al., Specific serum amino-acid profiles of trauma and septic children. *Clin. Nutr.* 7:165–170, 1988.

Malloy, M. H., and Rassin, D. K., Cysteine supplementation of total parenteral nutrition: the effect on beagle pups. *Ped. Res.,* 18(8):747–751, 1984.

Marklund, S., Nordensson, I., and Back, O., Normal CuZn superoxide dismutase, Mn superoxide dismutase, catalase and glutathione peroxidase in Werner's syndrome. *J. Geron.,* 36(4):405–409, 1981.

Martin, D., Willis, S., and Cline, D., N-Acetylcysteine in the treatment of human arsenic poisoning. *J. Am. Board Fam. Pract.,* 3:293–296, 1990.

Martin, R., Litt, M., and Marriott, C., The effect of mucolytic agents on the rheologic and transport properties of canine tracheal mucus. *Rev. Res. Dis.,* 121:495, 1980.

Martinez, E., and Domingo, P., N-acetylcysteine as chemoprotectant in cancer chemotherapy. *Lancet,* 338, July 27, 1991.

Martinez, F., Castillo, J., Leira, R., et al., Taurine levels in plasma and cerebrospinal fluid in migraine patients. *Headache J.,* 33(6), June 1993.

Martinez-Torres, C., Romano, E., and Layrisse, M., Effect of cysteine on iron absorption in man. *Amer. J. Clin. Nutr.,* 34:322–327, 1981.

McIntosh, C., Bakich, V., Trotter, T., Kwok, Y. N., Nishimura, E., Pederson, R., and Brown, J., Effect of cysteamine on secretion of gastrin and somatostatin from the rat stomach. *Gastroent.,* 86(5):834, 1984.

Meister, A., Selective modification of glutathione metabolism. *Science,* 220:43–478, 1983.

Melissinos, K. G., Delidou, A. Z., Varsou, A. G., Begietti, S. S., and Drivas, G. J., Serum and erythrocyte glutathione reductase activity in chronic renal failure. *Nephron,* 28:76–79, 1981.

Menon, K. K. G., and Natraj, C. V., Nutrients in the shadow-nutrients of substance. *J. Biosci.,* 6(4):459–474, 1984.

Merck Manual. Rahway, NJ: Merck, Sharp, and Dohme Research Laboratories.

Meydani, M., Dietary antioxidants modulation of aging and immune-endothelial cell interaction. *Mech. Aging Dev.,* 111:123–193, 1999.

Millard, W. J., Sagar, S. M., Landis, D. M. D., Martin, J. B., and Badger, T. M., Cysteamine: a potent and specific depletor of pituitary prolactin. *Science,* 217:452–454, 1982.

Miller, L. F., and Rumack, B. H., Clinical safety of high oral doses of acetylcysteine. *Sem. Oncol.,* 10(1):76–85, 1983.

Mills, B. J., Lindeman, R. D., and Lang, C. A., Differences in blood glutathione levels of tumor-implanted or zinc-deficient rats. *Amer. Inst. Nutr.,* III(9):1586–1592, 1981.

Moats, R. A., et al, Brain phenylalanine concentration in the management of adults with phenylketonuria. *Inherit. Metabolic Disorder,* Vol. 23(1), p.7–14, February 2000.

Morgan, L. R., Holdiness, M. R., and Gillen, L. E., N-acetylcysteine: its bioavailability and inter-action with ifosfamide metabolites. *Sem. Oncol.,* 10(1):56–61, 1983.

Morris, P. E., and Bernard, G. R., Significance of glutathione in lung disease and implications for therapy. *Am. J. Med. Sci.,* 307:119–127, 1994.

Mudd, S. H., Schnieder, J. A., Spielberg, S. P., Boxer, L., Oliver, J., Corash, L., and Sheetz, M., Genetic disorders of glutathione and sulfur amino-acid metabolism. *Ann. Int. Med.,* 9(3):330–346, 1980.

Mulders, T. M. T., Breimer, D. D., and Mulder, G. J., Glutathione conjugation in man. *Human Drug Metabolism.* Chapter 14. CRC Press, Inc., 1993.

Munthe, E., Kass, E., and Jellum, E., Intracellular glutathione correlating to clinical response in rheumatoid arthritis. *J. Rheumat.,* 7:14–19, 1981.

Murakami, M., and Webb, M., A morphological and biochemical study of the effects of L-cys-teine on the renal uptake and nephrotoxicity of cadmium. *Brit. J. Exp. Path.,* 62:115–130, 1981.

Murayama, K., and Kinoshita, T., Determination of glutathione on high performance liquid chromatography using N-chlorodansylamide (NCDA). *Analytical Letters,* 14(B15):1221–1232, 1981.

Nakagawa, Y., Hiraga, K., and Suga, T., Effects of butylated hydroxytoluene (BHT) on the level of glutathione and the activity of glutathione-S-transferase in rat liver. *J. Pharm. Dyn.,* 4:823–826, 1981.

Narkewicz, M. R., Caldwell, S., and Jones, G., Cysteine supplementation and reduction of total parenteral nutrition-induced hepatic lipid accumulation in the weanling rat. *Current Contents,* 23(33), August 14, 1995.

National Academy of Science. *Recommended Dietary Allowances.* 8:44, 1974.

Nielsen, F. H., Uhrich, K., and Uthus, E. O., Interactions among vanadium, iron, and cysteine in rats: growth, blood parameters, and organ wt/body wt ratios. *Biol. Trace Elem. Res.,* 6:117–132, 1984.

Noelle, R. J., and Lawrence, D. A., Determination of glutathione in lymphocytes and possible association of redox state and proliferative capacity of lymphocytes. *Biochem. J.,* 198:571–579, 1981.

Novi, A. A., Florke, R., and Stukenkemper, M., The effect of glutathione (GSH) on aflatoxin B1-induced tumors. Presented at *New York Academy of Science,* February 17, 1982.

———, Regression of aflatoxin B1-induced hepatocellular carcinomas by reduced glutathione. *Science,* 2121(5): 541–542, 1981.

Nutraletter. Glutathione. 2(2), October 1984.

Nutrition Reviews. Effects of lead on glutathione metabolism. 39(10):378–379, 1981.

Okuyama, S., and Mishina, H., Probable superoxide therapy of experimental cancer with D-penicillamine. *Tohoku J. Exp. Med.,* 135:215–216, 1981.

Oliver, I., et al., Prevention and dissolution of cystine stones by D-penicillamine. *Harefuah,* 84(1):11–12, 1973.

Olney, J. W., Ho, O. L., Rhee, V., and Schainker, B., Cysteine-induced brain damage in infant and fetal rodents. *Brain Res.,* 45:309–313, 1972.

Oppermann, R. V., Rolla, G., Johansen, J. R., and Assev, S. Thiol groups and reduced acidogenicity of dental plaque in the presence of metal ions *in vivo. Scand. J. Dent. Res.,* 88(5):389–396, 1980.

Orrenius, S., Ormstad, K., Thor, H., and Jewell, S. A., Turnover and functions of glutathione studied with isolated hepatic and renal cells. *Fed. Proc.,* 42(15):3177–3188, 1982.

Ovesen, L., Drug-nutrient interactions. *Drugs,* 18:278–298, 1979.

Pangborn, J., Building health with amino acids. *Nutrition for Optimal Health Association, Inc.* Conference on Amino Acids, Winnetka, IL, October 6, 1982.

Papaioannou, R., and Pfeiffer, C. C., Sulfite sensitivity—unrecognized threat: is molybdenum deficiency the cause? *J. Ortho. Psych.,* 13(2):105–110, 1984.

Parola, M., Paradisi, L., and Torrielli, M. V., Hepatic GSH concentration after treatment with non-steroidal anti-inflammatory agents during acute inflammation induced by carrageenan. *IRCS Med. Sci.,* 12:704–705, 1984.

Pekas, J. C., Larsen, G. L., and Fiel, V. J., Propachlor detoxication in the small intestine: cysteine conjugation. *J. Toxicol. & Environ. Health,* 5:653–662, 1979.

Penn, R. G., A theoretical approach to the management of paracetamol overdose. *J. Int. Med. Res.,* 4(4):98–104, 1976.

Peterson, R. G., and Rumack, B. H., Treating acute acetaminophen poisoning with acetylcysteine. *JAMA,* 237:2406–2407, 1977.

Pfeiffer, C. C., *Mental and Elemental Nutrients,* New Canaan, CT: Keats Publishing, Inc., 1975.

Pohlandt, F., Cystine: a semi-essential amino acid in the newborn infant. *Acta Paediatr. Scand.,* 63:801–804, 1974.

Prescott, L. F., Park, J., Ballantyne, A., Adriaenssens, P., and Proudfoot, A., Treatment of paracetamol (acetaminophen) poisoning with N-acetylcysteine. *Lancet,* August 1977.

Prohaska, J. R., and Gutsch, D. E., Development of glutathione peroxidase activity during dietary and genetic copper deficiency. *Bio. Trace Elem. Res.,* 5:35–45, 1983.

Puka-Sundvall, M., Brain injury after neonatal hypoxia-ischemia in rats: a role of cysteine. *Brain Res.,* Vol. 797(2), p.328–32, June 29, 1998.

Radak, K., and Kaneko, T., Regular exercise improves cognitive function and decreases oxidative damage in rat brain. *Neurochemistry International,* Vol. 38(1), p. 17–23, 2001.

Rafter, G. W., The effect of glutathione metabolism in human leukocytes. *Bio. Trace Element Res.,* 4:191–197, 1982.

Rasmussen, J. B., and Glennow, C., Reduction in days of illness after long-term treatment with N-acetylcysteine controlled release tablets in patients with chronic bronchitis. *Eur. Respir. J.,* 1:351–355, 1988.

Reim, M., Weidenfeld, E., and Santoso, B., Oxidized and reduced glutathione levels of the cornea *in vivo.* 211(2):165–175, 1979.

Renine, P. M., et al., Maternal hyperhomo-cysteinemia: a risk factor for neural tube defect? *Metabolism,* 43:1475–1480, 1994.

Revesz, L., and Edgren, M., Glutathione-dependent yield and repair of single-strand DNA breaks in irridiated cells. *Brit. J. Cancer*, 49(VI):55–60, 1984.

Riise, G. C., Larsson, S., Larsson, P., et al., The intrabronchial microbial flora in chronic bronchitis patients: a target for N-acetylcysteine therapy? *Eur. Respir. J.*, 7:94–101, 1994.

Roederer, M., Staal, F. J., Ela, S. W., et al., N-acetylcysteine: potential for AIDS therapy. *Pharmacology*, 46:121–129, 1993.

Rouzer, C. A., Scott, W. A., Griffith, O. W., Hamill, A. L., and Cohn, A. A., Arachidonic acid metabolism in glutathione-deficient macrophages. *Proc. Natl. Acad. Sci.*, 79(5):1621–1625, 1982.

————, et al., Depletion of glutathione selectively inhibits synthesis of leukotriene C by macrophages. *Proc. Natl. Acad. Sci.*, 78(4):2532–2536, 1981.

Rowe, L. D., Kim, H. L., and Camp, B. J., The antagonistic effect of L-cysteine in experimental hymenoxon intoxication in sheep. *Am. J. Vet. Res.*, 41(4):484, 1980.

Sakamoto, Y., Jigashi, T., and Tateishi, N., Glutathione storage, transport and turnover in mammals. *Annal. Biochem.*, 191(1), 1984.

Saunders, S. L., Shin, S. H., and Reifel, C. W., Cysteamine acts immediately to inhibit prolactin release and induce cellular changes in estradiol-primed male rats. *Neuroendocrin.*, 38:182–188, 1984.

Scammell, J. G., and Dannies, P. S., Depletion of pituitary prolactin by cysteamine is due to loss of immunological activity. *Endocrin.*, 114(3): 712–716, 1984.

Schwedes, U., Clemencon, G. H., Paschke, R., and Usadel, K. H., Effect of pentobarbital anesthesia and bile acids on cysteamine-induced duodenal and gastric ulcers in rats. *Scand. J. Gastroenterol.*, 19(92):121–124, 1984.

Scriver, C. R., Whelan, D. T., Clow, C. L., and Dallaire, L., Cystinuria: increased prevalence in patients with mental disease. *N. Engl. J. Med.*, 283:783–786, 1970.

Seiler, M., Szabo, S., Ourieff, S., McComb, D. J., Kovacs, K., and Reichlin, S., The effect of duodenal ulcerogen cysteamine on somatostatin and gastrin cells in the rat. *Exper. & Molecul. Pathol.*, 39:207–218, 1983.

Serougne, C., Ferezov, J., and Rukaj, A., Effects of excess dietary L-cystine on the rat plasma lipoproteins. *Ann. Nutr. Metab.*, 28:311–320, 1984.

Silvers, G. W., Maisel, J. C., Petty, T. L., Filley, G. F., and Mitchell, R. S., Increase of flow in excised emphysematous lungs following lavage with acetylcysteine or saline. *Amer. Rev. Resp. Dis.*, 110:170–175, 1974.

Simpkins, J. W., Estes, K. S., Millard, W. J., Sagar, S. M., and Martin, J. B., Cysteamine depletes prolactin in young and old hyperprolactinemic rats. *Endocrin.*, 112(5):1889–1891, 1983.

Skalka, H. W., and Parchal, J. T., Riboflavin and cataracts. *Amer. J. Clin. Nutr.*, 34(5):861–863, 1981.

Skovby, F., Rosenberg, L. E., and Thier, S. O., No effect of L-glutamine on cystinuria. *J. Med.*, 302(4), January 24, 1980.

Skullerud, K., Marstein, S., Schrader, H., Brundelet, P. J., and Jellum, E., The cerebral lesions in a patient with generalized glutathione deficiency. *Acta Neuropathol. (Berl.)*, 52:235–238, 1980.

Slavik, M., and Saiers, J. H., Phase I clinical study of acetylcysteine's preventing ifosfamide hematuria. *Seminars on Oncology*, 10(1):62–65, 1983.

Smith, A.C., James, R. C., Berman, M. L., and Harbison, R. D., Paradoxical effects of perturbation of intracellular levels of glutathione on halothane-induced hepatotoxicity in hyperthyroid rats. *Fundament. Appl. Toxicol.,* 4:221–230, 1984.

Smolin, L. A., and Benevenga, N. J., The use of cyst(e)ine in the removal of protein-bound homocysteine. *Am. J. Clin. Nutr.,* 39:730–737, 1984.

Sohler, A., Siegert, E., and Pfeiffer, C. C., Blood molybdenum level as a function of dietary molybdenum. *Trace Elements in Med.,* 1(2):50–53, 1984.

Sparnins, V. L., Venegas, P. L., and Wattenberg, L. W., Glutathione S-transferase activity: enhancement by compounds inhibiting chemical carcinogenesis and by dietary constituents. *NNCI,* 68(3):493–495, 1982.

Sprince, H., Parker, C. M., and Smith, G. G., Comparison of protection by L-ascorbic acid, L-cysteine, and adrenergic-blocking agents against acetaldehyde, acrolein, and formaldehyde toxicity: implications in smoking. *Agents & Actions,* 9(4):40–414, 1979.

Stampfer, M. J., Malinow, M. R., Willett, W. C., et al., A prospective study of plasma homo-cyst[e]ine and risk of myocardial infarction in U.S. Physicians. *JAMA,* 268(7), August 19, 1992.

Stefani, E. D., Boffetta, P., Deneo-Pellegrini, H., Mendilaharsu, M., Carzoglio, J. C., Ronco, A., and Olivera, L., Dietary antioxidants and lung cancer risk: a case-control study in Uruguay. *Nutr. Cancer,* 34:100–110, 1999.

Steiner, G., Mensal, H., Limbic, I., Onshore, F. K., and Bremer, H. J., Plasma glutathione per-oxidase after selenium supplementation in patients with reduced selenium state. *Euro. J. Ped.,* 138:138–140, 1982.

Stops, S. J., El-Rawhide, F. H., Lawson, T., Kobayashi, R. H., Wolf, B. G., and Potter, J. F., Changes in glutathione and glutathione metabolizing enzymes in human erythrocytes and lymphocytes as a function of age of donor. *Age,* 7(1):3–7, 1984.

Strudel, O., and Hoppenkamps, R., Relations between gastric glutathione and the ulcerogenic action of non-steroidal anti-inflammatory drugs. *Arch. Inter. de Pharmacodynamie et de Therapie,* 262(2):268–278, 1983.

Sturman, J. A., Gaull, G., and Raiha, N. C. R., Absence of cystathionase in human fetal liver: is cysteine essential? *Science,* 169:74–76, 1970.

Suarez, A., Ramirez-Tortosa, M., Gil, A., and Faus, M.J., Addition of vitamin E to long-chain polyunsaturated fatty-acid enriched diets protects neonatal tissue lipids against peroxidation in rats. *Eur. J. Nutr.,* 38:169–176, 1999.

Suarez, C., del Arco, C., Lahera, V., et al., N-acetylcysteine potentiates the antihypertensive effect of angiotensin converting enzyme inhibitors. *Current Contents,* 23(35), August 28, 1995.

Suter, P. M., Domeghetti, G., Schaller, M. D., et al., N-acetylcysteine enhances recovery from acute lung injury in man: a randomized, double-blind, placebo-controlled clinical study. *Chest,* 105:190–194, 1994.

Swaiman, K. F., Menkes, J. H., DeVivo, D. C., and Prensky, A.-L., Metabolic disorders of the central nervous system. In: *The Practice of Pediatric Neurology.* New York: C. V. Mosby Co., 1982, 472.

Szabo, S., and Reichlin, S., Somatostatin in rat tissues is depleted by cysteamine administration. *Endocrinology,* 109(6):2255–2257, 1981.

Tabet, N., Mantle, D., Walker, Z., and Orrell, M., Dietary and endogenous antioxidants in dementia. *Int. J. Geriatr. Psychiatry,* 16:639–641, 2001.

Tajimi, K., Kosugi, I., Okada, K, and Kobayashi, K., Effect of reduced glutathione on hemodynamic responses and plasma catecholamine levels during metabolic acidosis. *Crit. Care Med.,* 13(3):178–181, 1985.

Takeyama, H., Hoon, D. S. B,, Saxton, R. E., et al., Growth inhibition and modulation of cell markers of melanoma by S-allyl-cysteine. *Oncology,* 50:63–69, 1993.

Tateishi, N., Higashi, T., Naruse, A., Hikita, K., and Sakamato, Y., Relative contributions of sulfur atoms of dietary cysteine and methionine to rat liver glutathione and proteins. *J. Biochem.,* 90:1603–1610, 1981.

Taurine better than low-dose COQ10 for congestive heart disease. *Life Extension Update,* 6(10), October 1993.

Thomas, C. W., Scholz, R. W., Reddy, C. C., and Massaro, E. T., Inhibition of *in vitro* lipid peroxidation by reduced glutathione in rat liver microsomes. *Fed. Proc.,* 41(5), 1982.

Toft, B. S., and Hansen, H. S., Metabolism of prostaglandin E1 and of glutathione conjugate of prostaglandin A1 (GSH-prostaglandin A1) by prostaglandin in 9-ketoreductase from rabbit kidney. *Biochim. Biophys. Acta,* 574:33–38, 1979.

Tolgyesi, E., Coble, D. W., Fang, F. S., and Kairinen, E. O., A comparative study of beard and scalp hair. *J. Soc. Cosmet. Chem.,* 34(11):361–382, 1983.

Torchiana, M. L., Pendelton, R. G., Cook, P. G., Hanson, C. A., and Clineschmidt, B. V., Apparent irreversible H2-receptor blocking and prolonged gastric antisecretory activities of 3-N-{3-[3-(1-piperidinomethyl) phenoxy]propyl} amino-1, 2, 5-thiadiazole-1-oxide (L-643, 441)(1). *J. Pharma. Exper. Therap.,* 224(3):514–519, 1983.

Trachtman, H., Del Pizzo, R., Struman, J. A., et al., Taurine and osmoregulation. *AJDC,* 142, November 1988.

Trizna, Z., Schantz, S. P., and Hsu, T. C., Effects of N-acetyl-L-cysteine and ascorbic acid on mutagen-induced chromosomal sensitivity in patients with head and neck cancers. *Am. J. Surg.,* 162, October 1991.

Tucker, E. M., Young, J. D., and Crowley, C., Red cell glutathione deficiency: clinical and biochemical investigations using sheep as an experimental model system. *Brit. J. Haemat.,* 48:403–415, 1981.

Unverferth, D. V., Mehegan, J. P., Nelson, R. W., Scott, C. C., Leier, C. V., and Hamlin, R. L., The efficacy of N-acetylcysteine in preventing doxorubicin-induced cardiomyopathy in dogs. *Sem. Oncol.,* 10(1),2–6, 1983.

Uren, J. R., and Lazarus, H., L-cyst(e)ine requirements of malignant cells and progress toward depletion therapy. *Cancer Trea. Rep.,* 63(6):1073–1079, 1979.

Van Mansom, I., Van Tinteren, H., Stewart, F. A., et al., Effect of N-acetylcysteine on photofrin-induced skin photosensitivity in patients. *Current Contents* (Lasers in Surgery and Medicine), 16 (4), 1995.

Vecchiarelli, A., Dottorini, M,, Petrella, D., et al., Macrophage activation by N-acetyl-cysteine in COPD patients. *Chest,* 105:806–811, 1994.

Walcher, F., Marzi, I., Flecks, U., et al., N-acetylcysteine failed to improve early microcirculatory alterations of the rat liver after transplantation. *Current Contents,* 23(31), July 31, 1995.

Wang, Y. D., An experimental study of chemical debridement of full-thickness burn in rabbits by N-acetylcysteine. *Chung Hua Cheng Hsing Shao Shang Wai Ko Tsa Chih,* 7:45–47, 1991.

Wazir, R., Wilson, R., and Sherman, A. D., Plasma serine to cysteine ratio as a biological marker for psychosis. *Brit. J. Psychiat.,* 143:69–73, 1983.

Wehrenberg, W. B., Benoit, R., Baird, A., and Guillemin, R., Inhibitory effects of cysteamine on neuroendocrine function. *Regulatory Peptides,* 6:137–145, 1983.

Wendel, A., Feuerstein, S., and Konz, K.-H., Drug-induced lipid peroxidation in mouse liver. In: *Functions of Glutathione in Liver and Kidney,* eds. Sies and Wendel. New York: Springer-Verlag, 1978, 189–190.

Whitcomb, D. C., Sossenheimeer, M. J., and Rakela, J., Management of acetaminophen ingestion in the outpatient setting. *JCOM,* 2(4), July/August 1995.

Yamamoto, K., Kawashima, T., and Migita, S., Gluthione-catalyzed disulfide-linking of C9 in the membrane attack complex of complement. *J. Biol. Chem.,* 257(15):8573–8576, 1982.

Yamanouchi Pharmaceutical Co., Ltd. *Tathion.* 5(2):3–18, 1984.

Yarbro, W., et al., eds. N-acetylcysteine: A significant chemoprotective adjunct. Chicago: *Seminars on Oncology* fimp (1) (Suppl.), 1983.

Yim, C. Y., Hibbs, Jr., J. B., McGergor, J. R., et al., Use of N-acetyl cysteine to increase intracellular glutathione during the induction of antitumor responses by IL-2. *J. Immunol.,* 152:5796–5805, 1994.

Yoshimura, K., Iwauchi, Y., Sugiyama, S., Kuwamura, T., Odaka, Y., Satoh, T., and Kitagawa, H., Transport of L-cysteine and reduced glutathione through biological membranes. *Research Commun. Chem. Path. Pharm.,* 37(2): 171–186, 1982.

Zala, G., Flury, R., Wust, J., et al., N-acetylcysteine improves eradication of Helicobacter pylori by omeprazole/amoxicillin in cigarette smokers. *Current Contents,* 124(31–32), August 9, 1994.

Zandwijk, N., N-acetylcysteine for lung cancer prevention. *Chest,* 107(5), May 1995.

Zlotkin, S. H., Bryan, H., and Anderson, G. H., Cysteine supplementation to cysteine-free intravenous feeding regimens in newborn infants. *Amer. J. Clin. Nutr.,* 34:914–923, 1981.

Zmuda, J., and Friedenson, B., Changes in intracellular glutathione levels in stimulated and unstimulated lymphocytes in the presence of 2-mercaptoethanol or cysteine. *J. Immunol.,* 130(1):362–364, 1983.

Chapter 8: Taurine

Alvarez, J. G., and Storey, B. T., Taurine, hypotaurine, epinephrine and albumin inhibit lipid peroxidation in rabbit spermatozoa and protect against loss of motility. *Biol. Repro.,* 29:548–555, 1983.

Ament, M., Taurine supplementation in total parenteral nutrition. *Amer. Col. of Nutr. and Travenol Labs Conference,* Deerfield, IL: September 6, 1984.

Arzate, M. E., Ponce, H., and Pasantes-Morales, H., Antagonistic effects of taurine and 4-aminopyridine on guinea pig ileum. *J. Neurosci. Res.,* 11:271–280, 1984.

Atlas, M., Bahl, J. J., Roeske, W., and Bressler, R., *In vitro* osmoregulation of taurine in fetal mouse hearts. *J. Mol. Cell. Cardiol.,* 16:311–320, 1984.

Azari, J., Brumbaugh, P., and Huxtable, R., Prophylaxis by taurine in the hearts of cardiomyopathic hamsters. *J. Mol. Cell. Cardiol.,* 12:1353–1366, 1980.

Azuma, J., Sawamura, A., Awata, N., Hasegawa, H., Ogura, K., Harada, H., Ohta, H., Yamauchi, K., and Kishimoto, S., Double-blind randomized crossover trial of taurine in congestive heart failure. *Cur. Thera. Resrch.,* 34(4):543–557, 1983.

———, Hasegawa, H., Awata, N., Sawamura, A., Harada, H., Ogura, K., Yamauchi, K., and

Kishimoto, S., Taurine for treatment of congestive heart failure in humans. In: *Sulfur Amino Acids: Biochemical & Clinical Aspects.* New York: Alan R. Liss, Publishers, 1983, 61–72.

Bankier, A., Turner, M., and Hopkins, I. J., Pyridoxine dependent seizures—a wider clinical spectrum. *Arch. Dis. Child.,* 58:415–418, 1983.

Barbeau, A., Inoue, N., Tsukada, Y., and Butterworth, R. F., The neuropharmacology of taurine. *Life Sci.,* 17:669–678.

Baskin, S. I., Klekotka, S. J., Kendrick, Z. V., and Bartuska, D. G., Correlation of platelet taurine levels with thyroid function. *J. Endocrinol. Invest.,* 2:245, 1979.

———, Leibman, A. J., De Witt, W. S., Orr, P. L., Tarzy, N. T., Levy, P., Krusz, J. C., Dhopesh, V. P., and Schraeder, P. L., Mechanism of the anticonvulsant action of phenytoin: regulation of central nervous system taurine levels. *Neurology,* p. 331, April 1978.

———, Leibman, A. J., and Cohn, E. M., Possible functions of taurine in the central nervous system. *Adv. Biochem. Psychopharma.,* 15:153–164, 1976.

Klekotka, S. J., Kendrick, Z. V., and Bartuska, D.-G., Correlation of platelet taurine levels with thyroid function. *J. Endocrinol. Invest.,* 2:245, 1979.

Bergamini, L., Mutani, R., Delsedime, M., and Durelli, L., First clinical experience on the antiepileptic action of taurine. *Eur. Neur.,* 11:261–269, 1974.

Bonhaus, D. W., and Huxtable, R. J., Seizure-susceptibility and decreased taurine transport in the genetically epileptic rat. *Neurochem. Inter.,* 6(3):365–368, 1984.

———, The transport, biosynthesis and biochemical actions of taurine in a genetic epilepsy. *Neurochem. Inter.,* 5:413–419, 1983.

Bousquet, P., Feldman, J., Bloch, R., and Schwartz, J., Tag antagonizes the central cardiovascular effects of taurine. *Eur. J. Pharmacol.,* 98:269–273, 1984.

Broquist, H. P., Amino acid metabolism. *Nutr. Reviews,* 34(10):289, 1976.

Buff, S., and et al., Taurine and hypotaurine in spermatozoa and epididymal fluid of cats. *Journal of Reproduction and Fertility Supplements,* 57, 93–5, 2001.

Burnham, W. M., Albright, P., and Racine, R. J., The effect of taurine on kindled seizures in the rat. *Can. J. Physiol. Pharmacol.,* 56:497–500, 1978.

Carruthers-Jones, D. I., and Van Gelder, N. M., Influence of taurine dosage on cobalt epilepsy in mice. *Neurochem. Resrch.,* III:115–123, 1978.

Collins, G. G. S., The rates of synthesis, uptake and disappearance of [14 C]-taurine in eight areas of the rat central nervous system. *Brain Res.,* 76:447–459, 1974.

Collu, R., Charpenet, G., and Clermont, M. J., Antagonism by taurine of morphine induced growth hormone secretion. *Le Journal Canadien des Sciences Neurologiques,* 5(1):139–142, 1978.

Contreras, E., and Tamayo, L., Effects of taurine on tolerance to and dependence on morphine in mice. *Arch. Inter. de Pharma. et de Thera.,* 267(2):224–231, 1983.

Cortijo, J., and et al., Effects of taurine on pulmonary responses to antigen in sensitized Brown-Norway rats. *European Journal of Pharmacology,* 431(1), 111–7, November 2001.

Crass, M. F., and Lombardini, J. B., Loss of cardiac muscle taurine after acute left ventricular ischemia. *Life Sci.,* 21:951–958, 1978.

———, Release of tissue taurine from the oxygen-deficient perfused rat heart (40082). *Proceed. Soc. Exper. Biol. Med.,* 157:486–488, 1978.

De Luca, A., and et al., Taurine and skeletal muscle ion channels. *Advanced Experience Medical Biology,* 483, 45–56, 2000.

Dorvil, N. P., Yousef. I. M., Tuchweber, B., and Roy, C. C., Taurine prevents cholestasis induced by lithocholic acid sulfate in guinea pigs. *Amer. J. Clin. Nutr.,* 37:221–232, February 1983.

Dove, R. S., Nutritional therapy in the treatment of heart disease in dogs. *Alternative Medicine Review,* Suppl. S38–45, September 6, 2001.

Eppler, B., Dawson, R., Dietary taurine manipulations in aged male Fischer 344 rat tissue: taurine concentration, taurine biosynthesis, and oxidative markers. *Biochemical Pharmacology,* 62(1), 29–39, July 1, 2001.

Erberdobler, H. F., Egan, B. M., and et al., Effect of intravenous taurine on endotoxin-induced acute lung injury in sheep. *European Journal of Surgery,* 167(8), 575–80, August 2001.

Greulich, H. G., and Trautwein, E., Determination of taurine in foods and feeds using an amino acid analyzer. *J. Chromato.,* 245:332–334, 1983.

———, Determinations of taurine in milk and infant formula diets. *Eur. J. Pediatr.,* 142: 133–134, 1984.

Felig, P., Wahren, J., and Ahlborg, G., Uptake of individual amino acids by the human brain. *Pros. Soc. Exp. Biol. Med.,* 142:230–232, 1973.

———, Nagy, S. U., and Csaba, G., Effect of glutathione (gamma-L-glutamyl-taurine) on the serum glucocorticoid and estriol level in rats. *Endokrinologie,* 79(3):437–438, 1982.

Torok, O., and Csaba, G., Effect of glutataurine, a newly discovered parathyroid hormone on rat thymus cultures. *Acta Morphol. Acad. Sci. Hung.,* 26(2):87–94, 1978.

———, Madarasz, B., Sudar, F., and Csaba, G., Effect of glutataurine on the pineal gland of the rat. *Acta Morphol. Acad. Sci. Hung.,* 28(3):233–242, 1980.

———, Torok, O., and Csaba, G., Effect of glutataurine on vitamin A and prednisolone treated thymus cultures. *Acta Morphol. Acad. Sci. Hung.,* 26(2):75–85, 1978.

———, Fekete, M., Kadar, T., and Telegdy. G., Effect of intraventricular administration of glutathione on norepinephrine, dopamine and serotonin turnover in different brain regions in rats. *Acta Physiol. Hungarica,* 61(3):163–167, 1983.

Flemstrom, G., Briden, S., and Kivilaakso, E., Stimulation by BW775C and inhibition by cysteamine of duodenal epithelial alkaline secretion suggest a role of endogenous prostaglandin in mucosal protection. *Scand. J. Gastroenterol.,* 19(92):101–105, 1984.

Franconi, F., Stendardi, I., Matucci, R., Failli, P., Bennardini, F., Antonini, G., and Frosini, M., and et al., Effects of taurine and some structurally related analogues on the central mechanism of thermoregulation: a structure-activity relationship study. *Advanced Experience Medical Biology,* 483, 283–92, 2000.

Frosini, M., and et al., The possible role of taurine and GABA as endogenous cryogens in the rabbit: changes in CSF levels in heat-stress. *Advanced Experience Medical Biology,* 483, 335–44, 2000.

Gaull, G. E., Taurine in the nutrition of the human infant. *Acta Paediat. Scand.,* 269:38, 1982.

———, Is taurine an essential nutrient in man? *Amer. Coll. Nutr. & Travenol Labs Confer.,* Deerfield, IL: September 1984.

Goodman, H. O., Connolly, B. M., McLean, W., and Resnick, M., Taurine transport in epilepsy. *Clin. Chem.,* 26(3):414–419, 1980.

Giotti, A., Inotropic effect of taurine in guinea-pig ventricular strips. *Eur. J. Pharm.,* 102:511–514, 1984.

Gorby, W. G., and Martin, W. G. The synthesis of taurine from sulfate VIII. The effect of potassium (38580). *Proc. Soc. Exper. Biol. Med.,* 148:544–549, 1975.

Gordon, S. M., Does the alcoholic's remedy come in a pill? *Behavior Healthy Tomorrow,* 10(4), SR29–30, August 2001.

Hamosh, M., Breastfeeding: unraveling the mysteries of mother's milk. *Medscape Women's Health,* 1(9), 4, September 1996.

Hansen, S. H., The role of taurine in diabetes and the development of diabetic complications. *Diabetes Metab Res Review,* 17(5), 330–46, September–October 2001.

Hardison, W. G. M., Wood, C. A., and Proffitt, J. H., Quantification of taurine synthesis in the intact rat and cat liver (39744). *Proc. Soc. Exper. Biol. Med.,* 155:55–58, 1977.

Hayes, K. C., Taurine requirement in primates. *Nutr. Rev.,* 43(3):65–70, 1985.

————, Stephan, Z. F., and Sturman, J. A., Growth depression in taurine-depleted infant monkeys. *J. Nutr.,* 110(10):2058–2064, 1980.

Hernandez, J., Artillo, S., Serrano, M. I., and Serrano, J. S., Further evidence of the anti-arrhythmic efficacy of taurine in the rat heart. *Res. Commun. Chem. Patho. Pharma.,* 43(2):343–346, 1984.

Hill, L. J., and Martin, W. G., The synthesis of taurine from sulfate V. regulatory modifiers of the chick liver enzyme system (37629). *Proc. Soc. Exp. Biol. & Med.,* 144:530–531, 1973.

Hsu, J. M., and Anthony, W. L., Zinc deficiency and urinary excretion of taurine-35S and inorganic sulfate-35S following cystine-35S injection in rats. *J. Nutr.,* 100(10):1189–1196, 1970.

Huxtable, R., and Chubb, J., Adrenergic simulation of taurine transport by the heart. *Science,* 198(10):409–411, 1977.

————, and Bressler, R., Elevation of taurine in human congestive heart failure. *Life Sci.,* 14:1353–1359, 1974.

————, and Laird, H., The prolonged anticonvulsant action of taurine on genetically determined seizure-susceptibility. *Can. J. Neuro. Sci.,* V,215–221, 1978.

Ikeda, H., Effects of taurine on alcohol withdrawal. *Lancet,* 509, September 3, 1977.

Iwata, H., Nakayama, K., Matsuda, T., and Baba, A., Effect of taurine on a benzodiazepine-GABA-chloride inonophore receptor complex in rat brain membranes. *Neurochem. Res.,* (4):535–544, 1984.

Izumi, K., Donaldson, J., Minnich, J. L., and Barbeau, A., Ouabain-induced seizures in rats: suppressive effects of taurine and gamma-amino butyric acid. *Can. J. Physiol. Pharmacol.,* 51:885–889, 1973.

Kakee, A., and et al., Efflux of a suppressive neurotransmitter, GABA, across the blood-brain barrier. *Journal Neurochemistry,* 79(1), 100–8, October 2001.

Kang, Y.S., Taurine transport mechanism through the blood-brain barrier in spontaneously hypertensive rats. *Advanced Experience Medical Biology,* 483, 321–4, 2000.

Kerai, M. D., Reversal of thanol-induced hepatic steatosis and lipid peroxidation by taurine. *Alcohol,* 34(4), 529–41, July–August 1999.

Kerai, M. D., and et al, Taurine: protective properties against ethanol-induced hepatic steatosis and lipid peroxidation during chronic ethanol consumption in rats. *Amino Acids,* 15(1–2), 53–76, 1998.

Kibayashi, E., and et al., Daily dietary taurine intake in Japan. *Advanced Experience Medical Biology,* 483, 137–42, 2000.

Kim, K. S., Kurokawa, M., Kimura, T., and Sezaki, H., Effect of taurine on the gastric absorption of drugs: comparative studies with sodium lauryl sulfate. *J. Pharm. Dyn.,* 5:509–514, 1982.

Kimura, T., Yamashita, S., Kim, K. S., and Sezaki, H., Electrophysiological approach to the action of taurine on rat gastric mucosa. *J. Pharm. Dyn.,* 5:495–500, 1982.

Kirschmann, J. D., and Dunne, L. J., *Nutrition Almanac.* New York: McGraw-Hill Book Co., 1984.

Kohashi, N., and Katori, R., Decrease of urinary taurine in essential hypertension. *Japan. Heart J.,* January 1983.

Kohashi, N., Okabayashi, T., Hama, J., and Katori, R., Decreased urinary taurine in essential hypertension. In: *Sulfur Amino Acids: Biochemical and Clinical Aspects,* pp. 73–87.

Kondo, Y., and et al., Taurine reduces atherosclerotic lesion development in apolippoprotein E-deficient mice. *Advanced Experience Medical Biology,* 483, 193–202, 2000.

Kontro, P., Effects of cations on taurine, hypotaurine, and GABA intake in mouse brain slices. *Neurochem. Res.,* 7(11):1391–1401, 1982.

———, and Oja, S. S., Taurine and synaptic transmission. *Med. Bio.,* 61:79–82, 1983.

Kuriyama, K., Huxtable, N. J., and Iwata, H., Cardiovascular actions of sulfur amino acids. In: *Sulfur Amino Acids: Biochemical and Clinical Aspects,* 104–124.

Lake, N., Taurine depletion of lactating rats: effects on developing pups. *Neurochem. Res.,* 8(7):881–887, 1983.

Lampson, W. G., Kramer, J. H., and Schaffer, S. W., Potentiation of the actions of insulin by taurine. *Can. J. Physiol. Pharmacol.,* 61:457–463, 1983.

Lefauconnier, J.-M., Urban, F., and Mandel, P., Taurine transport into the brain in rat. *Biochimie,* 60:381–387, 1978.

Lehmann, A., and Hamberger, A., Inhibition of cholinergic response by taurine in frog isolated skeletal muscle. *J. Pharm. Pharmacol.,* 36:59–61, 1984.

Leibfried, M. L., and Bavister, B. D., The effects of taurine and hypotaurine on *in vitro* fertilization in the golden hamster. *Gamete Res.,* 4:57–63, 1981.

Lombardini, J. B., and Prien. S. D., Taurine binding by rat retinol membranes. *Exp. Eye Res.,* 37:239–250, 1983.

Mantovani, J., et al., Effects of taurine on seizures and growth hormone release in epileptic patients. *Arch. Neur.,* 36:672–674, 1979.

Marnela, K.-M., and Kontro, P., Free amino acids and the uptake of binding of taurine in the central nervous system of rats treated with gaunidinoethanesulphonate. *Neurosci.,* 12(1):323–328, 1984.

———, Timonen, M., and Lahdesmaki, P., Mass spectrometric analyses of brain synaptic peptides containing taurine. *J. Neurochem.,* 43(6):650–653, 1984.

Martin, W. G., Truex, R. C., Tarka, S., Gorby, W., and Hill, L., The synthesis of taurine from sulfate VI. Vitamin B-6 deficiency and taurine synthesis in the rat (38450). *Proc. Soc. Exper. Biol. Med.,* 147:835–838, 1974.

Meizel, S., Lui, C. W., Working, P. K., and Mrsny, R. J., Taurine and hypotaurine: their effects on motility, capacitation and the acrosome reaction of hamster sperm *in vitro* and their presence in sperm and reproductive tract fluids of several mammals. *Develop. Growth & Differ.,* 22(3):483–494, 1980.

Messiha, F. S., Taurine, Analogues and ethanol elicited responses. *Brain Res. Bull.,* 4:603–607, 1979.

Militante, J. D., and Lombardini J. B., Characterization of taurine uptake in the rat retina. *Advanced Experience Medical Biology,* 483, 477–85, 2000.

Mutani, R., Bergamini, L., Delesedime, M., and Durelli, L., Effects of taurine in chronic experimental epilepsy. *Brain Res.,* 79:330–332, 1974.

———, Monaco, F., Durelli, L., and Delsedime, M., Levels of free amino acids in serum and cerebrospinal fluid after administration of taurine to epileptic and normal subjects. *Epilepsia,* 16:765–769, 1975.

Nakagawa, K., and Kuriyama, K., Effect of taurine on alteration in adrenal functions induced by stress. *Japan. J. Pharmacol.,* 25:737–746, 1975.

Newman, W. H., Frangakis, C. J., Grosso, D. S., and Bressler, R.-A. Relation between myocardial taurine content and pulmonary wedge pressure in dogs with heart failure. *Physiolog. Chem. Physics,* 9(3):259–263, 1977.

Nutrition Reviews. Taurine function revealed by its nutritional requirement in the kitten. 37:121–123, 1979.

Obrosova, I. G., Taurine counteracts oxidative stress and nerve growth factor deficit in early experimental diabetic neuropathy. *Exp. Neurol.,* 172(1), 211–9, November 2001.

Oja, S. S., and Kontro, P., Free amino acids in epilepsy: possible role of taurine. *Acta Neuro. Scand.,* 93(67):5–20, 1983.

Okamoto, E., Rassin, D. E., Zucker, C. L., Salen, G. S., and Heird, W., Role of taurine in feeding the low-birth-weight infant. *J. Ped.,* 104(6):936–940, 1984.

———, Kimura, H., and Sakai, Y., Evidence for taurine as an inhibitory neurotransmitter in cerebella stellate interneurons: selective antagonism by TAG. *Brain Res.,* 265:163–168, 1983.

———, Effects of taurine and GABA on Ca spikes and Na spikes in cerebellar purkinje cells *in vitro:* intrasomatic study. *Brain Res.,* 260:240–259, 1983.

———, Ionic mechanisms of the action of taurine on cerebella purkinje cell dendrites *in vitro:* intradendritic study. *Brain Res.,* 260:261–269, 1983.

———, Taurine-induced increase of the Cl-conductance of cerebella purkinje cell dendrites *in vitro.* *Brain Res.,* 259:319–323, 1983.

Paakkari, P., Paakkari, I., Karppanen, H., Halmekoski, J., and Paasonen, M. K., Cardiovascular and ventilatory effects of taurine and homotaurine in anaesthetized rats. *Med. Bio.,* 60:316–322, 1982.

Pecci, L., Hypotaurine and superoxide dismutase: protection of the enzyme against inactivation by hydrogen peroxide and peroxidation to taurine. *Advanced Experience Medical Biology,* 483, 163–8, 2000.

Perry, T. L., Currier, R. D., Hansen, S., and Maclean, J., Aspartate-taurine imbalance in dominantly inherited olivopontocerebellar atrophy. *Neurology,* 257, March 1977.

———, Bratty, P. J. A., Hansen, S., Kennedy, J., Urquhart, N., and Dolman, C. L., Hereditary mental depression and Parkinsonism with taurine deficiency. *Arch. Neurol.,* 32(2):108–113, 1975.

———, Segments. *J. of Neuro. Res.,* 11:303–311, 1984.

Pettegrew, J. W., and et al., Effects of chronic lithium administration on rat brain phosphatidylinositol cycle constituents, membrane phospholipids and amino acids. *Bipolar Disorders,* 3(4), 189–201, August 2001.

Quilligan, C. J., Hilton, F. K., and Hilton, M. A., Taurine in hearts and bodies of embryonic through early postpartum CF mice. *Pro. Soc. Exper. Bio. & Med.,* 177:143–150, 1984.

Rassin, D. K., et al., Taurine and other free amino acids in milk of man and other mammals. *Early Human Devel.,* II:1–13, 1978.

Rigo, J., and Senterre, J., Is taurine essential for the neonates? *Bio. Neonate,* 32:73–76, 1977.

Rose, S. J., et al., Taurine fluxes in insulin dependent diabetes mellitus and rehydration in streptozotocin treated rats. *Advanced Experience Medical Biology,* 483, 497–501, 2000.

Ruiz-Feria, C. A., Taurine, cardiopulmonary hemodynamics, and pulmonary hypertension syndrome in broilers. *Poult Science,* 80(11), 1607–18, November 2001.

Salceda, R., and Pasantes-Morales, H., Uptake, release and binding of taurine in degenerated rat retinas. *J. Neurosi. Res.,* 8:631–642, 1982.

———, Carabez, A., Pacheco, P., and Pasantes-Morales, H., Taurine levels, uptake and synthesizing enzyme activities in degenerated rat retina. *Exp. Eye Res.,* 28:137–146, 1979.

Salmon, R. J., Laurent, M., and Thierry, J. P., Effect of taurocholic acid feeding on methyl-nitro-N-nitroso-guanidine induced gastric tumors. *Cancer Letters,* 22:315–320, 1984.

Samuels, S., Early life nutritional deprivation: persistent alteration of blood and urine amino acids in mice (37504). *Proc. Soc. Exper. Biol. Med.,* 143:1215–1217, 1973.

Sanberg, P. R., and Willow, M., Dose-dependent effects of taurine on convulsions induced by hypoxia in the rat. *Neuroscience Letters,* 16:297–300, 1980.

Sanderson, S. L., and et al., Effects of dietary fat and L-carnitine on plasma and whole blood taurine concentrations and cardiac function in healthy dogs fed protein-restricted diets. *American Journal Vet. Res.,* 62(10), 1616–23, October 2001.

Savoldi, F., and Tartara, A., Effects of taurine on acute epilepsy in rabbits. *Il Farmaco-Ed. Pr.,* 31(1):27–34, 1977.

Sawamura, A., Azuma, J., Harada, H., Hasegawa, H., Ogura, K., Scandurra, R., Politi, L., Dupre, S., Moriggi, M., Barra, D., and Cavallini, D., Comparative biological production of taurine from free cysteine and from cysteine bound to phosphopantothenate. *Bul. Molecular Biol. & Med.,* 2(12):172–177, 1977.

Schaffer, S., Taurine-deficient cardiomyopathy: role of phospholipids, calcium, and osmotic stress. *Advanced Experience Medical Biology,* 483, 57–69, 2000.

Schaffer, S., and Koesis, J. J., Taurine-research surges after 150 years. *Amer. Pharm.,* XIX:36–38, 1979.

Science. Salt-free salt. March. 8, 1985.

Sebring, L. A., and Huxtable, R. J., Cardiovascular actions of taurine. In: *Sulfur Amino Acids: Biochemical & Clinical Aspects,* 1983.

Sgaragli, G., Carla, V., Magnani, M., and Galli, A., Hypothermia induced in rabbits by intracerebroventricular taurine: specificity and relationships with central serotonin (5-HT) systems. *J. Pharma. Exper. Ther.,* 219(3): 778–785, 1981.

Shimada, M., Shimono, R., Watanabe, M., Imahayashi, T., Ozaki, H. S., Kihara, T., Yamaguchi, K., and Niizeki. S., Distribution of 35S-taurine in rat neonates and adults. *Histochem.,* 80:225–230, 1984.

Smayda, R., *Contemporary Review of Therapeutic Benefits of the Amino Acid Taurine.* www.mgwater.com.

Sperelakis, N., and Kishimoto, S., Protection by oral pretreatment with taurine against the negative inotropic effects of low-calcium medium on isolated perfused chick heart. *Cardiovas. Res.,* 17(10):620–626, 1983.

Stanbury, J. B., Wyngaarden, J. B., and Fredrickson, D. S., *The Metabolic Basis of Inherited Disease.* New York: McGraw-Hill Book Co., 1978.

Stephan, Z. F., Armstrong, M. J., and Hayes, K. C., Bile lipid alterations in taurine-depleted monkeys. *Amer. J. Clin. Nutr.,* 34(2):204–210, 1981.

Stipanuk, M. H., Kuo, S. M., Hirschberger, L. I., Changes in maternal taurine levels in response to pregnancy and lactation. *Life Sci.,* 35(11):1149–1156, 1984.

————, and Kuo, S. M., Effect of vitamin B6 deficiency on cysteinesulfinate decarboxylase activity and taurine concentration in tissues of rat dams and their offspring. *Life Sci.:* 30(3): 667, 1984.

Sturman, J. A., and Cohen, P. A., Cystine metabolism in vitamin B6 deficiency: evidence of multiple taurine pools. *Biochem. Med.,* 5(3):245-268, 1971.

————, Rassin, D. K., and Gaull, G. E., Taurine in development. *Life Sci.,* 21:1–22, 1977.

————, Taurine in developing rat brain: changes in blood-brain barrier. *J. Neurochem.,* 32:811–816, 1979.

————, Rassin, D. K., Hayes, K. C., and Gaull, G. E., Taurine deficiency in the kitten: exchange and turnover of (35S) taurine in brain, retina, and other tissues. *J. Nutr.,* CVIII:1462–76, 1978.

————, Taurine in nutrition. *Comp. Thera.,* III:59–65, 1977.

————, Taurine pool sizes in the rat: effects of vitamin B6 deficiency and high taurine diet. *J. Nutr.,* 103:1566–1580, 1973.

Tachiki, K. H., Hendrie, H. C., Kellams, J., and Aprison, M. H., A rapid column chromatographic procedure for the routine measurement of taurine in plasma of normal and depressed patients. *Clin. Chim. Acta,* 75:455–465, 1977.

Takahashi, K., and Ohyabu, Y., Taurine prevents ischemia damage in cultured neonatal rat cardiomyocytes. *Advanced Experience Medical Biology,* 483, 109–16, 2000.

Tallen, H. H., Jacobson, E., Wright, C. E., Schneidman, K., and Gaull, G. E., Taurine uptake by cultured human lymphoblastoid cells. *Life Sci.,* 33:1853–1860, 1983.

The Orlando Sentinel. Chemical in lobsters may control epilepsy. February 10, 1985.

Thompson, D. E., and Vivian, V. M., Dietary-induced variations in urinary taurine levels of college women. *J. Nutr.,* 107(4):673–679, 1977.

Toth, E., and Lajtha, A., Brain protein synthesis rates are not sensitive to elevated GABA, taurine or glycine. *Neurochem. Res.,* 9(2):173–180, 1984.

Urquhart, N., Perry, T. L., Hansen, S., and Kennedy, J., Passage of taurine into adult mammalian brain. *J. Neurochem.,* 22:871–872, 1974.

Usdin, E., Hamburg, D. A., and Barchas, J. D., eds., Hereditary mental depression with taurine deficiency. In: *Neuroregulators and Psychiatric Disorders.* Oxford: Oxford University Press, 1978.

van Gelder, N. M., A central mechanism of action for taurine: osmoregulation, bivalent cations, and excitation threshold. *Neurochem. Res.,* 8(5):687–699, 1983.

————, Sherwin, A. L., Sacks, C., and Andermann, F., Biochemical observations following administration of taurine to patients with epilepsy. *Brain Res.,* 94:297–306, 1975.

Vinton, N., Laidlaw, S., Wu, S., Ament, M., and Kopple, J., Plasma and platelet taurine concentrations in children receiving home total parenteral nutrition (TPN) and healthy children. *ACN,* Vol. 41, April 1985.

Voaden, M. J., Hussain, A. A., and Chan, I. P. R., Studies on retinitis pigmentosa in man. I. Taurine and blood platelets. *Brit. J. Opthal.,* 66(12):771–775, 1982.

Wada, J. A., Osawa, T., Wake, A., and Corcoran, M. E., Effects of taurine on kindled amygdaloidal seizures in rats, cats, and photosensitive baboons. *Epilepsia,* 16:229–234, 1975.

Watt, S. M., and Simmonds, W. J., Effects of four taurine-conjugated bile acids on mucosal uptake and lymphatic absorption of cholesterol in the rat. *J. Lip. Res.,* 25:448–455, 1984.

Wessberg, P., Hedner, T., Hedner, J., and Jonason, J., Effects of taurine and a taurine antagonist on some respiratory and cardiovascular parameters. *Life Sci.,* 33:1649–1655, 1983.

Whittle, B., and Smith, J. T., Effect of dietary sulfur on taurine excretion by the rat. *J. Nutr.,* 104(6):666–670, 1974.

Wu, J. Y., and et al., Mode of action of taurine and regulation dynamics of its synthesis in the CNS. *Advanced Experience Medical Biology,* 483, 35–44, 2000.

Yamaguchi, K., Shigehisa, S., Sakakibara, S., Hosokawa, Y., and Ueda, I. Cysteine metabolism *in vivo* of vitamin B6-deficient rats. *Biochim. et Biophys. Acta,* 381:1–8, 1975.

Yamamoto, H. A., McCain, H. W., Izumi, K., Misawa, S., and Way, E. L., Effects of amino acids, especially taurine and gamma-aminobutyric acid (GABA), on analgesia and calcium depletion induced by morphine in mice. *Euro. J. Pharma.,* 71(2/3):177–184, 1981.

Yamori, Y., Wang, H., Ikeda, K., Kihara, M., Nara, Y., and Horle, R., Role of sulfur amino acids in the prevention and regression of cardiovascular diseases. In: *Sulfur Amino Acids: Biochemical & Clinical Aspects,* 103–116.

Yarbrough, G. G., Singh, D. K., and Taylor, D. A., Neuropharmacological characterization of a taurine antagonist. *J. Pharm. Exper. Ther.,* 219(3):604–613, 1981.

Zemlyanoy, A., et al., The treatment of ammonia poisoning by taurine in combination with a broncholytic drug. *Advanced Experience Medical Biology,* 483, 627–30, 2000.

SECTION FOUR

Chapter 9: Arginine and Its Metabolites

Abou-Mohamed, G., Kaesemeyer, W. H., Caldwell, R. B., Caldwell, R. W., Role of L-arginine in the vascular action and development of tolerance to nitroglycerin. *Br. J. Pharmacol.,* 130(2):211–18, May 2000.

Akashi, K., Miyake, C., Yokota, A., Citrulline, a novel compatible solute in drought-tolerant wild watermelon leaves, is an efficient hydroxyl radical scavenger. *FEBS Lett.* 508(3):438–42, November 23, 2001.

Anderson, H. L., Cho, E. S., Krause, P. A., Hanson, K. C., Krause, G. F., and Wixom, R. L., Effects of dietary histidine and arginine on nitrogen retention of men. *J. Nutr.,* 107:2067–2068, 1977.

Barbeau, A., *Metabolic Ataxias: Taurine and Neurological Disorders.* New York: Raven Press, 1978, 403–411.

Barbul, A., Rettura, G., Levenson, S. M., and Seifter, E., Arginine: a thymotropic and wound-healing promoting agent. *Surgical Forum,* XVIII:101–103, October 1977.

———, and Seifter, E., Wound-healing and thymotropic effects of arginine: a pituitary mechanism of action. *Amer. J. Clin. Nutr.,* 37:786, 1983.

Barziza, D. E., Buentello, J. A., Gatlin, 3rd, D. M., Dietary arginine requirements of juvenile red drum (Sciaenops ocellatus) based on weight gain and feed efficiency. *J. Nutrit.,* 130(7):1796–9, July 2000.

Batshaw, M. L.. and Brusilow, S. W., Treatment of hyperammonemic coma caused by inborn errors of urea synthesis. *J. Ped.,* 97(6):893–900, 1980.

Batshaw, M. L., Wachtel, R. C., Thomas, G. H., Starrett, A., Bennett, M. J., Dear, P. R. F., McGinlay, J. M., and Gray, R. G. F., Acute neonatal citrullinaemia. *J. Inher. Metab. Dis.,* 7:85, 1984.

Beck, P., Eaton, R. P., Arnett, D. M., and Alsever, R. N., Effect of contraceptive steroids on arginine-stimulated glucagon and insulin secretion in women: I-lipid physiology. *Metabolism,* 24(9):1055–1065, 1975.

Bergamini, S., Rota, C., Canali, R., Staffieri, M., Daneri, F., Bini, A., Giovannini, F., Tomasi, A., Iannone, A., N-acetylcysteine inhibits *in vivo* nitric oxide production by inducible nitric oxide synthase. *Nitric Oxide,* 5 (4):349–60, August 2001.

Biegon, A., and Terlou, M., Arginine-vasopressin binding sites in rat brain: a quantitative autoradiographic study. *Neurosc. Letters,* 44(3), 1984.

Bradley, P. M., El-Fiki, F.. and Giles, K. L., Polyamines and arginine affect somatic embryo genesis of daucus carota. *Plant Sci. Let.,* 34:397–401, 1984.

Bratusch-Marrain, P., Bjorkman, O., Hagenfeldt, L., Waldhausl, W., and Wahren, J., Influence of arginine on splanchnic glucose metabolism in man. *Diabetes,* 28(2):126–131, February 1979.

Brusilow, S. W., and Batshaw, M. L., Arginine therapy of arginiosuccinase deficiency. *Lancet,* January 1979, pp. 124–126.

——, Wachtel, R. C., Thomas, G. H., and Starrett, A., Arginine-responsive asymptomatic hyperammonemia in the premature infant. *J. Pediat.,* 105(1): 86–91, 1984.

Bushinsky, D. A., and Gennari, J., Life-threatening hyperkalemia induced by arginine. *Ann. Int. Med.,* 89(5):632–634, 1978.

Buttlaire, D. H., and Cohn, M., Characterization of the active site structures of arginine kinase-substrate complexes. Water proton magnetic relaxation rates and electron paramagnetic resonance spectra of manganous-enzyme complexes with substrates and of a transition state. *Analog. J. Biol. Chem.,* 249(18):5741–5748, 1974.

Casaneuva, F. F., Villanueva, L., Cabranes, J. A., Cabexas-Cerrato, J., and Fernandez-Cruz, A., Cholinergic mediation of growth hormone secretion elicited by arginine, clonidine, and physical exercise in man. *J. Clin. Endocrin. & Metabol.,* 526–530, 1984.

Cederbaum, S. D., Shaw, K. N. F., Spector, E. B., Verity, M. A., Snodgrass, P.J., Sugarman, G. I., Hyperargininemia with arginase deficiency. *Pediat. Res.,* 13:827–833, 1979.

——, Shaw, K. N. F., and Valente, M., Hyperarginemia. *J. Ped.,* 90(4):569–573, 1977.

Cherrington, A. D., and Vranic, M., Effect of arginine on glucose turnover and plasma free fatty acids in normal dogs. *J. Amer. Diabetes Assoc.,* 22(7):537–543, 1973.

D'Hooge, R., Marescau, B., Qureshi, I. A., and De Deyn, P.P., Impaired cognitive performance in ornithine transcarbamylase-deficient mice on arginine-free diet. *Brain Resources,* 876(1–2), 1–9, September 8 2000.

Davila, N., Alcaniz, J., Salto, L., Estrada, J., Barcelo, B., Baumann, G., Serum growth hormone-binding protein is unchanged in adult panhypopituitarism. *J. Clin. Endocrinol. Metab.,* 79(5), 1347–50, November 1994.

Devlin, T. M., *Textbook of Biochemistry.* New York: John Wiley & Sons, 1982, p. 553.

Drago, F., Continella, G., Alloro, M. C., Auditore, S., and Pennisi, G., Behavioral effects of arginine in male rats. *Pharmacol. Res. Comm.,* 16(9):899–908, September 1984.

Easter, R. A., and Baker, D. H., Arginine and its relationship to the antibiotic growth response in swine. *J. Animal Sci.,* 45(1):108–112, 1977.

Endres, W., Schaller, R., and Shin, Y. S., Diagnosis and treatment of argininaemia. Characteristics of arginase in human erythrocytes and tissues. *J. Inher. Metab. Dis.,* 7:8 1984.

Ferrero, E., Casale, G., and De Nicola, P., Serum glucagon after arginine infusion in aged and young subjects. *J. Amer. Ger. Soc.,* XXVIII (6):285–287, 1980.

Frankel, B. J., Gerich, J. E., Fanska, R. E., Gerritsen, G. C., and Grodsky, G. M., Responses to arginine of the perfused pancreas of the genetically diabetic Chinese hamster. *Diabetes,* 24(3):272–279, 1975.

Fraschini, F., Ferioli, M. E., Nebuloni, R., and Scalabrino, G., Pineal gland and polyamines. *J. Neural. Trans.,* 48:209–221, 1980.

Fraser, G. E., Nut consumption, lipids, and risk of coronary event. *Clinical Cardiology,* 22(7 Suppl.), III1 1–5, July 1999.

Gelehrter, T. D., and Rosenberg, L. E., Ornithine transcarbamylase deficiency. *New. Eng. J. Med.,* 292:351–352, 1975.

Giroux, I., Kurowska, E. M., Freeman, D. J., and Carroll, K.K., Addition of arginine but not glycine to lysine plus methionine-enriched diets modulates serum cholesterol and liver phospholipids in rabbits. *Journal of Nutrition,* 129(10):1807–13, October 1999.

Goldstein, R. E., Marks, S. L., Cowgill, L. D., Kass, P. H., Rogers, Q. R., Plasma amino acid profiles in cats with naturally acquire chronic renal failure. *Am. J. Vet. Res.,* 60(1): 109–13, January 1999.

Grazi, E., Magri, E., and Balboni, G., On the control of arginine metabolism in chicken kidney and liver. *Eur. J. Biochem.,* 60:431–436, 1975.

Greco, A. V., Altomonte, L., Chirlanda, G., Rebuzzi, A. G., Manna, R., and Bertoli, A., Serum gastrin in portal and peripheral veins after arginine in man. *Acta Heptao-Gastroenterologica,* 26(2):97–101, 1979.

Haas, D., Matsumoto, H., Moretti, P., Stalon, V., and Mercenier, A., Arginine degradation in pseudomonas aeruginosa mutants blocked in two arginine catabolic pathways. *Mol. Gen. Genet.,* 193:437–444, 1984.

Harper, H. A., *Review of Physiological Chemistry,* 12th ed. Los Altos, CA: Lange Medical Pub., 1969.

Hashimoto, E., Kobayaski, T., and Yamamura, H., Mg2+ counteracts the inhibitory effect of spermine on liver phosphorylase kinase. *Biochem. Biophys. Res. Comm.,* 121(1):271–276, 1984.

Hassan, A. S., and Milner, J. A., Alterations in liver nucleic acids and nucleotides in arginine efficient rats. *Metabolism,* 30(8):739–744, 1981.

Hawkins, P., Steyn, C., McCGarrigle, H. H., Calder, N. A., Saito, T., Stratford, L. L., Noakes, D. E., and Hansona, M. A., Cardiovascular and hypothalamic-pituitary-adrenal axis development in late gestation fetal sheep and young lambs following modest maternal nutrient restriction in early gestation. *Reproductive Fertility Development,* 12(7–8), 443–56, 2000.

Honda, T., Amino acid metabolism in the brain with convulsive disorders. Part I: free amino acid patterns in the brain of el mouse with convulsive seizure. *Brain Dev.,* 6:17–21, 1984.

————, Part II: The effects of anticonvulsants on convulsions and free amino acid patterns in the brain of el mouse. *Brain Dev.*, 6:22–6, 1984.

Hutchinson, S. J., Reitz, M. S., Sudhir, K., Sievers, R. E., Zhu, B. Q., Sun, Y. P., Chou, T. M., Deedwania, P. C., Chatterjee, K., Glantz, S. A., Parmley, W. W., Chronic dietary L-arginine prevents endotheliatl dysfunction secondary to environmental tobacco smoke in normocholesterolemic rabbits. *Hypertension,* 29(5): 1186–91, May 1997.

Igarashi, K., Sugiyama, Y., Kasuya, F., Inoue, H., Matoba, R., Castagnoli, N., Analysis of citrulline in rat brain tissue after perfusion with haloperidol by liquid chromatography-mass spectrometry. *J. Chromatogr. B. Biomed. Sci. Appl.,* 746(1):33–40, September 1 2000.

Ikeda, Y., Young, L. H., Scalia, R., Lefer, A. M., Cardioprotective effects of citrulline in ishcemia reperfusion injury via a non-nitric oxide-mediated mechanism. *Methods Find Exp. Clin. Pharmacol.,* 22(7):563–71, September 2000.

Ito, T. Y., Trant, A. S., Polan, M. L., A double-blind placebo-controlled study of arginmax, a nutritional supplement for enhancement of female sexual function. *J. Sex Marital Therapy,* 27(5), 541–9, October–December 2001.

Job, J. C., Donnadieu, M., Garnier, P. E., Evain-Brion, D., Roger, M., and Chaussain, J. L., Ornithine stimulation test: correlation with subsequent response to hGH therapy. Evaluation of growth hormone secretion. *Pediat. Adolesc. Endocr.,* 12:86–102, 1983.

Josefsberg, Z., Laron, Z., Doron, M., Keret, R., Belinski, Y.. and Weismann, I., Plasma glucagon response to arginine infusion in children and adolescents with diabetes mellitus. *Clin. Endocrin.,* 4:487–492, 1975.

————, Kauli, R., Keret, R., Brown, M., Bialik, O., Greenberg, D., and Laron, Z., Tests for hGH secretion in childhood: comparison of response of growth hormone to insulin hypoglycemia and to arginine in children with constitutional short stature in different pubertal stages. *Pediat. Adolesc. Endocr.,* 12:66–74, 1983.

Jungling, M. L., and Bunge, R. G., The treatment of spermatogenic arrest with arginine. *Fertility & Sterility,* 27(3):282–283, 1976.

Kang, S.-S., Wong, P. W. K., and Melyn, M. A., Hyperargininemia: effect of ornithine and lysine supplementation. *J. Ped.,* 103(5):763–765, 1983.

Keller, D. W., and Polakoski, K. L., L-arginine stimulation of human sperm motility *in vitro. Bio. Repro.,* 13, 1975.

Kelly, J. J., Willimason, P., Martin, A., Whitworth, J. A., Effects of oral L-arginine on plasma nitrate and blood pressure in cortisol-treated humans. *J. Hypertens.,* 19(2):263–8, February 2001.

Khalilov, E. M., Torkhovskaya, T. I., Ivanov, A. S., Shingerey, M. V., Perepelitsa, V. N., Sergienko, V. I., and Lopukhin, Y. M., Dynamics of lipoprotein alterations in blood of patients with peripheric atherosclerosis after haemosorption. *Voprosy Meditsinskoi Khimii,* 30(6):24–27, 1984.

Kline, J. L., Hug, G., Schubert, W. K., and Berry, H., Arginine deficiency syndrome: its occurrence in carbamyl phosphate synthetase deficiency. *Am. J. Dis. Child.,* 135:437–441, 1981.

Khawaja, J. A., Nittyla, J., and Lindholm, D. B., The effect of magnesium deficiency on the polyamine content of different rat tissues. *Nutr. Rep. Inter.,* 29(4):903–910, 1984.

Kratzer, F. H., and Earl, L., Effect of arginine deficiency on normal and dystrophic chickens. *Soc. Exper. Biol. Med.,* 148:656–659, 1975.

Kraus, H., Stubbe, P., and von Berg, W., Effects of arginine infusion in infants: increased urea synthesis associated with unchanged ammonia blood levels. *Metabolism,* 25(11):1241–1247, 1976.

Krieger, L., Diseases for which non-inheritable gene therapy might be considered. *Amer. Med. News,* December 28, 1984, p. 19.

Kritchevsky, D., Tepper, S. A., Czarnecki, S. K., Klurfeld, D. M., and Story, J. A., Effects of animal and vegetable protein in experimental atherosclerosis. In: *Current Topics in Nutrition & Disease. Animal and Vegetable Proteins in Lipid Metabolism and Atherosclerosis,* Vol. 8. New York: Alan R. Liss, 1983, 85–100.

Kuiper, M. A., Teerlin, T., Visser, J. J., Bergmans, P. L., Scheltens, P., Wolters, E. C., Characterization of L-arginine transporters in rat renal inner medullary collecting duct. *Am. J. Physiol. Regul. Interg. Comp. Physiol.,* 278(6)R1506–12, June 2000.

Laitinen, S. I., Laitinen, P. H., and Pajunen, E. I., The effect of testosterone on the half-life of ornithine decarboxylase-mRNA in mouse kidney. *Biochem. Internat.,* 9(1):45–50, 1984.

Langdon, R. C., Fleckman, P., and McGuire, J., Calcium stimulates ornithine decarboxylase activity in cultured mammalian epithelial cells. *J. Cell. Physiol.,* 118:39–44, 1984.

Laron, Z., Tikva, P., and Butenandt, O., Evaluation of growth hormone secretion. *Pediat. Adoles. Endocr.,* 1983.

———, Topper, E., and Gil-Ad, I., Oral clonidine—a simple, safe and effective test for growth hormone secretion. Evaluation of growth hormone secretion. *Pediat. Adolesc. Endocr.,* 12:103–115, 1983.

Lawand, N. B., McNearney, T., Westlund, K. N., Amino acid release into the knee joint: key role in nociception and inflammation. *Pain,* 86(102): 69–74, May 2000.

Leonard, J.V., The nutritional management of urea cycle disorders. *Journal of Pediatrics,* 138 (1 Suppl.):S40–4,discussion S44–5, January 2001.

Mahan, L. K., Stump, S. E., *Food, Nutrition and Diet Therapy,* 10th Edition, 2000.

Chaitow, L., *Amino Acids in Therapy: A* Guide to the Therapeutic Application of Protein Constituents, *1988.*

Mailinow, M. R., McLaughlin, P., Bardana, E. J., and Craig, S., Elimination of toxicity from diets containing alfalfa seeds. Fd. Chem. Toxic., *22(7):583–587, 1984.*

Martin, J. B., Evaluation of growth hormone secretion: physiology and clinical application. Proceedings of a *Workshop of the International Growth and Develop. Assoc.,* Hinterzarten, 1983.

Mashiter, K., Harding, P. E., Chou, M., Mashiter, G. D., Stout, J., Diamond, D., and Field, J. B., Persistent pancreatic glucagon but not insulin response to arginine in pancreatectomized dogs. *Endocrinology,* 96(3):678–693, 1975.

Massara, F., Martelli, S., Ghigo, E., Camanni, F., and Molinatti, G. M., Arginine induced hypophosphatemia and hyperkalemia in man. *Diabete & Metabolisme,* 5:297–300, 1979.

McCabe, B. J., Horn, G., Kendrick, K. M., GABA, taurine and learning: release of amino acids from slices of chick brain following imprinting. *Neuroscience,* 105(2):317–24, 2001.

McDermott, J. R., Studies on the catabolism of NG-methylarginine, NG, NG-dimethylarginine and NG, NG-dimethylarginine in the rabbit. *Biochem. J.,* 154:179–184, 1976.

McInnes, R. R., Arshinoff, S. A., Bell, L., Marliss, E. B., and McCulloch, J. C., Hyperornithinaemia and gyrate atrophy of the retina: improvement of vision during treatment with a low-arginine diet. *Lancet,* pp. 513–518, March 1981.

Menard, H. A., Lapointe, E., Rochdi, M. D., Zhou, Z. J., Insights into rheumatoid arthritis derived from the Sa immune system. *Arthritis Res.,* 2(6):429–32, 2000.

Miller, J. A., Man-made growth factors work in volunteers. *Science News,* Vol. 123, 1983.

Milner, J. A., Prior, R. L., and Visek, W. J., Arginine deficiency and orotic aciduria in mammals. *Proc. Soc. Exper. Bio. Med.,* 150:282–288, 1975.

——, and Stepanovich, L. V., Inhibitory effect of dietary arginine on growth of Ehrlich ascites tumor cells in mice. *J. Nutr.,* 109:489–493, 1979.

——, and Visek, W. J., Dietary protein intake and arginine requirements in the rat. *J. Nutr.,* 108(3), 1978.

——, and Visek, W. J., Orotic aciduria in the female rate and its relation to dietary arginine. *J. Nutr.,* 108:1281–1288, 1978.

——, Mechanism for fatty liver induction in rats fed arginine deficient diets. *J. Nutr.* 109(4):663–670, 1979.

——, Wakeling, A. E., and Visek, W. J., Effect of arginine deficiency on growth and intermediary metabolism in rats. *J. Nutr.,* 104:1681–1689, 1974.

Moore, P., and Swendseid, M. E., Dietary regulation of the activities of ornithine decarboxylase and S-adenosylmethionine decarboxylase in rats. *J. Nutr.,* 113:1927–1935, 1983.

Morris, J. G., and Rogers, Q. R., Ammonia intoxication in the near-adult cat as a result of a dietary deficiency of arginine. *Science,* 199:431–432, 1978.

——, Arginine: an essential amino acid for the cat. *J. Nutr.,* 108: 1944–1953, December 1978.

Msall, M., Batshaw, M. L., Suss, R., Brusilow, S. W., and Mellits, E. D., Neurologic outcome in children with inborn errors of urea synthesis. *New Eng. J. Med.,* 310:1500–1505, 1984.

Navarro, A., and Grisolia, S., ATP and other purine nucleotides stimulate the inactivation of ornithine transcarbamylase by broken lyosomes. *Fed. European Biochem. Soc.,* 167(2):259–262, 1984.

Nelin, L. D., Hoffman, G. M., L-Arginine infusion lowers blood pressure in children. *J. Pediat.,* 139(5):747–9, November 2001.

Nielsen, F. H., Uthus, E. O., and Cornatzer, W. E., Arsenic possibly influences carcinogenesis by affecting arginine and zinc metabolism. *Biol. Trace Elem. Res.,* 5:389–397, 1983.

Nishimura, M., Yoshimura, M., and Takahashi, H., Role of brain L-arginine in central regulation of blood pressure. *Nippon Rinsho,* 58 Suppl. 1:41–5, January 2000.

Nutrition Reviews. Arginine: An acutely essential amino acid for the near-adult cat. 37(3):86–87, 1979.

——, Arginine as an essential amino acid in children with argininosuccinase deficiency. 37(4): 112–113, 1979.

——, Orotic aciduria and species specificity. 42(8): 292–294, 1984.

Otani, S., Matsui, I., Kuramoto, A., and Morisawa, S., Induction of ornithine decarboxylase in guinea-pig lymphocytes and its relations to phospholipid metabolism. *Biochim. Biophys. Acta,* 800:96–101, 1984.

Owczarczyk, B., and Barej, W., The different activities of arginase, arginine synthetase, ornithine transcarbamoylase and delta-ornithine transaminase in the liver and blood cells of some farm animals. *Comp. Biochem. Physiol.,* 50B:555–558, 1975.

Paschen, W., Polyamine metabolism in different pathological states of the brain. *Mol. Chem. Neuropathol.,* 16(3):241–71, June 1992

Pau, M. Y., and Milner, J. A., Dietary arginine and sexual maturation of the female rat. *J. Nutr.,* 112(10):1834–1842. 1982.

————, Dietary arginine deprivation and delayed puberty in the female rate. *J. Nutr.,* 114:112–118, 1984.

Pearson, D., and Shaw, S., *Life Extension.* New York: Warner Books, Inc., 1982, p. 477.

Peracchi, M., Cavagnini, Pinto, M., Bulgheroni, P., and Panerai, A. E., Effect of minophylline on growth hormone and insulin responses to arginine in normal subjects. *Hormone Metabolic Res.,* 7(5):437–438, 1975.

Pernet, P., Coudray-Lucas, C., Le boucher, J., Schlegal, L., Giboudeau, J., Cynober, L., and Aussel, C., Is the L-arginine-nitric oxide pathway involved in endotoxemia-indiced muscular hyper catabolism in rats? *Metabolism,* 48(2):190–3, February 1999.

Peters, H., Border, W. A., Noble, N. A., From rats to man: a perspective on dietary L-arginine supplementation in human renal disease. *Nephrol Dial Transplant,* 14(7):1640–50, July 1999.

Petrack, B., Czernik, A. J., Ansell, J., and Cassidy, J., Potentiation of arginine-induced glucagon secretion by adenosine. *Life Sci.,* 28:2611–2615, 1981.

Pontiroli, A. E., Viberti, G., and Pozza, G., Growth hormone response to arginine in normal subjects and in patients with chemical diabetes and effect of clofibrate and of metergoline. *Proc. Soc. Exper. Bio. Med.,* 155:160–163, 1977.

Provinciali, M., Montenovo, A., Di Stefano, G., Colombo, M., Daghetta, L., Cairati, M., Veroni, C., Cassino, R., Della Torre, F., and Fabris, N., Effect of zinc or zinc plus arginine supplementation on antibody titre and lymphocyte subsets after influenza vaccination in elderly subjects: a randomized controlled trial. *Age Ageing,* 27(6), 715–22, November 1998.

Pryme, I. F., The effects of orally administered L-arginine HCl on the development of myeloma tumors in BABL/C mice following the injection of single cell suspensions. *Cancer Letter,* 5:19–23, 1978.

Pryor, J. P., Blandy, J. P., Evans, P., and Usherwood, M., Controlled clinical trial of arginine for infertile men with oligozoospermia. *Brit. J. Urol.,* 50:47–50, 1978.

Pui, Y. M. L., and Fisher, H., Factorial supplementation with arginine and glycine on nitrogen retention and body weight gain in the traumatized rat. *J. Nutr.,* 109(2):240, 1979.

Rice, D. W., Schulz, G. E., and Guest, J. R., Structural relationship between glutathione reductase and lipoamide dehydrogenase. *J. Mol. Biol.,* 174(3):483–496, 1984.

Roseeuw, D. I., Marcelo, C. L., and Voorhees, J. J., Magnitude of ornithine decarboxylase induction by epidermal mitogens: effect of the assay technique. *Arch. Dermatol Res.,* 276:139–146, 1984.

Rosenthal, G. A., Dahlman, D. L., and Janzen, D. H., A novel means for dealing with L-canavanine, a toxic metabolite. *Science,* 192(4):256–257, 1976.

————, Hughes, C. G. and Janzen, D. H. L-canavanine, a dietary nitrogen source for the seed predator Caryedes brasiliensis (Bruchidae). *Science,* 217(7):353–355, 1982.

Roth, V. H., Influence of alimentary zinc deficiency on nitrogen elimination and enzyme activities of the urea cycle. *J. Anim. Physiol. Anim. Nutr. (Berl.),* 85(1–2): 45–52, February 2001.

Rozhin, J., Wilson, P. S., Bull, A. W., and Nigro, N. D., Ornithine decarboxylase activity in the rat and human colon. *Cancer Res.,* 44(8):3226–3230, 1984.

Ryzhenkov, V. E., Schanygina, K. I., Chistyakova, A. M., Miroshkina, V. N., Parfenova, N. S., and Kulushnikova, N. M., Action of arginine on the lipid and lipoprotein content in blood serum of animals. *Voprosy Meditsinskoi Khimi,* 30(6):76–80, September/October 1984.

Sasaki, Y., Matsui, M., Taguchi, M., Suzuki, K., Sakurada, S., Sato, T., Sakurada, T., and Kisara, K., D-arg2-darmorphin tetrapeptide analogs: a potent and long-lasting analgesic activity after subcutaneous administration. *Biochem. Biophys. Res. Commun.*, 120(1):214–218, 1984.

Sato, T., Sakurada, S., Sakurada, T., Furuta, S., Nakata, N., Kisara, K., Sasaki, Y., and Suzuki, K., Comparison of the antiociceptive effect between D-arg containing dipeptides and tetrapeptides in mice. *Neuropeptides,* 4:269–279, 1984.

Schachter, A., Goldman, J. A., and Zukerman, Z., Treatment of oligospermia with the amino acid arginine. *J. Urol.,* 110:311–313, 1973.

Schuber, F., and Lambert, C., Metabolism of ornithine and arginine in Jerusalem artichoke tuber tissue. Relationship with the biosynthesis of polyamines. *Physiol. Veg.,* 12(4):571–584, 1974.

Science. Salt-free salt. March 1985 p. 8.

Seidel, E. R., Haddox, M. K., and Johnson, L. R., Polyamines in the response to intestinal obstruction. *Am. J. Physiol.,* 246:G649–G653, 1984.

Seifter, E., Rettura, G., Barbul, A., and Levenson, S. M., Arginine: an essential amino acid for injured rats. *Surgery,* 84(2):224–230, 1978.

Seiler, N., Bolkenius, F. N., Polyamine reutilization and turnover in brain. *Neurochem. Res.,* 10(4): 529–44, April 1985.

Shih, V. E., Urea cycle disorders and other congenital hyperammonemic syndromes. In: *The Metabolic Basis of Inherited Disease.* Stanbury, J. B., Wyngaarden, J. B., and Fredrickson, D. S., eds. New York: McGraw-Hill Book Co., 1978.

Sizonenko, P. C., Rabinovitch, A., Schneider, P., Paunier, L., Wollheim, C. B., and Zahnd, G., Plasma growth hormone, insulin, and glucagon responses to arginine infusion in children and adolescents with idiopathic short stature, isolated growth hormone deficiency, panhypopituitarism, and anorexia nervosa. *Pediat. Res.,* 9:733–738, 1975.

Smirnov, Y. V., and Lukienko, P. I., The protective effect of alpha-tocopherol on the hydroxylating system in liver endoplasmic reticulum membranes against the injuring action of hyper baric oxygenation. *Voprosy Meditsinskoi Khimii,* 30(6):51–52, 1984.

Snyder man, S. E., Sandarac, C., Chen, W. J., Norton, P.M., and Phansalkar, S. V., Argininemia. *J. Ped.,* 90(4):563–568, 1977.

———, Mendecki, J., Weinzweig, J., Levenson, S. M., Shen, R.-N., and Rettura, G., Influence of supplemental vitamin A (VA) and arginine (ARC) in mice inoculated with C3HBA tumor cells. *J. Amer. Coll. Nutr.,* 3(3), 1984.

———, Norton, P. M., and Goldstein, F., Argininemia treated from birth. *J. Ped.,* 95(1):61–63, 1979.

Solomon, S. S., Duckworth, W. C., Jallepalli, P., Bobal, M. A., and Ramamurthi, I., The glucose intolerance of acute pancreatitis. *Diabetes,* 29(1):22–26, 1980.

———, et al., L-arginine as treatment for cystic fibrosis: state of the evidence. *Ped.,* 47:384, 1972.

Sporn, M. B., Dingman, W., Defalco, A., and Davies, R. K., Formation of urea from arginine in the brain of the living rat. *Nature,* 183:1520–1521, 1959.

Stanbury, J. B., Wyngaarden, J. B., and Frederickson, D. C., eds., *The Metabolic Basis of Inherited Disease.*

Stern, W. C., Miller, M., Jalowiec, J. E., Forbes, W. B., and Morgane, P. J., Effects of growth hormone on brain biogenic amine levels. *Pharmacol. Biochem. Behav.,* 3:1115–1118, 1975.

Sturman, J. A., and Kremzner, L. T., Polyamine biosynthesis and vitamin B-6 deficiency. Evidence for pyridoxal phosphate as coenzyme for S-adenosylmethionine decarboxylase. *Biochim. Biophys. Acta,* 372:162–170, 1974.

Sugano, M., Dietary protein-dependent modification of serum cholesterol level in rats. *Ann. Nutr. Metab.,* 28:192–199, 1984.

Sugiura, M., Shafman, T., Mitchell, T., Griffin, J., and Kufe, D., Involvement of spermidine in proliferation and differentation of human promyelocytic leukemia cells. *Blood,* 63(5): 1153–1158, 1984.

Takeda, Y., Tominaga, T., Tei, N., Kitamura, M., Taga, S., Murase, J., Taguchi, T., and Miwatani, T., Inhibitory effect of L-arginine on growth of rat mammary tumors induced by 7, 12-dimethylbenz(a)anthracene. *Cancer Res.,* 35:2390–2393, 1975.

Terpstra, A. H. M., Hermus, R. J. J., and West, C. E., Dietary protein and cholesterol metabolism in rabbits and rats. In: *Current Topics in Nutrition & Disease. Animal and Vegetable Proteins in Lipid Metabolism and Atherosclerosis,* pp. 19–49.

Thomsen, H. G., Plasma glucagon, insulin and blood glucose after various amino acids, hexoses, intestinal hormones, tolubutamide, exercise and food. *Diabetologia,* 6:66, 1979.

Toyota, T., Kudo, M., and Goto, Y., Insulin and growth hormone secretion stimulated by intravenous administration of arginine in the low insulin responders (prediabetes). *Tohohu J. Exp. Med.,* 123:359–364, 1977.

Valhouny, G. V., Chalcarz, W., Satchithanandam, S., Adamson, I., Klurfeld, D. M., and Kritchevsky, D., Effect of soy protein and casein intake on intestinal absorption and lymphatic transport of cholesterol and oleic acid. *Amer. J. Clin. Nutr.,* 40:1156–1164, 1984.

Van Venrooij, W. J., Pruijn, G. J., Citrullination: a small change for a protein with great consequences for rheumatoid arthritis. *Arthritis Res.,* 2(4):249–52, 2000.

Visek, W. J., Ammonia metabolism, urea cycle capacity and their biochemical assessment. *Nutr. Rev.,* 37(9): 273–282, 1979.

———, Conditional deficiencies of ornithine or arginine. Amer. Col. Nutr. conference, *Conditionally Essential Nutrients,* September 5, 1984.

———, Orotic acid as a diagnostic indicator of heptotoxicity. Amer. Col. Nutr. conference, *Conditionally Essential Nutrients,* September 6, 1984.

Wallace, H. M., Caslake, R., Polyamines and colon cancer. *Eur. J. Gastroenterol Hepatol.,* 13(9):1033–9, September 2001.

Wang, M., Kopple, J. D., and Swendseid, M. E., Effects of arginine-devoid diets in chronically uremic rats. *J. Nutr.,* 107(4) 495–501, 1977.

Weisburger, J. H., et al., Prevention of arginine glutamate of the carcinogenicity of acetamide in rats. *Appl. Pharma. Toxicol.,* 14:163–175, 1969.

Weldon, V. V., Gupta, S. K., Klingensmith, G., Clarke, W. L., Duck, S. C., Haymond, M. W., and Pagliara, A. S., Evaluation of growth hormone release in children using arginine and L-dopa in combination. *J. Ped.,* 87(4):540–544, 1975.

Wen, C., Li, M., Fraser, T., Wang, J., Turner, S. W., Whitworth, J. A., L-arginine partially reverses established adrenocorticotrophin-induced hypertension and nitric oxide deficiency in the rat. *Blood Press,* 9(5):298–304, 2000.

White, A., et al., *Principles of Biochemistry.* 6th ed. New York: McGraw-Hill, Book Co., 1978.

Wideman, L., Weltman, J. Y., Patrie, J.T., Bowers, C. Y., Shah, N., Story, S., Veldhuis, J. D., Weltman, A., Synergy of L-arginine and growth hormone (GH) releasing peptide-2 on GH release:

influence of gender. *Am. Journal Phsyiolo. Regul. Intergr. Comp. Physiol.,* 279(4), R1455–66, October 2000.

Wiechert, P., Mortelmans, J., Lavinha, F., Clara, R., Terheggen, H. G., and Lowenthal, A., Excretion of guandidino-derivates in urine of hyperargininemic patients. *J. Genet. Hum.,* 24(1)61–72, 1976.

Wiesinger, H., Arginine metabolism and the synthesis of nitric oxide in the nervous system. *Prog. Neurbiol.,* 64(4):365–91, July 2001.

Wilson, M. J., and Hatfield, D. L., Incorporation of modified amino acids into proteins *in vivo. Biochim. Biophys. Acta,* 781:205–215, 1984.

Wu, G., Meininger, C. J., Kanabe, D. A., Bazer, F. W., and Rhoads, J. M., Arginine nutrition in development, health and disease. *Current Opinion on Clinical Nutrition Metabolism Care,* 3(1):59–66, January 2000.

Wu, V. S., and Byus, C. V., A role for ornithine in the regulation of putrescine accumulation and ornithine decarboxylase activity in Reuber H35 hepatoma cells. *Biochim. Biophys. Acta,* 804(1):89–99, 1984.

Yoneda, T., Yoshikawa, M., Fu, A., Tsukaguchi, K., Okamoto, Y., Takenaka, H., Plasma levels of amino acids and hypermetabolism in patients with chronic obstructive pulmonary disease. *Nutrition,* 17(2):95–9, February 2001.

Yudkoff, M., Nissim, I., Pereira, G., and Segal, S., Urinary excretion of dimethylarginines in premature infants. *Biochem. Med.,* 32:242–251, 1984.

Zieve, L., Conditional deficiencies of ornithine or arginine. Amer. Col. of Nutrition conference, *Conditionally Essential Nutrients,* September 5, 1984.

Zollner, H., Ornithine uptake by isolated hepatocytes and distribution within the cell. *Int. J. Biochem.,* 16(6): 681–685, 1984.

Zumtobel, V., and Senkal, M., Relevance of preoperative nutritional therapy for postoperative outcome. *Langenbecks Arch. Chir. Suppl. Kongressbd.,* 115, 592–5, 1998.

SECTION FIVE

Chapter 10: Glutamic Acid, Gamma-Aminobuutyric Acid, and Glutamine

Antonaccio, M. J., Central GABA receptor stimulants as potential novel antihypertensive agents. *Drug Dev. Res.,* 4(3):315–330, 1984.

Aoki, T. T., et al., Plasma amino acid concentration in the overtraining syndrome: possible effects on the immune system. *Med. Sci. Sports Exerc.,* 24(12):1353, 1992.

Baraldi, M., Caselgrandi, E., and Santi, M., Effect of zinc on specific binding of GABA to rat brain. *Neurol. & Neurobiol.,* 11:59–72, 1983.

Bartholim, G., GABA systems, GABA receptor agonists and dyskinesia. *New Directions in Tardive Dyskinesia Res.,* 21:143–154, 1983.

Bigelow, J. C., Brown, D. S., and Wightman, R. M., Gamma-aminobutyric acid stimulates the release of endogenous ascorbic acid from rat striatal tissue. *J. Neurochem.,* 42(2):412–419, 1984.

Bizzi, A., Veneroni, E., Salmona, M., and Garattini, S., Kinetics of monosodium glutamate in relation to its neurotoxicity. *Toxicology Letters,* 1:123–130, 1977.

Bonhaus, D. W., and Huxtable, R. J., The transport, biosynthesis and biochemical actions of taurine in a genetic epilepsy. *Neurochem. Inter.,* 5:413–419, 1983.

Brand, K., Williams, J. F., and Weidemann, M. J., Glucose and glutamine metabolism in rat thymocytes. *Biochem. J.,* 221:471–475, 1984.

Brenner, H. J., et al., *Disturbance of Amino Acid Metabolism: Clinical Chemistry and Diagnosis.* Baltimore, MD: Urban and Schwarzenberg, Inc., 1981.

Btaiche, I. F., and Woster, P. S., Gabapentin and Lamotrigine: novel antiepileptic drugs. *Am. J. Health-Syst. Pharm.,* Vol. 52, January 1, 1995.

Butterworth, R. F., Hamel, E., Landerville, F., and Barbeau, A., Amino acid changes in thiamine-deficient encephalopathy: some implications for the pathogenesis of Friedreich's ataxia. *Le J. Canad. des Sci. Neurol.,* 6(2):217–222, 1979.

Cave, L. J., The brain's unsung cells. *Bioscience,* 33(10):614–615, 618, 1983.

Cheng, S.-C., and Brunner, E. A., Rat brain synaptosomes. In: *Glutamine, Glutamate, and GABA in the Central Nervous System.* Hertz, L., Kvamme, E., McGeer, E. G., and Schousboe, A., eds., New York: Alan R. Liss, Inc., 1983, 653–668.

Cohen, P. G., The metabolic basis for the genesis of seizures: the role of the potassium-ammonia axis. *Med. Hypotheses,* 13:199–204, 1984.

Collier, D. A., GABA A: modulating sensitivity to drugs and alcohol. *Mol. Psychiatry,* 5(1):10, January 2000.

Cooper, A. J. L., Vergara, F., and Duffy, T. E., Cerebral glutamine synthetase. In: *Glutamine, Glutamate, and GABA in the Central Nervous System,* pp. 77–94.

DeFeudis, F. V., Gamma-aminobutyric acid and cardiovascular function. *Experientia,* 39:845–849, 1983.

Denman, R. B., and Wedler, F. C., Association-dissociation of mammalian brain glutamine synthetase: effects of metal ions and other ligands. *Archiv. Biochem. Biophys.,* 232(2):427–440, 1984.

De Young, L., Ballaron, S., and Epstein, W., Transglutaminase activity in human and rabbit ear comedogenesis: a histochemical study. *J. Invest. Dermatol.,* 82(3):275–279, 1984.

Duvilanski, B. H., Manes, V. M., Diaz, M. D. C., Seilicovich, A., and Debeljuk, L., Serum prolactin levels and GABA-related enzymes in the hypothalamus and anterior pituitary during maturation in the rat. *Neuroendocrinol. Let.,* 6(4), 1984.

Ebert, A. G., The dietary administration of L-monosodium glutamate, DL-monosodium glutamate and L-glutamic acid to rats. *Toxicol. Let.,* 3:71–78, 1979.

———, MSG. *JAMA,* 233(3):224–225, 1975.

Esaky, R. L., Brownstein, M. J., and Long, R. T., Alpha-melanocyte-stimulating hormone: reduction in adult rat brain after monosodium glutamate treatment of neonates. *Science,* 205(8):827–828, 1979.

Fahr, M. J., Kornbluth, J., Blossom, S., et al., Glutamine enhances immunoregulation of tumor growth. *J. Parental & Enteral Nutr.,* 18(6), 1994.

Fariello, R. G., and Golden, G. T., Homotaurine: a GABA agonist with anticonvulsant effects. *GABA Neurotransmission: Brain Research Bulletin,* 5(2):691–699, 1980.

Fincle, L. P., Experiments in treating alcoholics with glutamic acid and glutamine. New York: Symposium on the *Biochemical and Nutritional Aspects of Alcoholism,* October 2, 1984. Sponsored by the Christopher D. Smithers Foundation and the Clayton Foundation Biochemical Institute of the University of Texas at Austin.

Fonnum, F., Storm-Mathisen, J., and Divac, I., Biochemical evidence for glutamate as neurotransmitter in corticostriatal and corticothalamic fibres in rat brain. *Neuroscience,* 6(5):863–873, 1981.

———, and Engelsen, B., Transmitter and metabolic glutamate in the brain. In: *Glutamine, Glutamate, and GABA in the Central Nervous System,* pp. 241–248.

French, J. A., Vigabatrin. *Epilepsia,* 40 Suppl. 5:S11–6, 1999.

Fricchione, G. L. Neuroleptic catatonia and its relationship to psychogenic catatonia. *Biol. Psych.,* 20:304–313, 1985.

Fuchs, E., Mansky, T., Stock, K. W., Vijayan, E., and Wuttke, W., Involvements of catecholamines and glutamate in GABAergic mechanism regulatory to luteinizing hormone and prolactin secretion. *Neuroendocrinology,* 38:484–489, 1984.

Gahwiler, B. H., Maurer, R., and Wuthrich, H. J., Pitrazepin, novel GABA antagonist. *Neurosci. Let.,* 45:311–316, 1984.

Garattini, S., Evaluation of the neurotoxic effects of glutamic acid. *Nutr. Brain,* 4:79–124, 1979.

Ghadimi, H., Kumar, S., and Abaci, F., Studies on monosodium glutamate ingestion: 1. biochemical explanation of Chinese restaurant syndrome. *Biochem. Med.,* 5(5):447–456, 1971.

Ghezzi, P., Salmona, M., Recchia, M., Dagnino, G., and Garattini, S., Monosodium glutamate kinetic studies in human volunteers. *Toxicology Letters,* 5:417–421, 1980.

Giacobini, E., and Guitierrez, M. del C., In: *Glutamine, Glutamate, and GABA in the Central Nervous System,* pp. 571–580.

Gillis, R. A., Yamada, K. A., DiMicco, J. A., Williford, D. J., Segal, S. A., Hamosh, P., and Norman, W. P., Central gamma-aminobutyric acid involvement in blood pressure control. *Fed. Proc.,* 43(1):32–38, January 1984.

Grachev, I. D., Fredrickson, B. E., Apkarian, A. V., Abnormal brain chemistry in chronic back pain: an *in vivo* proton magnetic resonance spectroscopy study. *Pain* 89(1):7–18, December 2000.

Greenamyre, J. T., Penney, J. B., Young, A. B., D'Amato, C. J., Hicks, S. P., Shoulson, I., Alterations in L-glutamate binding in Alzheimer's and Huntington's diseases. *Science,* 227(3): 1496–1498, 1985.

Guinard, M., Francon, A., Vacheron, M. J., Michel, G., Enzymatic preparation of an immunostimulant, the disaccharide-dipeptide, from a bacterial peptidolycan. *Euro. J. Biochem.,* 143(2):359–362, 1984.

Haefliger, W., Revesz, L., Maurer, R., Romer, D., and Buscher, H. H., Analgesic GABA agonists. Synthesis and structure-activity studies on analogues and derivatives of muscimol and THIP. *Eur. J. Med. Chem. Chim. Ther.,* 2:150–156, 1984.

Hamberger, A., Berthold, C.-H., Karlsson, B., Lehmann, A., and Nystrom, B., Extracellular GABA, glutamate and glutamine *in vivo*—perfusion-dialysis of the rabbit hippocampus. In: *Glutamine, Glutamate, and GABA in the Central Nervous System,* pp. 473–492.

Haray, P. E., Madsen, J. J., Thurston, O. G., et al., Oral glutamine supplementation benefits jejunum but not ileum. *Can. J. Gastroenterol.,* 8(2), March/April 1994.

Hattori, H., and Wasterlain, C. G., Excitatory amino acids in the developing brain: ontogeny, plasticity, and excitotoxicity. *Pediatr. Neurol.,* 6:219–228, 1990.

Haug, M., Simler, S., Ciesielski, L., Mandel, P., and Moutier, R., Influence of castration and brain GABA levels in three strains of mice on aggression towards lactating intruders. *Physiol. & Behav.,* 32:767–770, 1984.

Hertz, L., Yu, A. C. H., Potter, R. L., Fisher, T. E., and Schousboe, A., *Glutamine, Glutamate, and GABA in the Central Nervous System,* pp. 327–342.

Honda, T., Amino acid metabolism in the brain with convulsive disorders. Part I: free amino acid patterns in the brain of el mouse with convulsive seizure. *Brain Dev.,* 6:17–21, 1984.

Hosli, L., and Hosli, E., Glutamate neurotransmission at the cellular level. In: *Glutamine, Glutamate, and GABA in the Central Nervous System,* pp. 441–456.

Huxtable, R., Azari, J., Reisine, T., Johnson, P., Yamamura, H., and Barbeau, A., Regional distribution of amino acids in Friedreich's ataxia brains. *Le J. Canad. des Sci. Neurol,* 6(2):255–258, 1979.

Joy, R. M., Albertson, T. E., Stark, L. G., An analysis of the actions of progabide, a specific GABA receptor agonist, on kindling and kindled seizures. *Exper. Neuro.,* 83(1):144–154, 1984.

Kalviainen, R., Cognitive effects of GABAergic antiepileptic drugs. *Electroencephalogr. Clin. Neurophysiol. Suppl.,* 50:458–64, 1999.

Kamatchi, G. L., Bhakthavatsalam, P., Chandra, D., and Bapna, J. S., Inhibition of insulin hyperphagia by gamma aminobutyric acid antagonists in rats. *Life Sci.,* 34(23):2297–2302, 1984.

Kamrin, R. P., and Kamrin, A. A., The effects of pyridoxine antagonists and other convulsive agents on amino acid concentrations of the mouse brain. *J. Neurochem.,* 6:219–225, 1961.

Kardos, J., Recent advance in GABA research. *Neurchem. Int.,* 34 (5):353–8, May 1999.

Kirkendol, P. L., Pearson, J. E., and Robie, N. W., The cardiac and vascular effects of sodium glutamate. *Clin. Exper. Pharmacol. Physiol.,* 7:617–625, 1980.

Kizer, J. S., Nemeroff, C. B., and Youngblood, W. M., Neurotoxic amino acids and structurally related analogs. *Pharmacological Rev.,* 29:301–318, 1978.

Krogsgaard-Larsen, P., GABA agonists: structural, pharmacological, and clinical aspects, In: *Glutamine, Glutamate, and GABA in the Central Nervous System,* pp. 537–558.

Kuriyama, K., Kanmori, J., and Yoneda, Y., Functional alterations in central GABA neurons induced by stress. In: *Glutamine, Glutamate, and GABA in the Central Nervous System,* pp. 559–570.

Lahdesmaki, P., and Pajunen, A., Effect of taurine, GABA and glutamate on the distribution of Na+ and K+ ions between the isolated synaptosomes and incubation medium. *Neurosci. Let.,* 4:167–170, 1977.

Lai, J. C. K., Leung, T. K. C., and Lim, L., Brain regional distributions of glutamic acid decarboxylase, choline acetyltransferase, and acetylcholinesterase in the rat: effects of chronic manganese chloride administration after two years. *J. Neurochem.,* 36(4):1443–1448, 1981.

Lipton, S. A., Rosenberg, P. A., and Epstein, F. H., Excitatory amino acids as a final common pathway for neurologic disorders. *New Eng. J. Med.,* 330:613–622, March 3, 1994.

Liron, Z., Roberts, E., and Wong, E., Verapamil is a competitive inhibitor of gamma-aminobutyric acid and calcium uptake by mouse brain subcellular particles. *Life Sci.,* 36(4):321–328, 1985.

Loscher, W., and Siemes, H., Valproic acid increases gamma-aminobutyric acid in CSF of epileptic children. *Lancet,* p. 225, July 28, 1984.

MacDonald, J. F., Nistri, A., and Padjen, A. L., Neuronal depressant effects of diethylester derivatives of excitatory amino acids. *Can. J. Physiol. Pharmacol.*, 55:1387–1390, 1977.

Maggi, C. A., Manzini, S., and Meli, A., Evidence that GABA receptors mediate relaxation of rat duodenum by activating intramural nonadrenergic-non-cholinergic neurones. *J. Autonomic Pharmacol.*, 4(2):77–86, June 1984.

Maitre, M., and Mandel, P., Proprietes permettant d'attribuer au gamma-hydroxybutyrate la qualite de neurtransmetteur du systeme nerveux central. *C. R. Acad. Sc. Paris*, 298(III), 1984.

McBride, W. J., Hal, P. V., Chernet, E., Patrick, J. T., and Shapiro, S., Alterations of amino acid transmitter systems in spinal cords of chronic paraplegic dogs. *J. Neurochemistry*, 42: 1625–1631, 1984.

McBurney, R. N., and Crawford, A. C., Amino acid synergism at synapses. *Fed. Proc.*, 38(7):2080–2083, 1979.

McGeer, E. G., McGeer, P. L., and Thompson, S., GABA and glutamine enzymes. In: *Glutamine, Glutamate, and GABA in the Central Nervous System*, pp. 3–18.

McGehee, D. S., Heath, M. J. S., Gelber, S., et al., Nicotine enhancement of fast excitatory synaptic transmission in CNS by presynaptic receptors. *Science*, Vol. 269, September 22, 1995.

McLean, G., Neurotoxicity and axonal transport. *Trends Pharmacol. Sci.*, 5(6):243, 1984.

———, Granata, A. R., and Reis, D. J., Glutamatergic mechanisms in the nucleus tractus solitarius in blood pressure control. *Fed. Proc.*, 43(1):39–46, 1984.

Meldrum, B., Taking up GABA again. *Nature*, Vol. 376, July 13, 1995.

Meldrum, B. S., and Chapman, A. G., Excitatory amino acids and anticonvulsant drug action. In: *Glutamine, Glutamate, and GABA in the Central Nervous System*, pp. 625–642.

Michaelis, E. K., Freed, W. J., Galton, N., et al., Glutamate receptor changes in brain synaptic membranes from human alcoholics. *Neurochemical Research*, 15(11):1055–1063, 1990.

Moffet, A., and Scott, D. F., Stress and epilepsy—the value of a benzodiazepine-dorazepam. *J. Neurol. Neurosurg. Psychiat.*, 47(2), 1984.

Monaco, F., Mutani, R., Durelli, L., and Delsedime, M., Free amino acids in serum in patients with epilepsy: significant increase in taurine. *Epilepsia*, 16:245–249, 1975.

Mondrup, K., and Pedersen, E., The clinical effect of the GABA agonist progabide on spasticity. *Acta Neurolog. Scand.*, 69(4):200–206, 1984.

———, The effects of the GABA agonist progabide on stretch and flexor reflexes and on voluntary power in spastic patients. *Acta Neurolog. Scand.*, 69(4):191–199, 1984.

Monosodium Glutamate: A symposium. Sponsored by Quartermaster Food and Container Institute for the Armed Forces and Associates, March 4, 1948.

Moreadith, R. W., and Lehninger, A. L., The pathways of glutamate and glutamine oxidation by tumor cell mitochondria. *J. Biol. Chem.* 259(10):6215–6221, 1984.

Morgan, I. G., and Dvorak, D. R., In: *Glutamine, Glutamate, and GABA in the Central Nervous System*, pp. 287–296.

Naito, S., and Ueda, T., Adenosine triphosphate-dependent uptake of glutamate into protein I-associated synaptic vesicles. *J. Biol. Chem.*, 258(2):696–699, 1983.

———, Characterization of glutamate uptake into synaptic vesicles. *J. Neurochem.*, 99–109, 1985.

Neuhauser-Berthold, M., Wirth, S., Hellmann, U., et al., Utilization of N-acetyl-L-glutamine during long-term parenteral nutrition in growing rats: significance of glutamine for weight and nitrogen balance. *Clin. Nutr.,* 7:145–150, 1988.

New Scientist. Senile dementia—a case of loose connections. November 21, 1984.

Nguyen, T. T., and Sporn, P., Liquid chromatographic determination of flavor enhancers and chloride in food. *J. Assoc. Offic. Analyt. Chem.,* 67(4):747–751, 1984.

Nicklas, W. J., Relative contributions of neurons and glia to metabolism of glutamate and GABA. In: *Glutamine, Glutamate, and GABA in the Central Nervous System,* pp. 219–232.

Norenberg, M. D., Immunohistochemistry of glutamine synthetase. In: *Glutamine, Glutamate, and GABA in the Central Nervous System,* pp. 95–112.

Nutrition Reviews. Monosodium glutamate—studies on its possible effects of the central nervous system. 28(5):124–129, 1967.

Olney, J. W., Labruyere, J., and De Gubareff, T., Brain damage in mice from voluntary ingestion of glutamate and aspartate. *Neurobehav. Toxicol.,* 2:125–129, 1980.

Olney, J. W., Trying to get glutamine out of baby food. *Current Contents,* No. 34, August 20, 1990.

Ho, O. L., Brain damage in infant mice following oral intake of glutamate, aspartate or cysteine. *Nature,* 227(5258): 609–610, 1970.

Owen, G., The feeding of diets containing up to 4 percent monosodium glutamate to rats for 2 years. *Toxicol. Let.,* 1:221–226, 1978.

———, The feeding of diets containing up to 10 percent monosodium glutamate to beagle dogs for 2 years. *Toxicol. Let.,* 1:217–219, 1978.

Pangalos, M. N., Malizia, A. L., Francis, P. T., et al., Effect of psychotropic drugs on excitatory amino acids in patients undergoing psychosurgery for depression. *Brit. J. Psychiatry,* 160: 638–642, 1992.

Pekkov, A. A., Zhukova, O. S., Ivanova, T. P., Zanin, V. A., Berezov, T. T., and Dobrynin, Y. V., Effect of preparations of glutamin(asparagin)ase from microorganisms on DNA synthesis in tumor cells. *Bull. Exp. Biol. Med.,* 96(9), 1983.

Perry, T. L., Hansen, S., and Kloster, M., Huntington's chorea: deficiency of gamma-aminobutyric acid in brain. *New Eng. J. Med.,* 288(2):337–342, 1973.

———, Levels of glutamine, glutamate, and GABA in CSF and brain under pathological conditions. In: *Glutamine, Glutamate, and GABA in the Central Nervous System,* pp. 581–594.

Peterson, D. W., Collins, J. F., and Bradford, H. F., Transmitter amino acids and their antagonists in epilepsy. In: *Glutamine, Glutamate, and GABA in the Central Nervous System,* pp. 643–652.

Petroff, O. A., Hyder, F., Rothman, D. L., Mattson, R. H., Effects of gabapentin on brain GABA, homocarnosine and pyrrolidinone in epilepsy patients. *Epilepsia,* 41(6): 675–80, June 2000.

Pettigrew, J. D., and Daniels, J. D., Gamma-aminobutyric acid antagonism, in visual cortex: different effects on simple, complex, and hypercomplex neurons. *Science,* 182(10):81–82, 1973.

Petty, F., and Sherman, A. D., Plasma GABA levels in psychiatric illness, *J. Affect. Dis.,* 6(2):131–138, 1984.

Pfeiffer, C. C. (with Hasegawa, A. T.), The pharmacology of glutamic acid. *Modern Hospital,* April 1948.

Pizzi, W. J., Unnerstall, J. R., and Barnhart, J. E., Neonatal monosodium glutamate administration increases susceptibility to chemically-induced convulsions in adult mice. *Neurobehav. Toxicol.*, 1:169–173, 1979.

Pizzi, W. J., Barnhart, J. E., and Fanslow, D. J., Monosodium glutamate administration to the newborn reduces reproductive ability in female and male mice. *Science*, 196(4):452–454, 1977.

Unnerstall, J. R., Reproductive dysfunction in male rats following neonatal administration of monosodium L-glutamate. *Neurobehav. Toxicol.*, 1:1–4, 1979.

Plaitakis, A., and Ber, S., Involvement of glutamate dehydrogenase in degenerative neurological disorders. In: *Glutamine, Glutamate, and GABA in the Central Nervous System*, pp. 609–618.

Plaitakis, A., and Ber, S., Oral glutamate loading in disorders with spinocerebellar and extrapyramidal involvement effect on plasma glutamate, aspartate and taurine. *Extrapyramidal Dis.*, 19:65–74, 1983.

Post, R. M., Ballenger, J. C., Hare, T. A., and Bunney, W. E., Lack of effect of carbamazepine on gamma-aminobutyric acid in cerebrospinal fluid. *Neurology*, 30(9):1008–1011, 1980.

Preuss, H. G., Gaydos, D. S., Aujla, M. S., Areas, J., and Vertuno, L. L., *In vitro* correlation of glutamine and glutamate renal ammoniagenesis during adaptation. *Renal Physiol. Basel.*, 7:321–328, 1984.

Pulce, C., Vial, T., Verdier, F., et al., The Chinese restaurant syndrome: a reappraisal of monosodium glutamate's causative role. *Adverse Drug React. Toxicol. Rev.*, 11(1):19–39, 1992.

Quinn, M. R., and Chan, M. M., Effect of vitamin B6 deficiency on glutamic acid decarboxylase activity in rat olfactory bulb and brain. *J. Nutr.*, 109(10):1694–1702, 1979.

Rajeswari, T. S., and Radha, E., Metabolism of the glutamate group of amino acids in rat brain as a function of age. *Mech. Ag. & Dev.*, 24(2):139–150, 1984.

Reif-Lehrer, L., A questionnaire study of the prevalence of Chinese restaurant syndrome. *Fed. Proc.*, 36(4):1617–1623, 1977.

Stemmermann, M. G. Monosodium glutamate intolerance in children. *New Eng. J. Med.*, 293(12):1204, 1975.

————, Possible significance of adverse reactions to glutamate in humans. *Fed. Proc.*, 35(9):2205–2212, 1976.

Ribeiro, Jr., H., Ribeiro, T., Mattos, A., et al., Treatment of acute diarrhea with oral rehydration solutions containing glutamine. *Am. Col. Nutr.*, 13(3):251–255, 1994.

Roberts, E., GABA neurons in the mammalian central nervous system: model for a minimal basic neural unit. *Neurosci. Let.*, 47:195–200, 1984.

Roth, R. H., Formation and regional distribution of gamma-hydroxybutyric acid in mammalian brain. *Biochem. Pharma.*, 19:3013–3019, 1970.

Suhr, Y. Mechanism of the gamma-hydroxybutyrate-induced increase in brain dopamine and its relationship to "sleep". *Biochem. Pharmacol.*, 19:3001–3012, 1970.

Sadasivudu, B., Rao, T. I., and Murthy, C. R., Acute metabolic effects of ammonia in mouse brain. *Neurochem. Res.*, 2:639–655, 1977.

Schachter, S. C., Tiagabine. *Epilepsia*, 40 Suppl. 5:S17–22, 1999.

Schousboe, A., Larsson, O. M., Drejer, J., Krogsgaard-Larsen, P., and Hertz, L., Cultured neurons and astrocytes. In: *Glutamine, Glutamate, and GABA in the Central Nervous System,* pp. 297–316.

Shank, R. P., and Campbell, G. L., Metabolic precursors of glutamate and GABA. In: *Glutamine, Glutamate, and GABA in the Central Nervous System,* pp. 355–370.

Simpson, J. C., Amino acid levels in schizophrenia and celiac disease: another look. *Biol. Psych.,* 17(11):1353–1357, 1982.

Smith, R. J., Glutamine metabolism and its physiologic importance. *J. Parenteral & Enteral Nutr.,* 14:40S–44S, 1990.

Wilmore, D. W. Glutamine nutrition and requirements. *J. Parenteral & Enteral Nutr.,* 14: 94S–99S, 1990.

Stone, T. W., and Perkins, M. N., Ethylenediamine as a GABA-mimetic. *Trends Pharma. Sci.,* 5(6):241–242, 1984.

Sytinsky, I. A., and Soldatenkov, A. T., Neurochemical basis of the therapeutic effect of gamma-aminobutyric acid and its derivatives. *Prog. in Neurobio.,* 10:89–133, 1978.

Szerb, J. C., Mechanisms of GABA release. In: *Glutamine, Glutamate, and GABA in the Central Nervous System,* pp. 457–472.

Talley, N. J., Why do functional gastrointestinal disorders come and go? *Digest. Dis. & Sci.,* 39(4), April 1994.

Talman, W. T., Perrone, M. H., and Reis, D. J., Evidence for L-glutamate as the neurotransmitter of baroreceptor afferent nerve fibers. *Science,* 209(8):813–814, 1980.

Tanaka, Y., Miyazaki, M., Tsuda, M., et al., Blindness due to non-ketotic hyperglycinemia: report of a 38-year-old, the oldest case to date. *Internal Med.,* 32(8), August 1993.

Tapia, R., Regulation of glutamate decarboxylase activity. In: *Glutamine, Glutamate, and GABA in the Central Nervous System,* pp. 113–128.

Taulbee, P., Solving the mystery of anxiety. *Sci. News,* Vol. 124, July 16, 1983.

Tews, J. K., Rogers, O. R., Morris, J. G., and Harper, A. E., Effects of dietary protein and GABA on food intake, growth and tissue amino acids in cats. *Physiol. Behav.,* 32(2):30–33, 1984.

Thaker, G. K., Hare, T. A., and Tamminga, C. A., GABA system—clinical research and treatment of tardive dyskinesia. *Mod. Prob. Pharmacopsychiatry,* 21:155–167, 1983.

Tildon, J. T., Glutamine: a possible energy source for the brain, In: *Glutamine, Glutamate, and GABA in the Central Nervous System,* pp. 415–430.

Van Gelder, N. M., Taurine, the compartmentalized metabolism of glutamic acid, and the epilepsies. *Can. J. Physiol. Pharmacol.,* 56:362–373, 1978.

Verity, M. A., Neurotoxins and environmental poisons. *Cur. Opin. Neurol. & Neurosurg.* 5:401–405, 1992.

Vinnars, E., Ideal amino acid profile in post-operative TPN. *Brit. J. Clin. Pract.,* 41(12):S63, 1988.

Wade, A., and Reynolds, J. E. F., eds., *The Extra Pharmacopoeia.* London: The Pharmaceutical Press, June 1977.

Wernerman, J., Luo, J. L., Hammarqvist, F., Glutathione status in critically-ill patients: possibility of modulation by antioxidants. *Proc. Nutr. Soc.,* 58(3):677–80, August 1999.

Wenthold, R. J., and Altschuler, R. A., Immunocytochemistry of aspartate aminotransferase and glutaminase. In: *Glutamine, Glutamate, and GABA in the Central Nervous System,* pp. 33–50.

Whitman, R. M., Re-evaluation of a glutamate-vitamin-iron preparation (L-glutavite) in the treatment of geriatric chronic brain syndrome, with special reference to research design. *J. Amer. Geriatrics Soc.,* 14(8):859–870, 1966.

Wieraszko, A., Glutamic and aspartic acid as putative neurotransmitters—release and uptake studies on hippocampal slices. *Neurobiology of the Hippocampus:* 1981 International Symposium on Molecular, Cellular and Behavioral Neurobiology of the Hippocampus, held in Tegernsee, Federal Republic of Germany, September 28–October 2, 1981.

Wood, J. D., and Kurylo, E., Amino acid content of nerve endings (synaptosomes) in different regions of brain: effects of gabaculine and isonicotinic acid hydrazide. *J. Neurochem.,* 42(2):420–525, 1984.

Wood, P. L., Loo, P., Braunwalder, A., Yokoyama, N., and Cheney, D. L., *In vitro* characterization of benzodiazepine receptor agonists, antagonists, inverse agonists and agonist/antagonists. *J. Pharmacol. Exper. Therapeut.,* 231(3):572–576, 1984.

Wu, J.-Y., Immunocytochemical identification of GAB-ergic neurons and pathways. In: *Glutamine, Glutamate, and GABA in the Central Nervous System,* pp. 161–176.

Zukin, S. R., Amino acids: new therapy for schizophrenia. *Lifespanner,* NewsBriefs, 23.

Chapter 11: Proline and Hydroxyproline

Abraira, C., DeBartolo, M., Katzen, R., and Lawrence, A. M., Disappearance of glucagonoma rash after surgical resection, but not during dietary normalization of serum amino acids. *Amer. J. Clin. Nutr.,* 39(3):351–355, 1984.

Ananthanarayanan, V. S., Structural aspects of hydroxyproline-containing proteins. *J. Biomol. Struct. Dyn.,* 1(3), 1983.

Bates, C. J., Proline and hydroxyproline excretion and vitamin C status in elderly human subjects. *Clin. Sci. Molec. Med.,* 52(5):535–543, 1977.

Blake, R. L., Grillo, R. V., and Russell, E. S., Increased taurine excretion in hereditary hyperprolinemia of the mouse. *Life. Sci.,* 14:1285–1290, 1974.

Bruntrock, P., Jentzsch, K. D., Heder, G., Stimulation of wound healing, using brain extract with fibroblast growth factor (FGF) activity. I. Quantitative and biochemical studies into the formation of granulation tissue. *Exp. Pathol.,* 21(1): 46–53, 1982.

Chaitow, L., *Amino Acids in Therapy,* 1988.

Cherkin, A., Davis, J. L., and Garman, M. W., D-proline: stereospecificity and sodium chloride dependence of lethal convulsant activity in the chick. *Pharmacol. Biochem. Behav.,* 8:623–625, 1978.

Dingman, W., and Sporn, M. B., The penetration of proline and proline derivatives into brain. *J. Neurochem.,* 4:148–153, 1959.

Hacker, M. P., Newman, R. A., McCormack, J. J., and Krakoff, I.-H., Pharmacologic and toxicologic evaluation of thioproline: a proposed non-toxic inducer of reverse transformation. *Pharmacol.,* 22(3):452–453, 1980.

Hershenbich, D., Garcia-Tsao, G., Saldana, S. A., and Rojkind, M., Relationship between blood lactic acid and serum proline in alcoholic liver cirrhosis. *Gasteroenterol.,* 80:1012–1015, 1981.

Hyman, P. E., and Shapiro, L. J., Dietary hyperhydroxyprolinemia. *J. Ped.,* 104(4):595–596, 1984.

Ladd, K. F., Newmark, H. L., and Archer, M. C., N-nitrosation of proline in smokers and non-smokers. *JNCI,* 73(7):83–87, 1984.

Mendenhall, C. L., Chedid, A., and Kromme, C., Altered proline uptake by mouse liver cells after chronic exposure to ethanol and its metabolites. *Gut,* 25(2):138–144, 1984.

Morris, J. G., and Rogers, Q. R., Ammonia intoxication in the near-adult cat as a result of a dietary deficiency of arginine. *Science,* 199(1):431–432, 1978.

Myara, I., Charpentier, C., and Lemonnier, A., Prolidase and prolidase deficiency. *Life Sci.,* 34:1985–1998, 1984.

Pettit, L. D., and Formichka-Kozlowska, G. A., Suggested role for copper in the biological activity of neuropeptides. *Neurosci. Let.,* 50:53–56, 1984.

Reeds, P. J., Burrin, D. G., Stoll, B., Jahoor, F., Intestinal glutamate metabolism. *J. Nutrit.* (4S Suppl.):978S082S, April 2000.

Ribaya, J. D., and Gershoff, S. N., Effects of hydroxyproline and vitamin B6 on oxalate synthesis in rats. *J. Nutr.,* 111(7):1231–1239, 1981.

Scriver, C. R., Disorders of proline and hydroxyproline metabolism. *The Metabolic Basis of Inherited Disease,* eds. Stranbury, J. B., et al., New York: McGraw Hill Book Co., 1978, pp. 336–361.

Shaw, S., Warner, T. M., and Lieber, C. S., Frequency of hyperprolinemia in alcoholic liver cirrhosis: relationship to blood lactate. *Hepatology,* 4(2):295–300, 1984.

Sugden, M. C., Watts, D. I., West, P. S., and Palmer, T. N., Proline and hepatic lipogenesis. *Biochim. et Biophys. Acta,* 789(4):368–373, 1984.

Verch, R. L., Wallach, S., and Peabody, R. A., Automated analysis of hydroxyproline with elimination of non-specific reacting substances. *Clin. Chim. Acta,* 96:125–130, 1979.

Versaux-Botteri, C., and Legros-Nguyen, J., Evidence for a (3H)-L-proline effect on the number of dendritic spines on stellate neurons of the visual cortex in macaca. *C. R. Acad. Sc. Paris,* 298(III):577–582, 1984.

Chapter 12: Aspartic Acid and Asparagine

Abcouwer, S. F., Souba, W. W., Is glutamine a pretender to the throne? *Nutrition,* 15(1):71–2, January 1999.

Airakinsen, E. M., Oja, S. S., Marnela, K.-M., and Sihvola, P., Taurine and other amino acids of platelets and plasma in retinitis pigmentosa. *Ann. Clin. Res.,* 12:52–54, 1980.

Benevenga, N. J., and Steel, R. D., Adverse effects of excessive consumption of amino acids. *Ann. Rev. Nutr.,* 4:157–181, 1984.

Braillon, J., Guichard, M., and Herve, G., Aspartate transcarbamylase from human tumoral cell lines: accurate determination of michaelis constant for carbamylphosphate by intercept replots. *Cancer Res.,* 44(5):2251–2252, 1984.

Callicott, J. H., Bertolino, A., Egan, M. F., Mattay, V. S., Langheim, F. J., Weinberger, D. R., Selective relationship between prefrontal N-acetyl aspartate measures and negative symptoms in schizophrenia. *Am J Psychiatry,* 157(10):164–51, October 2000.

Chaitow, L., *Amino Acid in Therapy—A Guide to the Therapeutic Application of Protein Constituents,* 86, 1988.

Charlwood, J., Dingwall, C., Matico, R., Hussain, I., Johanson, K., Moore, S., Powell, D. J., Skehel, J. M., Ratcliffe, S., Clarke, B., Trill, J., Sweitzer, S., Camilleri, P., Characterization of the glycosylation of Alzheimer's beta-secretase protein Asp-2 expressed in a variety of cell lines. *J. Biol Chem.*, 276(20): 16739–48, May 18, 2001.

Choline metabolites in cognitively and clinically asymptomatic HIV+ patients. *Neurology*, 52(5):995–1003, March 23, 1999.

Croucher, M. J., Collins, J. F., and Meldrum, B. S., Anticonvulsant action of excitatory amino acid antagonists. *Science*, 216:899–901, 1982.

Darling, B. K., Abdel-Rahim, M., Moores, R. R., Chang, A. S., Howard, R. S., O'Neal, J. T., Brain excitatory amino acid concentrations are lower in the neonatal pig: a buffer against excito-toxicity? *Biol Neonate*, 80(4): 305–12, 2001.

Donazanti, B. A., and Uretsky, N. J., Magnesium selectivity inhibits N-methyl-aspartic acid-induced hypermotility after intra-accumbens injection. *Pharmacol. Biochem. & Behav.*, 20(2):243–246, 1984.

Forli, L., Pedersen, J. I., Bjortuft, Vatn, M., Kofstad, J., Boe, J., Serum amono acids in relation to nutritional status, lung function and energy intake in patients with advanced pulmonary disease. *Respir. Med.*, 94(9):868–74, September 2000.

Gebhard, O., and Veldstra, H., N-acetylaspartic acid. Experiments on biosynthesis and function. *J. Neurochem.*, 11:613–617, 1964.

Godfrey, D. A., Bowers, M., Johnson, B. A., and Ross, C. D., Aspartate aminotransferase activity in fiber tracts of the rat's brain. *J. Neurochem.*, 1450–1456, 1984.

Grachev, I. D., Spectroscopic brain mapping the N-acetyl aspartate to cognitive-perceptual states in chronic pain. *Mol. Psychiatry*, 6(2):124, March 2001.

Hess, R. A., and Thurston, R. J., Protein, cholesterol, acid phosphatase and aspartate amino-transaminase in the seminal plasma of turkeys (meleagris gallopavo) producing normal white or abnormal yellow semen. *Biol. Repro.*, 31:239–243, 1984.

Hollaar, L., Jansen, P. Y., van der Laarse, A., Dijkshoorn, N. J., Bogers, A. J. J. C., and Huysmans, H. A., Pyridoxal-5'-phosphate-induced stimulation of aspartate aminotransferase and its isoenzymes in human myocardial biopsies and autopsies. *Clin. Chim. Acta*, 139(1):47–54, 1984.

Honda, T., Amino acid metabolism in the brain with convulsive disorders. *Brain Dev.*, 6:17–21, 1984.

Iwata, H., Matsuda, T., Yamagami, S., Hirata, Y., and Baba, A., Changes of taurine content in the brain tissue of barbiturate-dependent rats. *Biochem. Pharmacol.*, 27:1955–1959, 1978.

Kawata, M., and Suzuki, K. T., The effect of cadmium, zinc, or copper loading on the metabolism of amino acids in mouse liver. *Toxicol. Let.*, 20:149–154, 1984.

Koyuncuoglu, E., et al., Antagonizing effect of aspartic acid on the development of physical dependence on and tolerance to morphine in the rat. *Arzneimittel Forschung*, XXXVII: 1676–1679, 1977.

Launcha, Jr., A. H., Recco, M. D., Abdalla, D. S., Curi, R., Effect of aspartate, asparagines, and carnitine supplementation in the diet on metabolism of skeletal muscle during a moderate exercise. *Physiol. Behav.*, 57(2):367–71, February 1995.

Logan, W. J., and Synder, S. H., High affinity uptake systems for glycine, glutamic and aspartic acids in synaptosomes of rat central nervous tissues. *Brain Res.*, 42:413–431, 1972.

MacDonald, J. F., and Schneiderman, J. H., L-aspartic acid potentials "slow" inward current in cultured spinal cord neurons. *Brain Res.*, 296(2):350–355, 1984.

McIntosh, J. C., and Cooper, J. R., Function of N-acetyl aspartic. *Nature*, 203(4945):658, 1964.

Netikova, J., and Pospisil, M., Effect of K and Mg aspartates on spleen erythropoiesis in mice. *Travail recu le agressologie,* 21(2):97–99, October 1979.

Perry, T. L., Currier, R. D., Hansen, S., and MacLean, J., Aspartate-taurine imbalance in dominantly inherited olivoponto-cerebellar atrophy. *Neurology,* March 1977, pp. 257–261.

Pipalova, I., and Pospisil, M., The effect of dietary administration of aspartic acid on thymus weight in C57 black mice. *Experientia,* 36:874–875, 1980.

Pizzi, W. J., Tabor, J. M., and Barnhart, J. E., Somatic, behavioral, and reproductive disturbances in mice following neonatal administration of sodium L-aspartate. *Pharmacol. Biochem. & Behav.,* 9:481–485, 1978.

Pospisil, M., Netikova, J., Pipalova, I., and Mikeska, J., Effect of K and Mg salts of aspartic acid on haemopoiesis and recovery from radiation damage in mice. *Folia Biologica (Praha),* 26:54–61, 1980.

Riveros, N., and Orrego, F., A study of possible excitatory effects of N-acetylaspartylglutamate in different *in vivo* and *in vitro* brain preparations. *Brain Res.,* 299(2), 1984.

Shank, R. P., Wang, M. B., and Freeman, A. R., Action of aspartate at lobster excitatory neuromuscular junctions. *Brain Res.,* 126:176–180, 1977.

Shimazaki, H., Karwoski, C. J., and Proenza, L. M., Aspartate-induced dissociation of proximal from distal retinal activity in the mudpuppy. *Vision Res.,* 24(6):411–425, 1984.

Simon, R. P., Swan, J. H., Griffiths, T., and Meldrum, B. S., Blockade of N-methyl-D-aspartate receptors may protect against ischemic damage in the brain. *Science,* 226:850–852, 1984.

Storm-Mathisen, J., and Opsahl, M. W., Aspartate and/or glutamate may be transmitters in hippocampal efferents to septum and hypothalamus. *Neurosc. Let.,* 9:65–70, 1978.

Wardlaw, J. M., Marshall, I., Wild, J., Dennis, M. S., Cannon, J., Lewis, S. C., Studies of acute ischemic stroke with proton magnetic resonance spectroscopy: relation between time from onset, neurological deficit, metabolite abnormalities in the infarct, blood flow, and clinical outcome. *Stroke,* 29(8):1618–24, August 1998

SECTION SIX
Chapter 13: Threonine

Barbeau, A., Roy, M., and Chouza, C., Pilot study of threonine supplementation in human spasticity. *Le Journal Canadien des Sci. Neurol.,* 9(2):141–145, 1982.

Chaitow, L., *Amino Acid in Therapy: A Guide to the Therapeutic Application of Protein Constituents.* 1988.

Dozier, 3rd, W. A., Moran, Jr., E. T., Kidd, M. T., Male and female broiler responses to low and adequate dietary threonine on nitrogen and energy balance. *Poult. Sci.,* 80(7) 926–70, July 2001.

Hetenyi, G., Anderson, P. J., and Kinson, G. A., Gluconeogenesis from threonine in normal and diabetic rats. *Biochem. J.,* 224(2), 1985.

Honda, T., Amino acid metabolism in the brain with convulsive disorders. Part 2: the effects of anticonvulsants on convulsions and free amino acid patterns in the brain of el mouse. *Brain Dev.,* 6:22–6, 1984.

Issa, A. M., Gauthier, S., Collier, B., Effects of calyculin A and okadaic acid on acetylcholine release and subcellular distribution in rat hippocampal formation. *J. Neurochem.,* 72(1): 166–73, January 1999.

Jozwik, M., Teng, C., Wilkening, R. B., Meschia, G., Tooze, J., Chung, M., Battaglia, F. C., Effects of branched-chain amino acids on placental amino acid transfer and insulin and glucagons release in the ovine fetus. *Am. J. Obstet. Gynecol.,* 185(2):487–95, August 2001.

Krieger, I., and Booth, F., Threonine dehydratase deficiency—a probable cause of non-ketotic hyperglycinaemia. *J. Inher. Metabolic Dis.,* 7(2):53–55, 1984.

Lotan, R., Mokady, S., and Horenstein, L., The effect of lysine and threonine supplementation on the immune response of growing rats fed wheat gluten diets. *Nutr. Reports Inter.,* 22(3):313–318, 1980.

Maher, T. J., and Wurtman, R. J., L-threonine administration increases ~0álycine concentrations in the rat central nervous system. *Life Sci.,* 26:1283–1286, 1980.

Nath, M., and Sanwal, G. G., Threonine (serine) dehydratase in mouse liver as a function of age. *Indian J. Biochem. Biophys.,* 21(1):68–69, 1984.

Nasset, E. S., Heald, F. P., Calloway, D. H., Margen, S., and Schneeman, P., Amino acids in human blood plasma after single meals of meat, oil, sucrose and whiskey. *J. Nutr.,* 109(4), 1979.

Titchenal, C. A., Rogers, Q. R., Indrieri, R. J., and Morris, J. G., Threonine imbalance, deficiency and neurologic dysfunction in the kitten. *J. Nutr.,* 110(12):2444–2459, 1980.

Chapter 14: Glycine

Abbey, L., E. Windsor, NJ: Health Extension Services, January 1985.

Aprison, M. H., Glycine as a neurotransmitter. *Psychopharmacology: a Generation of Progress.* Lipton, M.A., DiMascio, A., and Killam, K. F., eds., New York: Raven Press, 1978, pp. 333–346.

Barbeau, A., and Chouza, R. C., Pilot study of threonine supplementation in human spasticity. *Le Journal Canadien des Sci. Neurol.,* 9(2), 1982.

Barne, L., B15: the politics of ergogenicity. *The Physician and Sportsmedicine,* 7(11):17–18, 1979.

Castellano, C., and Pavone, F., Effects of DL-allyglycine, alone or in combination with morphine, on passive avoidance behavior in C57BL/6 mice. *Arch. Int. Pharmacodyn. Ther.,* 267(1):141–148, 1984.

Cohn, R. M., Yudkoff, M., Rothman, R., and Segal, S., Isovaleric acidemia: use of glycine therapy in neonates. *New Eng. J. Med.,* 299:996–999, 1978.

Cunningham, R., and Miller, R. F., Electrophysiological analysis of taurine and glycine action of neurons of the mudpuppy retina. 1. intracellular recording. *Brain Res.,* 197:123–138, 1980.

DeFeudis, F. V., Glycine-receptors in the vertebrate central nervous system. *Acta Physiol. Latinoam.,* 27:131–145, 1977.

Deutsch, S. I., Peselow, E. R., Banay-Schwartz, M., Gershon, S., Virgilio, J., Fieve, R., and Rotrosen, J., Effect of lithium on glycine levels in patients with affective disorders. *Am. J. Psychiatry,* 138(5):683–684, 1981.

Downs, R., with Van Baak, A., An interview about cells: glutathione. *Bestways,* (12):32–33, 1982.

Food Processing. Sweet tasting amino acid, glycine, enhances flavor and provides functional properties. July 1983.

Graber, C. D., Goust, J. M., Glassman, A. D., Kendall, R., and Loadholt, C. B., Immunomodulating properties of dimethylglycine in humans. *J. of Infect. Dis.,* 143(1):101–105, 1981.

Gundersen, C. B., Miledi, R., and Parker, I., Properties of human brain glycine receptors expressed in zenopus oocytes. *Proc. Royal Soc. London—Series B-Biological Sci.,* 221(1223): 221–234, 1984.

Hall, P. V., Smith, J. E., Lane, J., Mote, T., and Campbell, R., Glycine and experimental spinal spasticity. *Neurology,* 29(2):262–266, 1979.

Harvey, S. G., and Gibson, J. R., The effects on wound healing of three amino acids—a comparison of two models. *Brit. J. Dermatol,* III(27):171–173, 1984.

Herbert, V. N., N-dimethylglycine for epilepsy. *QD463,* 308(9):527, 1983.

Hydrick, C. R., and Fox, I. H., Nutrition and gout. Nutrition Reviews' *Present Knowledge in Nutrition.* Washington, D.C.: The Nutrition Foundation, Inc., 1984, pp. 740–752.

Josephson, E. M., *The Thymus, Myasthenia Gravis and Manganese.* New York: Chedney Press, 1961.

Kasai, K., Suzuki, H., Nakamura, T., Shiina, H., and Shimoda, S. I., Glycine stimulates growth hormone release in man. *Acta Endocrin.,* 93:283–286, 1980.

Kim, K. S., Kurokawa, M., Kimura, T., and Sezaki, H., Effect of taurine on the gastric absorption of drugs: comparative studies with sodium lauryl sulfate. *J. Pharm. Dyn.,* 5:509–514, 1982.

Kleinkopf, K. N., N-dimethylglycine hydrochloride and calcium gluconate (gluconic 15) and its effect on maximum oxygen consumption (Max Vo2) on highly conditioned athletes: a pilot study. College of S. Idaho, 1980.

Krieger, I., and Tanaka. K., Therapeutic effects of glycine in isovaleric acidemia. *Pediat. Res.,* 10:25–29, 1976.

Lauterburg, B. H., Vaishnav, Y., Stillwell, W. G., and Mitchell, J. R., The effects of age and glutathione depletion on hepatic glutathione turnover *in vivo* determined by acetaminophen probe analysis. *J. Pharmacol. Exp. Ther.,* 213(1):54–58, 1980.

Le Rudulier, D., Strom, A. R., Dandekar, A. M., Smith, L. T., and Valentine, R. C., Molecular biology of osmoregulation. *Science,* 224(6):1064–1068, 1984.

Levine, S. B., Myhre, G. D., Smith, G. L., and Burns, J. G., Effect of a nutritional supplement containing N, N-dimethylglycine (DMG) on the racing standardbred. *Equine Practice,* 4(3):17–19, 1982.

Loveday, K. S., and Seixas, G. M., A mutagenicity analysis of N, N-dimethylglycine hydrochloride. Burlington, VT: Bioassay Systems Corporation, 1981.

Mackenzie, C. G., Conversion of N-methyl glycines to active formaldehyde and serine. In: *A Symposium on Amino Acid Metabolism,* McElroy, W. D., and Glass, H. B., eds. Baltimore, MD: The Johns Hopkins Press, 1955, pp. 417–427.

———, and Frisell, W. R. The metabolism of dimethylglycine by liver mitochondria. *J. of Biol. Chem.,* 232:417–427, 1958.

Meduski, J. W., Meduski, J. D., Hyman, S., Kilz, R., Kim, S.-H., Thein, P., and Yoshimoto, R., Decrease of lactic acid concentration in blood of animals given N, N-dimethylglycine. *Pacific Slope Biochemical Conference,* U. of Ca., San Diego, July 7–9, 1980.

———, Nutritional evaluation of the results of the 157-day subchronical estimation of N, N-dimethylglycine toxicity carried out in the nutritional research laboratory, U. of S. Ca. School of Medicine. *Pacific Slope Biochemical Conference,* U. of Ca., San Diego, July 7–9 1980.

Meister, A., *Biochemistry of the Amino Acids: Volume II.* Boston, MA: Tufts University Press, 1984.

Myers, V. C., Prognostic significance of elevated blood creatinine. *J. Lab. & Clin. Med.,* 29(10):1001–1019, 1944.

Nizametidinova, G. A., Effectiveness of calcium pangamate introduced into vaccinated and X-irradiated animals. Kazan, U.S.S.R.: *Rep. Kazan Veterinary Inst.,* 112:100–104, 1972.

Nutritional Data, 6th ed. Some primary functions in amino acids. H. J. Heinz Co., 1972.

Nyhan, W. L., Nonketotic hyperglycinemia. *The Metabolic Basis of Inherited Disease,* Stanbury, J. B., et al., eds. New York: McGraw-Hill Book Co., 1978, p. 518.

Pearson, D., and Shaw, S., *The Life Extension Companion.* New York: Warner Books, 1983.

Perry, T. L., Hansen, S., Kennedy, J., and Wada, J. A., Amino acids in human epileptogenic foci. *Arch. Neurol.* 32(11):752–754, 1975.

Pui, Y. M. L., and Fisher, H., Factorial supplementation with arginine and glycine on nitrogen retention and body weight gain in the traumatized rat. *J. Nutr.* 109(2):240–246, 1979.

Pycock, C. J., and Kerwin, R. W., The status of glycine as a supraspinal neurotransmitter. *Life Sci.,* 28:2679–2686, 1981.

Raj, D. S., Ouwendyk, M., Francoeur, R., Pierratos, A., Plasma amino acid profile on nocturnal hemodialysis. *Blood Purif.* 18(2): 97–102, 2000.

Roach, E. S., Failure of N, N-dimethylglycine in epilepsy. *Ann. Neurol.,* 14(3):347, 1983.

———, and Carlin, L., N, N-dimethylglycine for epilepsy. *New Engl. J. Med.,* 1081–1082, October 21, 1982.

Rodger, J. C.. and Breed, W. G., Why so many mammalian spermatozoa—a clue from marsupials. *Proc. Royal Soc. of London, Series B—Biolog. Sci.,* 221(1223):221–234, 1984.

Rosenblat, S., Gaull, G. E., Chanley, J. D., Rosenthal, J. S., Smith, H., and Sarkozi, L., Amino acids in bipolar effective disorders: increased glycine levels in erythrocytes. *Am. J. Psychia.,* 136(5):672–674, 1979.

Ryzhenkov, V. E., Molokowsky, D. S., and Joffe, D. V., Hypolipidemic action of glycine and its derivatives. *Voprosy Meditsinskoi Khimii,* 30(2):78–80, 1984.

Sawada, S., and Yamamoto, C., Gamma-D-glutamyglycine and cis-2, 3-piperidine dicarboxylate as antagonists of excitatory amino acids in the hippocampus. *Exper. Brain Res.,* 55(2):351–358, 1984.

Schuberth, J., and Dahlberg, L., Antagonistic effects of isovalerate and glycine on plasma choline levels in rabbits. *Life Sci.,* 26:273–276, 1980.

Seifter, E., Rettura, G., Barbul, A., and Levenson, S. M., Arginine: An essential amino acid for injured rats. *Surgery,* (8)224–230, 1978.

Seiler, N., and Sarhan, S., Synergistic anticonvulsant effects and GABA-T inhibitors and glycine. *Arch. Pharma.,* 326(5):49–57, 1984.

Shetlar, M. D., Taylor, J. A., and Hom, K., Photochemical exchange reactions of thymine, uracil and their nucleosides with selected amino acids. *Photochem. Photobiol.,* 40(3):299–308, 1984.

Takeuchi, H., Isobe, M., Usui, S., and Muramatsu, K., Supplemental effects of arginine and methionine on growth, and on formations of urea and creatine of adrenalectomized rats fed high glycine diets. *Agr. Biol. Chem.,* 39(5):931–938, 1975.

Tavoloni, N., Sarkozi, L., and Jones, M. J. T., Choleretic effects of differently structured bile acids in the guinea pig. *Proc. Soc. Exper. Biol. & Med.,* 178:60–67, 1985.

Tomaszewski, A., Kleinrok, A., Zaczkiewicz, A., Gorny, D., and Billewiczstankiewicz, J., The influence of strychnine and glycine on the metabolism of acetylcholine in the rat striatum and hippocampus. *Polish J. Pharmacol. Pharma.*, 35(4):27, 1983.

Twin Laboratories, Inc. Predigested collagen protein. Deer Park, NY, 1984.

Yamamoto, H.-A., McCain, H. W., Izumi, K., Misawa, S., and Way, E. L., Effects of amino acids, especially taurine and gamma-aminobutyric acid (GABA), on analgesia and calcium depletion induced by morphine in mice. *Euro. J. Pharma.*, 71:177–184, 1981.

Yokota, F., Esashi, T., and Suzue, R., Nutritional anemia induced by excess methionine in rat and the alleviative effects of glycine on it. *J. Nutr. Sci. Vitaminol.*, 24:527–533, 1978.

Chapter 15: Serine

Aboaysha, A. M., and Kratzer, F. H., Serine utilization in the chick as influenced by dietary pyridoxine (40802). *Proc. Soc. Exper. Bio. & Med.*, 163:490–495, 1980.

Hiasa, Y., Enoki, N., Kitahori, Y., Konishi, N., and Shimoyama, T., DL-serine: promoting activity on renal tumorigenesis by N-ethyl-N-hydroxyethylnitrosamine in rats. *J. Nat. Cancer Inst.*, 73(1):297, 1984.

Hoeldtke, R.D., Cilmi, K. M., and Mattis-Graves, K., DL-threo-3,4-dihydroxyphenylserine does not exert a pressor effect in orthostatic hypotension. *Clin. Pharmacol. Therapeut.*, Brain Dev., 6:17–21, 1984.

Hoss, W., Abood, L. G., and Smiley, C., Enhancement of opiate binding to neural membranes with an ethyl glycolate ester of phosphatidyl serine. *Neurochem. Res.*, 2:303–309, 1977.

Hwang, D., Rhee, S. H., Receptor-mediated signaling pathways: potential targets of modulation by dietary fatty acids. *Am. J. Clin. Nutr.*, 70 (4): 545–56, October 1999.

Longnecker, D. S., Effect of pyridoxal deficiency on pancreatic DNA damage and nodule induction by azaserine. *Carcinogenesis*, 5(5):555–558, 1984.

Nemer, M. J., Wise, E. M., Washington, F. M., and Elwyn, D., The rate of turnover of serine and phosphoserine in rat liver. *J. Biol. Chem.*, 235(7):2063, 1980.

Nutri-Dyn Products, Inc. *Nutritional information about free form amino acids.* Niles, IL, 1984.

Pepplinkhuizen, L., Bruinvels, J., Blom, W., and Moleman, P., Schizophrenia-like psychosis caused by a metabolic disorder. *Lancet,* (4):454–456, 1980.

Pfeiffer, C. C., and Bacchi, D., Copper, zinc, manganese, niacin and pyridoxine in the schizophrenias. *J. Applied Nutr.*, 27(2,3):9–39, 1975.

Salina, P. C., Hall, A. C., Lithium and synaptic plasticity. *Bipolar Disorder,* 1(2): 87–90, December 1999.

Sauberlich, H. E., Implications of nutritional status on human biochemistry, physiology and health. *Clin. Biochem.*, 17(4):132–142, 1984.

Schouten, M. J., Bruinvels, J., Pepplinkhuizen, L., and Wilson, J.-H.-P., Serine and glycine-induced catalepsy in porphyric rats: an animal model for psychosis. *Pharmacol. Biochem. Behav.*, 19:245–250, 1983.

Science News. Cancer biochemistry data questioned. September 12, 1981, 165.

Smith, D. S., Incorporation of serine into the phospholipids of phosphatidylethanolamine-depleted tetrahymena. *Arch. Biochem. Biophysics,* 230(2):525–532, 1984.

Smith, I. K., and Cheema, H. K., Inhibition of serine transport into tobacco cells by chlorpromazine and A23187. *Bioch. Biophys. Acta,* 769:317–322, 1984.

Smythies, J. R., The transmethylation hypotheses of schizophrenia re-evaluated. *Trends in Neuroscience,* 7(2):45–47, 1984.

Sundaram, K. S., and Lev, M., L-cycloserine inhibition of sphingolipid synthesis in the anaerobic bacterium bacteroides levii. *Biochem. Biophys. Res. Commun.,* 119(2):814, 1984.

Suzuki, S., Yamatoya, H., Sakai, M., Kataoka, A., Furushiro, M., Kudo, S., Oral administration of soybean lecithin transphosphatidylated phosphatidylserine improves memory impairment in aged rats. *J. Nutr.,* 131 (11): 2951–6, November 2001.

Waziri, R., Wilson, R., and Sherman, A. D., Plasma serine to cysteine ratio as a biological marker for psychosis. *Brit. J. Psychiat.,* 143:69–73, 1983.

————, Wilcox, J., Sherman, A. D., and Mott, J., Serine metabolism and psychosis. *Psychiat. Res.,* 12:121–136, 1984.

Wilcox, J., Waziri, R., Sherman, A., and Mott, J., Metabolism of an ingested serine load in psychotic and nonpsychotic subjects. *Biol. Psych.,* 20:41–49, 1985.

Zurlo, J., Roebuck, B. D., Rutkowski, J. V., Curphey, T. J., and Longnecker, D. S., Effect of pyridoxal deficiency on pancreatic DNA damage and nodule induction by azaserine. *Carcinogenesis,* 5(5):555–558, 1984.

Chapter 16: Alanine

Alexander, A. N., Carey, H. V., Oral IGF-1 enhances nutrient and electrolyte absorption in neonatal piglet intestine. *Am. J. Physiol.,* 277(e Pt 1): G619–25, September 1999.

Bennet, W. M., Connacher, A. A., Jung, R. T., et al., Effects of insulin and amino acids on leg protein turnover in IDDM patients. *Diabetes,* 40(4), April 1991.

Berard, M. P., Hankard, R., Cynober L., Amino acid metabolism during total parental nutrition in healthy volunteers: evaluation of a new amino acid solution. *Clin. Nutr.,* 20 (5): 407–14, October 2001.

Buchman, A. L., Ament, M. E., and et al., Choline deficiency causes reversible hepatic abnormalities in patients receiving parenteral nutrition: proof of a human choline requirement: a placebo-controlled trial: JPEN. *J. Parenter Enteral Nutr.,* 25 (5):260–8, September–October 2001.

Caffara, P., and Santamaria, V., The effects of phosphatidylserine in patients with mild cognitive decline. An open trial. *Clin. Trials J.,* 24:109–114, 1987.

Cenacchi, T., Bertoldin, T., Farina, C., et al., Cognitive decline in the elderly: a double-blind, placebo-controlled multicenter study on efficacy of phosphatidylserine administration. *Aging* (Italy), 5:123–133, 1993.

Chiarla, C., Giovannini, I., Siegel, J. H., Boldrini, G., Castagneto, M., The relationship between plasma taurine and other amino acids levels in human sepsis. *J. Nutr.,* 130(9): 2222–7, September 2000.

Chow, F.-H. C., Dysart, M. I., Hamar, D. W., Lewis, L. D., and Udall, R. H., Alanine: a toxicity study. *Toxicol. & Applied Pharma.,* 37:491–497, 1976.

Crook, T., Petrie, W., Wells, C., et al., Effects of phosphatidylserine in Alzheimer's disease. *Psychopharmacol. Bull.,* 18:61–66, 1992.

Crook, T. H., Tinklenberg, J., Yesavage, J., et al., Effects of phosphatidylserine in age-associated memory impairment. *Neurology,* 41:644–649, 1991.

Delwaide, P. J., Gyselynck-Mambourg, A. M., Hurlet, A., et al., Double-blind randomized controlled study of phosphatidylserine in senile demented patients. *Acta Neurol. Scand.* (Denmark), 73:136–140, 1986.

Engel, R. R., Satzger, W., Gunther, W., et al., Double-blind cross-over study of phosphatidylserine vs. placebo in patients with early dementia of the Alzheimer type. *Eur. Neuropsychopharmacol.* (Netherlands), 1:149–155, 1992.

Funfgeld, E. W., Baggen, M., Nedwidek, P., et al., Double-blind study with phosphatidylserine (PS) in Parkinsonian patients with senile dementia of Alzheimer's type (SDAT). *Prog. Clin. Biol. Res.* 317:1235–1246, 1989.

Granata, Q., and DiMichele, J., Phosphatidylserine in elderly patients. An open trial. *Clin. Trials J.,* 24:99–103, 1987.

Gupta, M., Prabha, V., Changes in brain and plasma amino acids of mice intoxicated with methyl osocyanate. *J. Appl. Toxicol.,* 16(6): 469–73 November–December 1996.

Hagenfeldt, L., Dahlquist, G., Persson, B., Plasma amino acids in relation to metabolic control in insulin-dependent diabetic children. *Acta Pediatr. Scand.,* 78:278–282, 1989.

Hahn, R. G., Mantha, S., Rao, S. M., et al., Glycine absorption and visually evoked potentials. Huddinge University Hospital, Sweden, and Nizam's Institute of Medical Science, India.

Kew, S., Wells, S. M., Yaqoob, P., Wallace, F. A., Miles, E. A., Calder, P. C., Dietary glutamine enhances murine T-lymphocyte responsiveness. *J. Nutr.,* 129 (8): 1524–31, August 1999.

Lenox, R. H., McNamara, R. K., Papke, R. L., Manji, H. K., Neurobiology of lithium: an update. *J. Clin. Psychiatry,* 59 Suppl. 6:37–47, 1998.

Loeb, C.. Benassi, E., Bo, G. P., et al., Preliminary evaluation of the effect of GABA and phosphatidylserine in epileptic patients. *Epilepsy Res.* (Netherlands), 1:209–212, 1987.

Lombardi, G. F., Pharmacological treatment with phosphatidylserine of 40 ambulatory patients with senile dementia syndrome. *Minerva Med.* (Italy), 80:599–602, 1989.

Macciardi, F., Lucca, A., Catalano, M., et al., Amino acid patterns in schizophrenia: some new findings. *Psychiatry Res.,* 32:63–70.

Maggioni, M., Picotti, G. B., Bondiolotti, G. P., et al., Effects of phosphatidylserine therapy in geriatric patients with depressive disorders. *Acta Psychiatr. Scand.* (Denmark), 81:265–270, 1990.

Manning, A., MSG: just a taste is safe. *USA Today,* September 3, 1995.

Monteleone, P., Beinat, L., Tanzillo, C., et al., Effects of phosphatidylserine on the neuroendocrine response to physical stress in humans. *Neuroendocrinology,* 52:243–248, 1990.

Monteleone, P., Maj, M., Beinat, L., et al., Blunting by chronic phosphatidylserine administration of the stress-induced activation of the hypothalamo-pituitary-adrenal axis in healthy men. *Eur. J. Clin. Pharmacol.* (Germany), 42:385–388, 1992.

Nelson, J., Qureshi, I. A., Vasudevan, S., Mecanismes de l'effect de la serine et de la threonine sur l'ammoniagenese et la biosynthese de l'orotate chez la souris. *Clin. Invest. Med.,* 15(2):113–121.

Nosadini, R., Alberti, K. G. M. M., Johnston, D. G., Del Prato, S., Marescotti, C., and Duner, E., The antiketogenic effect of alanine in normal man: evidence for an alanine-ketone body cycle. *Metabolism,* 30(6):563–567, 1981.

Nutrition Reviews. Arginine as an essential amino acid in children with argininosuccinase deficiency. 37(4):112–113, April 1979.

Okamoto, K., and Sakai, Y., Localization of sensitive sites to taurine, gamma-aminobutyric acid, glycine and beta-alanine in the molecular layer of guinea-pig cerebellar slices. *Brit. J. Pharmac.,* 69:407–413, 1980.

Pangalos, M. N., Malizia, A. L., Francis, P. T., et al., Effect of psychotropic drugs on excitatory amino acids in patients undergoing psychosurgery for depression. *Brit. J. Psychiatry,* 160:638–642, 1992.

Quemener, V., Chamaillard, L., Brachet, P., et al., Involvement of polyamines in tumor growth: Antitumoral effects of polyamine deprivation. *Current Contents,* 23(37), September 11, 1995.

Rotter, V., Yakir, Y., and Trainin, N., Role of L-alanine in the response of human lymphocytes to PHA and CON *Ana. J. Immunol.,* 123(4):1726–1731, 1975.

Rudman, D., et al., Fasting plasma amino acids in elderly men. *Am. J. Clin. Nutr.,* 46:559–566, 1989.

Shaffer, J. E., and Kocais, J. J., Taurine mobilizing effects of beta alanine and other inhibitors of taurine transport. *Life Sci.,* 28:2727–2736, 1981.

Shuja, M., Abanamy, A., Khaleel, M., et al., The spectrum of acute Epstein-Barr virus infection in Saudi children. *Ann. Saudi Med.,* 12(5), 1992.

Singer, P., Cohen, J., Cynober, L., Effect of nutritional state of brain-dead organ donor on transplantation. Nutrition, 17 (11–12): 948–52, November–December 2001.

Tanaka, T., Imano, M., Yamashita, T., et al., Effect of combined alanine and glutamine administration on the inhibition of liver regeneration caused by long-term administration of alcohol. *Current Contents,* 23(35), August 28, 1995.

Tangkijvanich, P., Mahachai, V., Wittayalertpanya, S., Ariyawongsopon, V.. Short-term effects of branched-chain amino acids on liver function tests in cirrhotic patients. *Southeast Asian J. Trop. Med. Public Health,* 31 (1):152–7 March 2000.

Treem, W. R., and Watkins, J. B., Alanine inhibits taurocholate (TC) uptake in perfused rat liver. *J. Amer. Col. Nutr.,* 3(3), 1984.

Tremel, H., Kienly, B., Weilmann, L. S., et al., Glutamine dipeptide-supplemented parenteral nutrition maintains intestinal function in the critically ill. *Gastrointerology,* 107:1595–1601, 1994.

Wapnir, R. A., Zdanowicz, M. M., Teichberg, S., et al., Oral hydration solutions in experimental osmotic diarrhea: enhancement by alanine and other amino acids and oligopeptides. *Am. J. Clin. Nutr.,* 48:84–90, 1988.

William, H. E., and Smith, L. H., Primary hyperoxaluria. *The Metabolic Basis of Inherited Disease,* ed. Stanbury, J. B., et al., New York: McGraw-Hill Book Co., 1978, pp. 182–204.

Yarbrough, G. G., Singh, D. K., and Taylor, D. A., Neuropharmacological characterization of a taurine antagonist. *J. Pharma. & Exper. Thera.,* 219(3):604, 1981.

Yin, M., Ikejima, K., Arteel, G. E., Seabra, V., Bradford, B. U., Kono, H., Rusyn, I., Thurman, R. G., Glycine accelerates recovery from alcohol induced liver injury. *J. Pharmacol. Exp. Ther.,* 286 (2): 1014–9, August 1998.

Zanotti, A., Valzelli, L., Toffano, G., Chronic phosphatidylserine treatment improves spatial memory and passive avoidance in aged rats. *Psychopharmacology,* 99:316–321, 1989.

SECTION SEVEN

Chapter 17: Isoleucine, Leucine, and Valine

Albanese, A. A., Orto, L. A., and Zavattaro, N., Nutrition and metabolic effects of physical exercise. *Nutr. Report Int.,* 3(3):165–186, 1971.

Amino acid supplementation and exercise performance. *Townsend Letter for Doctors,* June 1995.

Arvat, E., Gianotti, L., Grottoli, S., et al., Arginine and growth hormone-releasing hormone restore the blunted growth hormone-releasing activity of hexarelin in elderly subjects. *J. Clin. Endoc. & Metab.,* 79(5), 1994.

Bailey, J. W., Miles, J. M., and Haymond, M. W., Effect of parenteral administration of short-chain triglycerides on leucine metabolism. *Am. J. Clin. Nutr.,* 558:912–916, 1993.

Bardocz, S., The role of dietary polyamines. *Eur. J. Clin. Nutr.,* 47:683–690, 1993.

Battistin, L., and Zanchin, G., The role of amino acids in hepatic encephalopathy. *Neurochem. Clin. Neurol.,* 315–326, 1980.

Bernardini, P., and Fischer, J. E., Amino acid imbalance and hepatic encephalopathy. *Ann. Rev. Nutr.,* 2:419–54, 1982.

Berry, H. K., Brunner, R. L., Hunt, M. M., et al., Valine, isoleucine, and lelucine. A new treatment for phenylketonuria. *AJDC,* Vol. 144, May 1990.

Bessman, S. P., The justification theory: the essential nature of the non-essential amino acids. *Nutr. Rev.,* 37(7):209–220, 1979.

Bialo, G., Iscra, F., Bosutti, A., Toigo, G., Ciocchi, B., Geatti, O., Gullo, A., and Guarnieri, G., Growth hormone decreases muscle glutamine production and stimulates protein synthesis in hypercatabolic patients. *Am. J. Physiol. Endocrinol. Metab.,* 279:E323–332, 2000.

Bijlsma, J. A., Rabelink, A. J., Kaasjager, K. A. H., et al., L-arginine does not prevent the renal effects of endothelin in humans. *J. Am. Soc. Nephrol.,* 5:1508–1516, 1995.

Bionostics, Inc., Sample Case Report. Lisle, Ill. June 1982.

Blackburn, G. L., et al., Branched-chain amino acid administration and metabolism during starvation, injury and infection. *Surgery,* 86:307, 1979.

Blonde-Cynober, F., Aussel, C., and Cynober, L., Abnormalities in branched-chain amino acid metabolism in cirrhosis: influence of hormonal and nutritional factors and directions for future research. *Clinical Nutrition,* 18:5–13, 1999.

Bowes, S. B., Benn, J. J., Scobie, I. N., et al., Leucine metabolism in patients with Cushing's syndrome before and after successful treatment. *Clin. Endocr.,* 39:591–598, 1993.

Brand, K., and Hauschildt, S., Metabolism of 2-oxo-acid analogues of leucine and valine in isolated rat hepatocytes. *Hoppe-Seyler's Z. Physiol. Chem. Bd.,* 365:463–468, April 1984.

Burns, R. A., Garton, R. L., and Milner, J. A., Leucine, isoleucine and valine requirements of immature beagle dogs. *J. Nutr.,* 114:204–209, 1984.

Cabre, E., and Gasull, M. A., Nutritional issue in cirrhosis and liver transplantation. *Current Opinion of Clinical Nutrition Metabolic Care,* 2:373–380, 1999.

Campollo, O., Sprengers, D., McIntyre, N., The BCAA/AAA ratio of plasma amino acids in three different groups of cirrhotics. *Rev. Inv. Clin.,* 44:513–518, 1992.

Cerra, F. B., et al., Branched-chains support postoperative protein synthesis. *Surgery,* 92:192, 1982.

Chakravarty, N., Effect of arachidonic acid metabolism on the release of histamine and SRS (leukotrienes) from guinea-pig lung. *Agents & Actions,* 14:429–434, 1984.

Cheraskin, E., Ringsdorf, W. M., and Medford, F. H., The "ideal" daily intake of threonine, valine, phenylalanine, leucine, isoleucine, and methionine. *J. Orthomol. Psych.,* 7(3):150–155, 1978.

Choi, Y. H., Fletcher, P. J., Harvey Anderson, G., Extracellular amino acid profiles in the paraventricular neucleus of the rat hypothalamus are influenced by diet composition. *Brain Res,* 892(2):320–8, February 2001.

Clowes, G. H. A., and Saravis, G. A., Muscle proteolysis in sepsis or trauma. *New Eng. J. Med.,* 494, August 25, 1983.

Coomes, J. S., McNaughton, L. R., Effects of branched-chain amino acids supplementation on serum creatine kinase and lactate dehydrogenase after prolonged exercise. *J. Sports Med. Phys. Fitness,* 40(3):240–6, September 2000.

Cusick, P. K., Koehler, K. M., Ferrier, B., and Hasekell, B. E., The neurotoxicity of valine deficiency in rats. *J. Nutr.,* 108(7):1200–1206, 1978.

Dufour, F., Nalecz, K. A., Nalecz, M. J., and Nehlig, A., Modulation of absence seizures by branched-chain amino acids: correlation with brain amino acid concentrations. *Neuroscience Resource,* 40:255–263, 2001.

Freund, H. R., Ryan, J. A., and Fischer, J. E., Amino acid derangements in patients with sepsis: treatment with branched-chain amino acid rich infusions. *Ann. Surg.,* 188:423, 1978.

Fuchs, D., Baier-Bitterlich, G., Wachter, H., et al., Nitric oxide and AIDS dementia. *New Eng. J. Med.,* 333(8):521–522, August 24, 1995.

Gaby, A. R., Steam inhalation for colds. *Townsend Letter for Doctors,* August/September 1988.

Goldberg, A. L., Factors affecting protein balance in skeletal muscle in normal and pathological states. In: *Amino Acids: Metabolism and Medical Applications.* Blackburn, G. L., Grant, J. P., and Young, V. R., eds., Littleton, MA: John Wright and PSG, 1983.

Hagihira, H., Ogata, M., Takedatsu, N., and Suda, M., Intestinal absorption of amino acids. *J. Biochem.,* 47(1):139–143, 1960.

Harper, A. E., Miller, R. H., and Block, K. P., Branched-chain amino acid metabolism. *Ann. Rev. Nutr.,* 4:409–54, 1984.

Hauschildt, S., and Brand, K., Comparative studies between rates of incorporation of branched-chain amino acids and their alpha-ketoanalogues into rat tissue proteins under different dietary conditions. *J. Nutr. Sci. Vitaminol.,* 30:143–152, 1984.

Hausmann, D. F., Nutz, V., Rommelsheim, K., et al., Anabolic steroids in polytrauma patients. Influence on renal nitrogen and amino acid losses: a double-blind study. *J. Parenteral & Enternal Nutr.,* 14-111–114, 1990.

Herlong, H. F., and Diehl, A. M., Branched-chain amino acids in hepatic encephalopathy. In: *Amino Acids: Metabolism and Medical Applications.*

Heyman, M. B., General and specialized parenteral amino acid formulations for nutrition support. *Perspectives in Practice,* 90(3), March 1990.

Hoffer, A., Editorial: Mega Amino Acid Therapy. Tyson & Assoc. Reseda, CA.

———, Mega amino acid therapy. *J. Ortho. Psych.,* 9(1):2–5, 1980.

Holdsworth, J. D., Clague, M. B., Wright, P. D., and Johnston, I. D. A., The effect of branched-chain amino acids on body protein breakdown and synthesis in patients with chronic liver disease. In: *Amino Acids: Metabolism and Medical Applications.*

Hutsin, S. M., and Harris, R.A., Introduction. Symposium: leucine as a nutritional signal. *Journal of Nutrition,* 131:839S–840S, 2001.

Jakobs, C., Sweetman, L., and Nyhan, W. L., Stable isotope dilution analysis of 3-hydroxyisovaleric acid in amniotic fluid: contribution to the prenatal diagnosis of inherited disorders of leucine catabolism. *J. Inher. Metab. Dis.,* 7:15–20, 1984.

James, J. H., Ziparo, V., Jeppsson, B., and Fischer, J. E., Hyperammonaemia, plasma amino acid imbalance, and blood-brain amino acid transport: a unified theory of portal-systemic encephalopathy. *Lancet,* 2:772–777, 1369, 1979.

Joseph, M. S., Brewerton, D., Reus, V. I., and Stebbins, G. T., Plasma L-tryptophan/neutral amino acid ratio and dexamethasone suppression in depression. *Psych. Res.,* 11:185–192, 1984.

Kiester, E. A., little fever is good for you. *Science,* 68–173, 1984.

Kinsbourne, M., and Woolf, L. I., Idiopathic infantile hypoglycaemia. *Arch. Dis. Child,* 34:166–170, 1959.

Kinura, T., Suzuki, S., and Yoshida, A., Effect of force-feeding of a valine-free diet on gastrointestinal function of rats. *J. Nutr.,* 105:257, 1975.

Klaire Laboratories, Inc. for Hypervalinemia and Disordered Metabolism of Beta-Amino Acids. Carlsbad, CA.

Laskin, D., The little molecule: gauging the effects. *Newsday,* August 24, 1993.

Laurent, B. C., Moldawer, L. L., and Young, V. R., Bistrian, B.-R., and Blackburn, G. L., Whole-body leucine and muscle protein kinetics in rats varying protein intakes. *Am. J. Physiol.,* 246:E444–E451, 1984.

Maddrey, W. C., Branched-chain amino acid therapy in liver disease. *J. ACN,* 3(3), 1984.

Manni, A., Wechter, R., Grove, R., et al., Polyamine profiles and growth properties of ornithine decarboxylase overexpressing MCF-7 breast cancer cells in culture. *Breast Cancer Res. & Treat.,* 34:45–53, 1995.

Marchesini, G., Bianchi, G., and Zoli, M., Oral BCAA in the treatment of chronic hepatic encephalopathy. *HEPAT,* 00813 (Bologna, Italy).

Medical World News. Parkinson's researchers try amino acid therapy. November 26, 1981.

Meguid, M. M., Landel, A., Lo, C.-C., Chang, C.-R., Debonis, D., and Hill, L. R., Branched-chain amino acid solutions enhance nitrogen accretion in postoperative cancer patients. In: *Amino Acids: Metabolism and Medical Applications.*

———, Schwarz, H., Matthews, D. W., Karl, I. E., Young, V. R., and Bier, D. M., *In vivo* and *in vitro* branched-chain amino acid interactions. In: *Amino Acids: Metabolism and Medical Applications.*

Mero, A., Leucine supplementation and intense training. *Sports Med.,* 27(6):347–58, June 1999.

Miller, G. M., Yatin, S. M., De La Garza, 2nd, R., Goulet, M., and Madras, B. K., Cloning of dopamine, norepinephrine and serotonin transporters from monkey brain: relevance to cocaine sensitivity. *Brain Resource Molecular Brain Resource,* 19:124–143, 2001.

Moldawer, L. L.. and Blackburn, G. L., Muscle proteolysis in sepsis or trauma. *New Eng. J. Med.,* 494, August 25, 1983.

Moser, S. A., Takach, M. D., Dritz, S. S., Goodband, R. D., Nelssen, J. L., Loughmiller, J. A., The effects of branched-chain amino acids on sow and litter performance. *J. Anim. Sci.,* 78(3):658–67, March 2000.

Moss, G., Elevation of postoperative plasma amino acid concentrations by immediate full enteral nutrition. *J. ACN,* 3:325–332, 1984.

Nachbauer, C. A., James, J. H., Edwards, L. L., Ghory, M. J., and Fischer, J. E., Infusion of branched-chain-enriched amino acid solutions in sepsis. *1984 Surgical Forum,* XXXV (147): 743–752, 1984.

Nissen, S. L., Van Huysen, C., and Haymond, M. W., Quantitation of branched-chain amino and alpha-ketoacids by HPLC. In: *Amino Acids: Metabolism and Medical Applications.*

———, Edwards, L. L., James, J. H., Ghory, M. J., and Fischer, J. E., Plasma and brain amino acids in surgical stress and sepsis: the effect of branched-chain amino acid infusion. *Amer. Col. Surg. Surgical Forum,* vol. XXV, 1984.

Nutrition Reviews, Muscle protein catabolism in cirrhotic patients reduced by branched-chain amino acids. 41(5):146–150, 1983.

———, An unsettled question: when and where are branched-chain amino acids used as fuel? 43(2):59–60, 1985.

———, Treatment of hepatic coma with an L-valine supplement to full parenteral nutrition. 39(3):125–127, 1981.

Nuwer, N., et al., Does modified amino acid total parenteral nutrition alter immune responses in high level surgical stress? *JPEN,* 7:521, 1983.

Paxton, R., and Harris, R. A., Regulation of branched-chain ketoacid dehydrogenase kinase. *Arch. Biochem. Biophys.,* 231(1):48–57, 1984.

Penz, A. M., Clifford, A. J., Rogers, Q. R., and Kratzer, F. H., Failure of dietary leucine to influence the tryptophan-niacin pathway in the chicken. *J. Nutr.,* 33–41, 1984.

Picciano, P. T., Johnson, B., Walenga, R. W., Donovan, M., Borman, B. J., Douglas, W. H. J., Kreutzer, D. L., Effects of D-valine on pulmonary artery endothelial cell morphology and function in cell morphology and function in cell culture. *Experimental Cell Res.,* 151(1):123–133, 1984.

Rakela, J., Fulminant hepatitis: treatment or management? *Mayo Clin. Proc.,* 58:690–692, 1983.

Reiser, S., Scholfield, D., Trout, D., Wilson, A., and Aparicio, P., Effect of glucose and fructose on the absorption of leucine in humans. *Nutr. Rep. Int.,* 30(1):151–162, 1984.

Riederer, P., Jellinger, K., Kleinberger, G., and Weiser, M., Oral and parenteral nutrition with L-valine: Mode of action. *Nutr. Metab.,* 24:209–217, 1980.

Riggs, T. R., Pote, K. G., Im, H.-S., Huff, D. W., Thyroxine-induced changes in the development of neutral amino acid transport systems of rat brain. *J. Neurochem.,* 1984, pp. 1260–1268.

Saito, T., Kobatake, K., Ozawa, H., et al., Aromatic and branched-chain amino acid levels in alcoholics. *Alcohol & Alcoholism,* 29(S1):133–135, 1994.

Satoh, T., Narisawa, K., Tazawa, Y., Suzuki, H., Hayasaka, K., Tada, K., and Kawakami, T., Dietary therapy in a girl with propionic acidemia: supplement with leucine resulted in catch-up growth. *Tohoku J. Exp. Med.,* 139:411–415, 1983.

Schauder, P., Herbertz, L., and Langenbeck, U., Serum branched-chain amino and keto acid response to fasting in humans. *Metabolism Clin. Exper.,* 34(1):58–61, 1985.

Shiota, T., Watanabe, A., Higashi, T., and Nagashima, H., Prevention of methionine and ammonia-induced coma by intravenous infusion of a branched-chain amino acid solution to rats with liver injury. *Acta Med. Okayama,* 38(5):479–482, 1984.

Siegel, J. H., et al., Physiological and metabolic correlations in human sepsis. *Surgery,* 86:163. 1979.

Sleeping sickness. *The Economist,* December 22, 1990.

Snyderman, S. E., Dietary and genetic therapy of inborn errors of metabolism: a summary. *Ann. N.Y. Acad. Sci.,* 477 (Mental Retardation), pp. 231–236.

Snyderman, S. E., Goldstein, F., Sansaricq, and Norton, P. M., The relationship between the branched-chain amino acids and their ketoacids in maple syrup urine disease. *Ped. Res.,* 18(9):851–853, 1984.

Soliman, A. T., Aref, M. K., Hassan, A. I., Defective arginine-induced insulin secretion in children with nutritional rickets. *Ann. Saudi Med.,* 8(5), 1988.

Staten, M. A., Bier, D. M., and Matthews, D. W., Regulation of valine metabolism in man: a stable isotope study. *Amer. J. Clin. Nutr.,* 40:1224–1234, 1984.

Stein, T. P., and Schluter, M. D., Plasma amino acids during human space flight. *Aviat. Space Environ. Med.,* 70:250–255, 1999.

Suzuki, T., Yuyama, S., Sasaki, A., Yamada, M., and Kumagai, R., Influence of excess leucine intake on the conversion of tryptophan to NAD in rats fed low protein diet. *Progress in Tryptophan and Serotonin Research,* 1984, pp. 599–602.

Tada, K., Wada, Y., and Arakawa, T., Hypervalinemia. *Amer. J. Dis. Child.,* 113, January 1967.

Takala, J., Klossner, J., Irjala, J., and Hannula, S., Branched-chain amino acids in surgically stressed patients. In: *Amino Acids: Metabolism and Medical Applications.*

Thurlow, R. J., Brown, J. P., Gee, N. S., Hill, D. R., Woodruff, G. N., [3H] Gabapentin may label a system L-like neutral amino acid carrier in brain, *Eur. J. Pharmacol.,* 247(3):341–5, November 1993.

Traber, J., Davies, M. A., Dompert, W. U., Glaser, T., Schuurman, T., and Seidel, P.-R., Brain serotonin receptors as a target for the putative anxiolytic TVX Q 7821 *Brain Res. Bul.,* 12:741–744, 1984.

Tsalikian, E., Howard, C., Gerich, J. E., and Haymond, M. W., Increased leucine flux in short-term fasted human subjects: evidence for increased proteolysis. *Am. J. Physiol.,* 247:E323–E327, 1984.

Uauy, R., Mize, C., Aargyle, C., et al., Metabolic tolerance to arginine: implications for the safe use of arginine salt-aztreonam combination in the neonatal period. *J. Ped.,* 118(6), June 1991.

Wachtel, U., Inherited amino acid metabolism disorders and their significance in infancy and childhood. *Ann. Saudi Med.,* 8(5), 1988.

Weisdorf, S. A., Shronts, E. P., Freese, D. K., Tsai, M. Y., and Cerra, F. B., Amino acid abnormalities in infants with non-correlated extra hepatic billiary atresia (EBA). *J. Am. Coll. Nutr.,* 3(3), 1984.

Wolfe, R. R., Protein supplements and exercises. *American Journal of Clinical Nutrition,* 72:551S–557S, 2000.

Yoshida, S., Kaibara, A., Ishibashi, N., and Shirouzu, K., Glutamine supplementation in cancer patients. *Nutrition,* 17:766–768, 2001.

SECTION EIGHT
Chapter 18: Lysine

Adour, K., Hilsinger, R., and Byl, F., Amer. Acad. Otolaryngology & Annual Meeting, Dallas, October 7–11, 1979.

Albanese, A. A., Higgons, R. A., Hyde, G. M., and Orto, L., Biochemical and nutritional effects of lysine-reinforced diets. *Am. J. Clin. Nutr.,* 3(3):121–128, 1955.

———, Some species and age differences in amino acid requirements. *Protein and Amino Acid Requirements of Mammals,* New York: Academic Press, Inc., 1950, 9.

———, Orto, L. A., and Savattaro, D. N., Nutritional and metabolic effects of physical exercise. *Nutr. Rep. Inter.,* 3(3):165, 1971.

Azzout, B., Chaez, M., Bois-Joyeux, B., and Peret, J., Gluconeogenesis from dihydroxyacetone in rat heatocytes during the shift from a low protein, high carbohydrate to a high protein, carbohydrate-free diet. *J. Nutr.,* 114(11), 1984.

Blough, H. A., and Giuntoli, R. L., Successful treatment of human genital herpes infections with 2-deoxy-D-glucose. *JAMA,* 241(26):2798–2801, 1979.

Broquist, H. P., Amino acid metabolism. *Nutr. Rev.,* 34(10):289– 292, 1976.

Carpenter, T. O., Levy, H. L., Holtrop, M. E., Shih, V. E., and Anast, C. S., Lysinuric protein intolerance presenting as childhood osteoporosis: clinical and skeletal response to citrulline therapy. *New Eng. J. Med.,* 312(1):290–294, 1985.

Cassandra confirmed? *JAMA,* 238(2):133–134, 1977.

Chang. Y.-F., Lysine metabolism in the human and the monkey: demonstration of pipecolic acid formation in the brain and other organs. *Neurochemical Res.,* 7(5):577–588, 1982.

Cline, T. R., Cromwell, G. L., Crenshaw, T. D., Ewan, R. C., Hamilton, C. R., Lewis, A. J., Mahan, D. C., Southern, L. L., Further assessment of the dietary lysine requirement of finishing gilts. *J. Anim. Sci.,* 78 (4):987–92, April 2000.

Cooper, J. R., Bloom, F. E., and Roth, R. H., *The Biochemical Bases of Neuropharmacology.* New York: Oxford University Press, 1982.

Di Salvo, J., Gifford, D., and Kokkinakis, A., Modulation of aortic protein phosphatase activity by polylysine. *Proc. Soc. Exper. Biol. Med.,* 177:24–32, 1984.

Douglas, A. E., Minto, L. B., Wilkinson, T. L., Quantifying nutrient production by the microbial symbiots in a aphid. *J. Exp. Biol.,* 204(Pt. 2):349–58, January 2001.

Fitzherbert, J. C., Genital herpes and zinc. *Med. J. Australia,* May 1979.

Friedman, M., Brandon, D.L., Nutritional and health benefits of soy proteins. *J. Agric. Food Chem.,* 49(3):1069–86, March 2001

Giacobini, E., Nomura, Y., and Schmidt-Glenewinkel, T., Pipecolic acid: organ, biosynthesis and metabolism in the brain. *Cellular & Molecular Biology,* 26:135–146, 1980.

Gilbert, D. N., Kohlhepp, S. J., and Kohnen, P. W., Failure of lysine to prevent experimental gentamicin nephrotoxicity. *J. Infect. Dis.,* 145(1):129, 1982.

Graham, G. G., Morales, E., Cordano, A., and Placko, R. P., Lysine enrichment of wheat flour: prolonged feeding of infants. *Amer. J. Clin. Nutr.,* 24:200–206, 1971.

Greenwood, R. H., Titgemeyer, E. C., Limiting amino acids for growing Holstein steers limit-fed soybean hull-based diets. *J. Amin. Sci.,* 78(7):1997–2004, July 2000.

Grendell, J. H., Tseng, H. C., and Rothman, S. S., Regulation of digestion. I. Effects of glucose and lysine on pancreatic secretion. *Amer. J. Physiol.,* 246(4):G445–G450, 1984.

Griffith, R. S., Norins, A. L., and Kagan, C., A multicentered study of lysine therapy in herpes simplex infection. *Dermatologica,* 156:257–267, 1978.

Grinstead, G. S., Goodband, R. D., Dritz, S. S., Tokach, M. D., Nelssen, J. L., Woodworth, J. C.,

Molitor, M., Effects of a whey protein product and spray-dried animal plasma on growth performance of weanling pigs. *J. Anim. Sci.*, 78(3):647–57, March 2000.

Gustafson, J. M., Dodds, S. J., Rudquist, J., Kelley, J., Ayers, S., and Mercer, P., Food intake and weight gain responses to graded amino acid deficiencies in rats. *Nutr. Rep. Inter.*, 30(11):1019–1026, 1984.

Hale, H. B., Garcia, J. B., Ellis, J. P., and Storm, W. F., Human amino acid excretion patterns during and following prolonged multistressor tests. *Aviation, Space & Environmental Med.*, 173, February 1975.

Hesse, H., Kreft, O., Maimann, S., Zeh, M., Willmitzer, L., Hofgen, R., Approaches towards understanding methionine biosynthesis in higher plants. *Amino Acids*, 20(3):281–9, 2001.

Honda, T., Amino acid metabolism in the brain with convulsive disorders. Part 2: the effects of anticonvulsants on convulsions and free amino acid patterns in the brain of el mouse. *Brain Dev.*, 6:22–6, 1984.

————, Amino acid metabolism in the brain with convulsive disorders. Part 3: free amino acid patterns in cerebrospinal fluid in infants and children with convulsive disorders. *Brain Dev.*, 6:27–32, 1984.

Jockenhoevel, S., Zund, G., Hoerstrup, S. P., Chalabi, K., Sachweh, J. S., Demircan, L., Messmer, B. J., Turina, M., Fibrin gel – advantages of a new scaffold in cardiovascular tissue engineering. *Eur. J. Cardiothorac Surg.*, 19(4):424–30, April 2001.

Kamoun, P. P., and Parvy, P. R., Analysis for free amino acids in pre-breakfast urine samples. *Clin. Chem.*, 27(5):783, 1981.

Khan-Siddiqui, L., and Bamji, M. S., Lysine-carnitine conversion in normal and undernourished adult men—suggestion of a nonpeptidyl pathway. *Amer. J. Clin. Nutr.*, 37(1):93–98, 1983.

Kirschmann, J. D., and Dunne, L. J., *Nutrition Almanac*, 2nd ed. Completely Revised and Updated. New York: McGraw-Hill Book Co., 1984.

Klandorf, H., Rathore, D. S., Iqbal, M., Shi, X., Van Dyke, K., Accelerated tissue aging and increased oxidative stress in broiler chickens fed allopurinol. *Comp. Biochem. Physiol. C. Toxicol. Pharmacol.*, 129(2):93–104, June 2001.

Klemesrud, M. J., Klopfenstein, T. J., Stock, R. A., Lewis, A. J., Herold, D. W., Effect of dietary concentration of metabolizable lysine on finishing cattle performance. *J. Anim. Sci.*, 78(4):1060–6, April 2000.

Konashi, S. K., Akiba, Y., Effects of dietary essential amino acid deficiencies on immunological variables in broiler chickens. *Br. J. Nutr.*, 83(4):449–56, April 2000.

Krajcovicova-Kudlackova, M., Simoncic, R., Bederova, A., Babinska, K., Beder, I., Correlation of carnitine levels to methionine and lysine intake. *Physiol. Res.*, 49(3):399–402, 2000.

Lamont, L. S., McCullough, A. J., Kalhan, S. C., Relationship between leucine oxidation and oxygen consumption during steady-state exercise. *Med. Sci. Sports Exerc.*, 33(2):237–41, February 2001.

Leeming, T. K., and Donaldson, W. E., Effect of dietary methionine and lysine on the toxicity of ingested lead acetate in the chick. *J. Nutr.*, 114(11):2155–2159, 1984.

Lotan, R., Mokady, S., and Horenstein, L., The effect of lysine and threonine supplementation on the immune response of growing rats fed wheat gluten diets. *Nutr. Rep. Inter.*, 22(9):313, 1980.

Malis, C. D., Racusen, L. C., Solez, K., and Whelton, A., Nephrotoxicity of lysine and of a single dose of aminoglycoside in rats given lysine. *J. Lab. Clin. Med.*, 103(5):660–676, 1984.

Markison, S., Thompson, B. L., Smith, J. C., Spector, A. C., Time course and pattern of compensatory ingestive behavioral adjustments to lysine deficiency in rats. *J. Nutr.,* 130(5):1320–8, May 2000.

McWeeny, D. J., The chemical behavior of food additives. *Proc. Nutr. Soc.,* 38:129, 1979.

Medical News, Herpes simplex virus and cervical cancer. *JAMA,* 238(10):1614–1615, 1977.

Metges, C. C., Contribution of microbial amino acids to amino acid homeostasis of the host. *J. Nutr.,* 130(7):1857S–64S, July 2000.

Millward, D. J., Fereday, A., Gibson, N. R., Pacy, P. J., Human adult amino acid requirements: [1–13C] leucine balance evaluation of the efficiency of utilization and apparent requirements for wheat protein and lysine compared with those for milk protein in healthy adults. *Am. J. Clin. Nutr.,* 72(1):112–21, July 2000.

Milman, N., Scheibel, J., and Jessen, O., Failure of lysine treatment in recurrent herpes simplex labialis. *Lancet,* October 28, 1978.

———, ———, and ———, Lysine prophylaxis in recurrent herpes simplex labialis: a double-blind, controlled crossover study. *Acta Dermatovener,* 60:85–87, 1979.

Mohn, S., Gillis, A. M., Moughan, P. J., de Lange, C. F., Influence of dietary lysine and energy intakes on body protein deposition and lysine utilization in the growing pig. *J. Amin. Sci.,* 78(6):1510–19, June 2000.

Niiyama, S., Koelker, S., Degen, I., Hoffmann, G. F., Happle, R., Hoffmann, R., Acrodermatitis acidemica secondary to malnutrition in glutaric aciduria type I. *Eur. J. Dermatol.,* 11(3):244–6, May–June 2001.

Nutrition Reviews. Accelerated remission of episodes of herpes labialis in response to a bioflavonoid-ascorbate supplement. 36(10):300–301, 1978.

———, The role of growth hormone in the action of vitamin B6 on cellular transfer of amino acids. 37(9):300–301, 1979.

Owen, K. Q., Nelssen, J. L., Goodband, R. D., Tokach, M. D., Friesen, K. G., Effects of dietary L-carnitine on growth performance and body composition in nursery and growing-finishing pigs. J. Anim. Sci., 79(6):1509–15, June 2001.

Peisker, M., Efficiency of a lysine-tryptophan blend as a tryptophan source in animal nutrition. *Adv. Exp. Med. Biol.,* 467:743–7, 1999.

Perez, J. F., Gernat, A. G., Murillo, J. G., Research notes: the effects of different levels of palm kernel meal in layer diets. *Poul. Sci.,* 79(1):77–9, January 2000.

Prevention, Lysine. 136, March 1983.

Rapp, F., and Kemeny. B. A., Oncogenic potential of herpes simplex virus in mammalian cells following photodynamic inactivation. *Photochem. & Photobiol.,* 25(4):335–338, 1977.

Reeds, P. J., Dispensable and indispensable amino acids for humans. *J. Nutr.,* 130(7):1835S–40S, July 2000.

Robinson, P. H., Caliper, W., Stiffen, C. J., Julian, W. E., Sato, H., Foiled, T., Ueda, T., Suzuki, H., Influence of abdominal infusion of high levels of lysine or motioning, or both, on luminal fermentation, eating behavior, and performance of lactating diary cow. *J. Amin. Sci.,* 78(4):1–67–77, April 2000.

Roesler, K. R., Rao, A. G., Rapid gastric fluid digestion and biochemical characterization of engineered proteins enriched in essential amino acids. *J. Agric. Food Chem.,* 49(7):3443–51, July 2001.

Roth, F. X., Eder, K., Rademacher, M., Kirchgessner, M., Influence of the dietary ration between sulphur containing amino acids and lysine on performance of growing-finishing pigs fed diets with various lysine concentrations. *Arch. Tierernahr.,* 53(2):141–55, 2000.

Rytel, M. W., Herpes simplex infections. *Drug Therapy,* 27–39, September 1976.

Saturday Evening Post. A free bag of high-lysine, whole-grain corn meal with each paid subscription or renewal. March 1984.

————, Purdue high-lysine corn recipes. 1983.

————, Servaas, C., Does L-lysine stop herpes? July/August 1982.

Shiehzadeh, S. A., Herbers, L. H., and Schalles, R. R., Inheritance of response to lysine-deficient diet by rats. *J. Heredity,* 63:119–121, May–June 1972.

Smiriga, M., Mori, M., Torii, K., Circadian release of hypothalamic norepinephrine in rats *in vivo* is depressed during early L-lysine deficiency. *J. Nutr.,* 130(6):1641–3, June 2000.

Staniar, W. B., Kronfeld, D. S., Wilson, J. A., Lawrence, L. A., Cooper, W. L., Harris, P. A., Growth of thoroughbreds fed a low-protein supplement fortified with lysine and threonine. *J. Anim. Sci.,* 79(8):2143–51, August 2001.

Swaiman, K. F., and Wright, F. S., Metabolic disorders of the central nervous system: diseases of amino acid metabolism and associated conditions. *The Practice of Pediatric Neurology,* Vol. 1, 2nd ed. St. Louis, MO: The C. V. Mosby Co., 1982.

Tennican, P.O., Carl, G. Z., and Chvapil, M., Antiviral activity of zinc-medicated collagen sponges against genital herpes simplex. *Cur. Chemoth.,* 363–366, 1978.

Wahba, A., Topical application of zinc-solutions: a new treatment for herpes simplex infections of the skin? *Acta Dermatovener,* 60:175–177, 1979.

Walser, M., Urea metabolism: regulation and sources of nitrogen. *Amino Acids: Metabolism and Medical Applications.*

Walter, W. M., Collins, W. W., and Purcell, A. E., Sweet potato protein. *J. Agric. Food Chem.,* 32:695, 1984.

Warren, W. A., Emmert, J. L., Efficacy of phase-feeding in supporting growth performance of broiler chicks during the started and finisher phases. *Poult. Sci.,* 79(5):764–70, May 2000.

Wolinsky, I., and Fosmire, G. J., Calcium metabolism in aged mice ingesting a lysine-deficient diet. *Gerontology,* 28:156–162, 1982.

Woodham, A. A., Cereals as protein sources. *Proc. Nutr. Soc.,* 36:137–142, 1977.

Yang, H., Foxcroft, G. R., Pettigrew, J. E, Johnston, L. J., Shurson, G. S., Costa, A. N., Zak, L. J., Impacts of dietary lysine intake during lactation on follicular development on oocyte maturation after weaning in primiparous sows. *J. Amin. Sci.,* 78(4):993–1000, April 2000.

Young, V. R., et al., Plasma amino acid response curve and amino acid requirements in young men: valine and lysine. *J. Nutr.,* 102(9):1159–1170, 1972.

Chapter 19: Carnitine

Adembri, C., Domenici, L. L., Formigli, L., et al., Ischemi-reperfusion of human skeletal muscle during aortoiliac surgery: effects of acetylcarnitine. *Histology & Histopathy,* 9(4):683–690, October 1994.

Alaoui-Talibi, Z., Bouhaddioni, N., and Moravec, J., Assessment of the cardiostimulant action of propionyl-L-carnitine on chronically volume-overloaded rat hearts. *Cardiovasc. Drugs & Ther.,* 7:357–363, 1993.

Angelucci, L., Ramacci, M. T., Taglialatela, G., et al., Nerve growth factor binding in aged rat central nervous system: effect of acetyl-L-carnitine. *J. Neurosci. Res.* (USA), 20(4):491–496, 1988.

APMA National Fax Network News. APMA obtains Dykstra Report: Highlights of recommendations of the Dietary Supplement Task Force. June 17, 1993.

Bell, F. P., DeLucia, A., Bryant, L. R., Patt, C. S., and Greenberg, H. S., Carnitine metabolism in Macaca arctoides: the effects of dietary change and fasting on serum triglycerides, unesterified carnitine, esterified (acyl) carnitine, and B-hydroxybutyrate. *Amer. J. Clin. Nutr.*, 36:115–121, 1982.

Bella, R., Biondi, R., Raffaele, R., et al., Effect of acetyl-L-carnitine on geriatric patients suffering from dysthymic disorders. *Int. J. Clin. Pharmacol. Res.*, 10:355–360, 1990.

Bertoni-Freddari, C., Fattoretti, P., Casoli, T., et al., Dynamic morphology of the synaptic junctional areas during aging: the effect of chronic acetyl-L-carnitine administration. *Brain Res.* (Netherlands), 656(2):359–366, 1994.

Bizzi, A., Cini, M., Garrattini, S., Mingardi, G., Licini, L., and Mecca, G., L-carnitine addition to haemodialysis fluid prevents plasma-carnitine deficiency during dialysis. *Lancet*, 1213:882, April 21, 1979.

Bonavita, E., Study of the efficacy and tolerability of L-acetylcarnitine therapy in the senile brain. *Int. J. Clin. Pharmacol. Ther. Toxicol.*, 24:511–516, 1986.

Borum, P. R., York, C. M., and Bennett, S. G., Carnitine concentration of red blood cells. *Amer. J. Clin. Nutr.*, 41:653–656, 1985.

———, et al., Carnitine content of liquid formulas and special diets. *Amer. J. Clin. Nutr.*, 32:2272–2276, 1979.

Broquist, H. P., Carnitine biosynthesis and function. *Fed. Proc.*, 41(12): 2840, 1982.

Calvani, M., et al., Action of acetyl-L-carnitine in neurodegeneration and Alzheimer's disease. *Ann. N.Y. Acad. Sci.* (USA), 663:483–486, 1992.

Carlsson, M., Forsberg, E., and Thorne, A., Observations during L-carnitine infusion in two long-term critically ill patients. *Clin. Physiol.*, 4:363–365, 1984.

Carta, A., et al., Acetyl-L-carnitine and Alzheimer's disease: pharmacological considerations beyond the cholinergic sphere. *Ann. N.Y. Acad. Sci.* (USA), 695:324–326, 1993.

———, and Calvani, M., Acetyl-L-carnitine: a drug able to slow the progress of Alzheimer's disease? *Ann. N.Y. Acad. Sci.* (USA), 640:228–232, 1991.

Chaitow, L., *Amino Acids in Therapy.* 75–77. 1988.

Chapoy, P. R., Angelini, C., Brown, W. J., Stiff, J. E., Shug, A. L., and Cederbaum, S. D., Systemic carnitine deficiency—a treatable inherited lipid-storage disease presenting as Reye's syndrome. *New Eng. J. Med.*, 303:1389, 1980.

Chazot, C., Laurent, G., Charra, B., Blanc, C., VoVan, C., Hean, G., Vanel, T., Terrat, J. C., Ruffet, M., Malnutrition in long-term haemodialysis survivors. *Nephrol. Dial. Transplant*, 16(1):61–9, January 2001.

Cipolli, C., and Chiari, G., Effects of L-acetylcarnitine on mental deterioration in the aged: initial results. *Clin. Ter.*, 132:479–510, 1990.

Cucinotta, D., Passeri, M., Ventura, S., et al., Multicenter clinical placebo-controlled study with acetyl-l-carnitine (LAC) in the treatment of mildly demented elderly patients. *Drug Dev. Res.* (USA), 14(3–4):213–216, 1988.

Davis, S., Markowska, A. L., Wenk, G. L., Barnes, C. A., Acetyl-L-carnitine: behavioral, electrophysiological and neurochemical effects. *Neurbiol. Aging,* 14(1):107–15, January–February 1993.

Dayanandan, A., Kumar, P., Kalaiselvi, T., et al., Effect of L-carnitine on blood lipid composition in atherosclerotic rats. *J. Clin. Biochem. & Nutr.,* 17:2, September 1994.

De Vivo, D. C., Bohan, T. P., Coulter, D. L., Dreifuss, F. E., Greenwood, R. S., Nordli, Jr., D. R., Shields, W. D., Stafstrop, C. E., Tein, I., L-carnitine supplementation in childhood epilepsy: current perspectives. *Epilepsia,* 39(11):1216–25, November 1998.

DeAngelis, C., Scarfo, C., Falcinelli, M., et al., Acetyl-L-carnitine prevents age-dependent structural alterations in rat peripheral nerves and promotes regeneration following sciatic nerve injury in young and senescent rats. *Exp. Neurol.* (USA), 128(1):103–114, 1994.

DeFalco, F. A., et al., Effect of the chronic treatment with L-acetylcarnitine in Down's syndrome. *Clin. Ther.,* 144:123–127, 1994.

Dimkovic, N., Erythropoietin-beta in the treatment of anemia in patients with chronic renal insufficiency. *Med. Pregl.,* 54(5–6):235–40, May–June 2001.

Dove, R. S., Nutritional therapy in the treatment of heart disease in dogs. *Altern. Med. Rev.,* 6 Suppl.:S38–45, September 2001.

Dowson, J. H., Wilton-Cox, H., Cairns, M. R., et al., The morphology of lipopigment in rat Purkinje neurons after chronic acetyl-L-carnitine administration. a reduction in aging-related changes. *Biol. Psychiatry* (USA), 32(2):179–187, 1992.

Felipo, V., Hermenegildo, C., Montoliu, C., Llansola, M., Minana, M. D., Neurotoxicity of ammonia and glutamate: molecular mechanisms and prevention. *Neurtoxicology,* 19(4–5):675–81, August–October 1998.

Felipo, V., Kosenko, E., Minana, M. D., Marcaida, G., Grisolia, S., Molecular mechanisms of acute ammonia toxicity and of its prevention by L-carnitine. *Adv. Exp. Med. Biol.,* 368: 65–77, 1994.

Fracarelli, M., Rocchi, L., and Calvani, M., Acute effects of carnitine in primary myopathies evaluated by quantitative electromyography. *Drugs Exptl. Clin. Res.,* X(6):413–420, 1984.

Gecele, M., Francesetti, G., and Meluzzi, A., Acetyl-L-carnitine in aged subjects with major depression: clinical efficacy and effects on the circadian rhythm of cortisol. *Dementia,* 2:333–337, 1991.

Geelen, S. N., Blazquez, C., Geelen, M. J., Sloet van Oldruitenborgh-Oosterbaan, M. M., Beynen A. C., High fat intake lowers hepatic fatty acid synthesis and raises fatty acid oxidation in aerobic muscle in Shetland ponies. *Br. J. Nutr.,* 86(1):31–6, July 2001.

Ghirardi, O., Milano, S., Ramacci, M. T., et al., Effect of acetyl-L-carnitine chronic treatment on discrimination models in aged rats. *Physiol. Behav.* (USA), 44(6):769–773, 1988.

Ghyczy, M., Boros, M., Electrophilic methyl groups present in the diet ameliorate pathological states induced by reductive and oxidative stress: a hypothesis. *Br. J. Nutr.,* 85(4):409–14, April 2001.

Guarnaschelli, C., Fugazza, G., and Pistarini, C., Pathological brain aging: evaluation of the efficacy of a pharmacological aid. *Drugs Exp. Clin. Res.,* 14:715–718, 1988.

Hahn, P., and Novak, M., How important are carnitine and ketones for the new born infant? *Fed. Proc.,* 44:2369–2373, 1985.

————, Allardyce, D. B., and Frohlich, J., Plasma carnitine levels during total parenteral nutrition of adult surgical patients. *Amer. J. Clin. Nutr.,* 36:569–572, 1982.

Hongu, N., Sachan, D. S., Caffeine, carnitine and choline supplementation of rats decreased body fat and serum leptin concentration as does exercise. *J. Nutr.*, 130(2):152–7, February 2000.

Hughes, R. E., Hurley, R. J., and Jones, E., Dietary ascorbic acid and muscle carnitine (B-OH-y-(trimethylamino) butyric acid) in guinea-pigs. *Brit. J. Nutr.*, 43:385–387, 1980.

Iannetti, E., Carpinteri, G., Trovato, G. M., Arterial hypertension in chronic kidney failure: a volume-dependent pathology or a disease due to malnutrition? *G. Ital. Cardiol.*, 29(3):284–90, March 1999.

Iliceto, S., Scrutinio, D., Bruzzi, P., et al., Effects of L-carnitine administration on left ventricular remodeling after acute anterior myocardial infarction: the L-Carnitine Ecocardiografia Digitalizzata Infarto Miocardioc (CEDIM) Trial. *Current Contents*, 23(35), August 28, 1995.

Imperato, A., Scrocco, M. G., Ghirardi, O., et al., *In vivo* probing of the brain cholinergic system in the aged rat: effects of long-term treatment with acetyl-l-carnitine. *Ann. N.Y. Acad. Sci.* (USA), 621:90–97, 1991.

Kanter, M. M., and Williams, M. H., Antioxidants, carnitine, and choline as putative ergogenic aids. *Int. J. Sport Nutr.*, 5:S120–S131, 1995.

Katz, M. I., Rice, L. M., Gao, C. L., Dietary carnitine supplements slow disease progression in a putative mouse model for hereditary ceroid-lipfuscinosis. 50(1):123–32, October 1997.

Keith, M. E., Ball, A., Jeejeebhoy, K. N., Kurian, R., Butany, J., Dawood, F., Wen, W. H., Madapallimattam, A., Sole, M. J., Conditioned nutritional deficiencies in the cardiomyopathic hamster heart. *Can. J. Cardiol.*, 17(4):449–58, April 2001.

Kelly, G. S., Insulin resistance: lifestyle and nutritional interventions. *Altern. Med. Rev.*, 5(2):109–32, April 2000.

Kendall, R. V. N., N-dimethylglucine and L-carnitine as performance enhancers in athletes. *Current Contents*, Comment, 22(38), September 19, 1994.

Kerner, J., Forseth, J. A., Miller, E. R., and Bieber, L. L., A study of the acetylcarnitine content of sows' colostrums, milk and newborn piglet tissues: demonstration of high amounts of iso-valeryl-carnitine in colostrum and milk. *J. Nutr.*, 114:854–861, 1984.

Khan, L., and Bamji, M. S., Tissue carnitine deficiency due to dietary lysine deficiency: triglyceride accumulation and concomitant impairment in fatty acid oxidation. *J. Nutr.*, 109:24–31, 1979.

Khan-Siddiqui, L., and Bamji, M. S., Lysine-carnitine conversion in normal and undernourished adult men—suggestion of a nonpeptidyl pathway. *Amer. J. Clin. Nutr.*, 37:93–98, 1983.

———, Plasma carnitine levels in adult males in India: effects of high cereal, low fat diet, fat supplementation, and nutrition status. *Am. J. Clin. Nutr.*, 33:1259–1263, 1980.

Kido, Y., Tamai, I., Ohnari, A., Sai, Y., Kagami, T., Nezu, J., Nikaido, H., Hashimoto, N., Asano, M., Tsuji, A., Functional relevance of carnitine transporter OCTN2 to brain distribution of L-carnitine and acetyl-L-carnitine across the blood-brain barrier. *J. Neurochem.*, 79(%):959–69, December 2001.

Kohjimoto, Y., Ogawa, T., Matsumoto, M., et al., Effects of acetyl-L-carnitine on the brain lipofuscin content and emotional behavior in aged rats. *J. Pharmacol.* (Japan), 48(3):365–371, 1988.

Koudelova, J., Mourek, J., Drahota, Z., Rauchova, H., Protective effect of carnitine of lipoperoxide formation in rat brain. *Physiol. Res.*, 43(6):387–9, 1994.

Krahenbuhl, S., Mang, G., Kupferschmidt, H., et al., Plasma and hepatic carnitine and coenzyme A pools in a patient with fatal, valproate induced hepatotoxicity. *Current Contents,* Comment, 23(31), July 31, 1995.

Krajcovicova-Kudlackova, M., Simoncic, R., Bederova, A., Babinska, K., Beder, I., Correlation of carnitine levels to methionine and lysine intake. *Physiol. Rev.,* 49(3):399–402, 2000.

Lee, J. S., Bruce, C. R., Spriet, L. L., Hawley, J. A., Interaction of diet and training on endurance performance in rats. *Exp. Physiol.,* 86(4):499–508, July 2001.

Leibovitz, B., *Carnitine the Vitamin BT Phenomenon.* New York: Dell Publishing Co., Inc., 1984.

Lien, T. F., Horng, Y. M., The effect of supplementary dietary L-carnitine on growth performance, serum components, carcase traits and enzyme activities in relation to fatty acid beta-oxidation of broiler chickens. *Br. Poult. Sci.,* 42(1):92–5, March 2001.

Lino, A., et al., Psycho-functional changes in attention and learning under the action of L-acetylcarnitine in 17 young subjects. A pilot study of its use in mental deterioration. *Clin. Ter.,* 140:569–573, 1992.

Makar, T. K., Cooper, A. J., Tofel–Grehl, B., Thaler, H. T., Blass, J. P., Carnitine, Carnitine acetyltrasferase, and glutathione in Alzheimer brain. *Neurochem. Res.,* 20(6):705–11, June 1995

Mayatepek, E., Kurczunski, T. W., and Hoppel, C. L., Long-term L-carnitine treatment in isovaleric acidemia. *Ped. Neur.,* 7(2), March-April 1991.

Montessuit, C., Papageorgiou, I., Tardy-Cantalupi, I., Rosenblatt-Velin, N., Lerch, R., Postischemic recovery of heart metabolism and function: role of mitochondrial fatty acid transfer. *J. Appl. Physiol.,* 89(1):111–9, July 2000.

Napoleone, P., Ferrante, F., Ghirardi, O., et al., Age-dependent nerve cell loss in the brain of Sprague-Dawley rats: Effect of long-term acetyl-L-carnitine treatment. *Arch. Gerontol. Geriatrs.* (Netherlands), 10(2):173–185, 1990.

Nasca, D., Zurria, G., Aguglia, E., Action of acetyl-L-carnitine with mianserine on depressed old people. *New Trends Clin. Neuropharmacol.* (Italy), 3(4):225–230, 1989.

Nutrition Reviews. Role of carnitine in branched-chain ketoacid metabolism. 39(11):406–407, 1981.

———, Cardiac carnitine-binding protein, 42(5):198–199, 1984.

———, Carnitine biosynthesis in rat and man: tissue specificity. 39(1):24–26, 1981.

Owen, K. Q., Nelssen, J. L., Goodband, R. D., Tokach, Friesen, K. G., Effects of dietary L-carnitine on growth performance and body composition in nursery and growing-finishing pigs. *J. Anim. Sci.,* 79(6):1509–15, June 2001.

Parnetti, L., et al., Multicentre study of L-alpha-glyceryl-phosphorylcholine vs. ST200 among patients with probable senile dementia of Alzheimer's type. *Drugs Aging,* 3:159–164, 1993.

Parnetti, L., Gaiti, A., Mecocci, P., et al., Effect of acetyl-L-carnitine on serum levels of cortisol and adrenocorticotropic hormone and its clinical effect in patients with dementia of Alzheimer type. *Dementia* (Switzerland), 1(3):165–168, 1990.

Pascale, A., Milano, S., Corsico, N., et al., Protein kinase C activation and anti-amnesic effect of acetyl-L-carnitine: *in vitro* and *in vivo* studies. *Aur. J. Pharmacol.,* 265:1–2, November 14, 1994.

Paulson, D. J., Schmidt, M. J., Traxler, J. S., Ramacci, M. R., and Shug, A. L., Improvement of myocardial function in diabetic rats after treatment with L-carnitine. *Metabolism,* 33(4):358–362, 1984.

Penn, D., Schmidt-Sommerfield, E., and Wolf, H., Carnitine deficiency in premature infants receiving total parenteral nutrition. *Early Human Devel.,* 23–24, 1980.

Pepine, C. J., Therapeutic potential of L-carnitine in cardiovascular disorders. *Clin. Ther.,* 13:2–21 (discussion 1), 1991.

Pillepich, J. A., Potential therapeutic applications of Propionyl-L-carnitine. 1993.

Pola, P., Tondi, P., Dal Lago, A., Serricchio, M., and Flore, R., Statistical evaluation of long-term L-carnitine therapy in hyperlipoproteinaemias. *Drugs Exptl. Clin. Res.,* IX(12):925–934,1983.

———, Savi, L., Serricchio, M., Dal Lago, A., Grilli, M., and Tondi, P., Use of physiological substance, acetyl-carnitine, in the treatment of angiospastic syndromes. *Drugs Exptl. Clin. Res.,* X(4):213–217, 1984.

Rabie, M. H., Szilagyi, M., Effects of L-carnitine supplementation of diets differing in energy levels on performance, abdominal fat content and yield and composition of edible meat of broilers. *Br. J. Nutr.,* 80(4):391–400, October 1998.

Rai, G., et al., Double-blind, placebo-controlled study of acetyl-L-carnitine in patients with Alzheimer's dementia. *Cur. Med. Res. Opin.,* 11:638–647, 1990.

———, Wright, G., Scott, L., et al., Double-blind, placebo-controlled study of acetyl-l-carnitine in patients with Alzheimer's disease. *Cur. Med. Res. Opin.* (United Kingdom), 11(10):638–647, 1989.

Ramacci, M. T., DeRossi, M., Lucreziotti, M. R., et al., Effect of long-term treatment with acetyl-L-carnitine on structural changes of aging rat brain. *Drugs Exp. Clin. Res.* (Switzerland), 14(9):593–601, 1988.

Rebouche, C. J., Effect of dietary carnitine isomers and -butyrobetaine on L-carnitine biosynthesis and metabolism in the rat. *J. Nutr.,* 113:1906–1913, 1983.

———, and Engel, A. G. Carnitine metabolism and deficiency syndromes. *Mayo Clin. Proc.,* 58:533–540, 1983.

———, Kinetic compartmental analysis of carnitine metabolism in the human carnitine deficiency syndromes. *J. Clin. Invest.,* 73:857–867, 1984.

Roe, C. R., Millington, D. S., Maltby, D. A., et al., L-carnitine therapy in isovaleric acidemia. *J. Clin. Invest.,* 74:2290–2295, December 1984.

Rosenthal, R. E., Williams, R., Bogaert, Y. E., et al., Prevention of postischemic canine neurological injury through potentiation of brain energy metabolism by acetyl-L-carnitine. *Stroke* (USA), 23(9):1312–1318, 1992.

Sachan, D. S., Rhew, T. H., and Ruark, R. A., Ameliorating effects of carnitine and its precursors on alcohol-induced fatty liver. *Amer. J. Clin. Nutr.,* 39:738–744, 1984.

Salvioli, G., and Neri, M., L-acetylcarnitine treatment of mental decline in the elderly. *Drugs Exp. & Clin. Res.,* ‹20(4):169–176, 1994.

Sandor, A., Pecsuvac, K., Kerner, J., and Alkonyi, I., On carnitine content of the human breast milk. *Pediatr. Res.,* 16:89–91, 1982.

Sano, M., et al., Double-blind parallel design pilot study of acetyl levocarnitine in patients with Alzheimer's disease. *Arch. Neurol.,* 49:1137–1141, 1992.

Sbriccoli, A., Carretta, D., Santarelli, M., Granato, A., Minciacchi, D.. An optimized procedure for prenatal ethanol exposure with determination of its effects on the central nervous system connections. *Brain Res. Protoc.,* 3(3):264–9, January 1999.

Scholte, H. R., Stinis, J. T., and Jennekens, F. G. I., Low carnitine levels in serum of pregnant women. *New Eng. J. Med.,* 299:1079–1080, 1979.

Seccombe, D., Burget, D., Frohlich, J., Hahn, P., Cleator, I., and Gourlay, R. H., Oral L-carnitine administration after jejunoileal by-pass surgery. *Interntl. J. Obesity,* 8:427–433, 1984.

Sershen, H., Harsing, Jr., L. G., Banay-Schwartz, M., et al., Effect of acetyl-L-carnitine on the dopaminergic system in aging brain. *J. Neurosci. Res.* (USA), 30(3):555–559, 1991.

Shug, A. L., Schmidt, M. J., Golden G. T., and Fariello, R. G., The distribution and role of carnitine in the mammalian brain. *Life Sci.,* 31:2869–2874, 1982.

Sinforiani, E., et al., Neuropsychological changes in demented patients treated with acetyl-l-carnitine. *Int. J. Clin. Pharmacol. Res.,* 10:69–74, 1990.

Slonim, A. E., Borum, P. R., Tanaka, K., Stanley, C. A., Kasselberg, A. G., Greene, H. L., and Burr. I. M., Dietary-dependent carnitine deficiency as a cause of nonketotic hypoglycemia in an infant. *J. Ped.,* 99(4):551–556, 1981.

Spagnoli, A., et al., Long-term acetyl-L-carnitine treatment in Alzheimer's disease. *Neurology,* 41:1726–1732, 1991.

Suzuki, G., Chen, Z., Sugimoto, Y., Fujii, Y., Kamei, C., Effects of histamine and related compounds on regional cerebral blood flow in rats. *Methods Find Exp. Clin. Pharmacol.,* 21(9):613–7, November 1999.

Taglialatela, G., Caprioli, A., Giuliani, A., Ghirardi, O., Spatial memory and NGF levels in aged rats: natural variability and effects of acetyl-L-carnitine treatment. *Exp. Gerontol.,* 31(5):577–87, September–October 1996.

Taglialatela, G., Angelucci, L., Ramacci, M. T., et al., Stimulation of nerve growth factor receptors in PC12 by acetyl-L-carnitine. *Biochem. Pharmacol.* (UK), 44(3):577–585, 1992.

Tempesta, E., et al., L-acetylcarnitine in depressed elderly subjects. A cross-over study vs. placebo. *Drugs Exp. Clin. Res.* 13:417–423, 1987.

————, et al., Role of acetyl-L-carnitine in the treatment of cognitive deficit in chronic alcoholism. *Int. J. Clin. Pharmacol. Res.,* 10:101–107, 1990.

Turcotte, L. P., Role of fats in exercise: types and quality. *Clin. Sports Med.,* 18(3):485–98, July 1999.

Vecchi, G. P., Chiari, G., Cipolli, C., et al., Acetyl-l-carnitine treatment of mental impairment in the elderly: evidence from multicentre study. *Arch. Gerontol. Geriatr.* (Netherlands), (Suppl. 2):159–168, 1991.

Vecchiet, L., DiLisa, F., Pieralisi, G., et al., Influence of L-carnitine administration on maximal physical exercise. *Eur. J. Appl. Physiol.,* 61:486–490, 1990.

Watanabe, S., Ajisaka, R., Masuoka, T., et al., Effects of L- and DL-carnitine on patients with impaired exercise tolerance. *Current Contents,* Comment, 23(31), July 31, 1995.

Weschler, A., Aviram, M., Levin, M., Better, O. S., and Brook, J. G., High dose of L-carnitine increases platelet aggregation and plasma triglyceride levels in uremic patients on hemodialysis. *Nephron,* 38:120–124, 1984.

White, H. L., and Scates, P. W., Acetyl-L-carnitine as a precursor of acetylcholine. *Neurochem. Res.* (USA), 15(6):597–601, 1990.

Witte, K. K., Clark, A. L., Cleland, J. G., Chronic heart failure and micronutrients. *J. Am. Coll. Cardiol.,* 37(7):1765–74, June 2001.

Chapter 20: Histidine

Adachi, N., and Itoh, Y., Direct evidence for increased continuous histamine release in the striatum of conscious freely moving rats produced by middle cerebral artery occlusion. *Journal of Cerebral Blood Flow Metabolism,* 12(3), 477–83, July 1992.

Anagnostrides, A. A., Christofides, N. D., et al., Peptide histidine isoleucine—a secretagogue in human jejunum. *Gut,* 25(4):381–385, 1984.

Aoyama, Y., and Kato, C., Suppressive effect of excess dietary histidine on the expression of hepatic metallothionein-1 in rats. *Bioscience Biotechnology Biochemistry,* 64(3), 588–91, March 2000.

Bizzi, A., Crane, R. C., Autilio-Gambetti, L., and Gambetti, P., Aluminum effect on slow axonal transport: a novel impairment of neurofilament transport. *J. Neurosci.,* 4(3):722–731, 1984.

Bunce, G. E., Nutrition and Cataract. *Nutr. Rev.,* 37(11):337–342, 1979.

Chiu, Y. N., Austic, R. E., and Rumsey, G. L., Effect of dietary electrolytes and histidine on histidine metabolism and acid base balance in rainbow trout (Salmo gairdneri). *Comp. Biochem. & Physiol.,* 78(4):777– 784, 1984.

Cho, E. S., Anderson, H. L., Wixom, R. L., Hanson, K. C., and Krause, G. F., Long-term effects of low histidine intake on men. *J. Nutr.,* 114(2):369–384, 1984.

Clairborne, B. J., and Selverston, A. I., Histamine as a neurotransmitter in the stomatogastric nervous system of the spiny lobster. *J. Neurosci.,* 4(3):708–721, 1984.

Clemens, R. A., Kopple, J. D., Swendseid, M. E., Metabolic effects of histidine-deficient diets fed to growing rats by gastric tube. *J. Nutr.,* 114(11):2138–2146, 1984.

Crush, K. G., Carnosine and related substances in animal tissues. *Comp. Biochem. Physiol.,* 34:3–30, 1970.

Dickerson, R. N., and et al., Effect of pentoxifylline on nitrogen balance and 3-methylhistidine excretion in parenterally fed edotoxemic rats. *Nutrition,* 17(7–8), 623–7, July–August 2001.

Dyme, I. Z., Horwitz, S. J., Bacchus, B., and Kerr, D. S., A case with resolution of myoclonic seizures after treatment with a low-histidine diet. *Am. J. Dis. Child.,* 137:256–258, 1983.

Gerber, D. A., Antirheumatic drugs, the ESR, and the hypohistinenemia of rheumatoid arthritis. *J. Rheumatol.,* 4:40–45, 1977.

———, Treatment of rheumatoid arthritis with histidine. *Arthritis & Rheum.* (abst.), 12:295, 1969.

———, Decreased concentration of free histidine in serum in rheumatoid arthritis, an isolated amino acid abnormality not associated with generalized hypoaminoacidemia. *J. Rheumat.,* 2(4):384–392, 1975.

———, Low free serum histidine concentration in rheumatoid arthritis: a measure of disease activity. *J. Clin. Invest.,* 55:1164–1173, 1975.

———, and Gerber, M. G., Specificity of a low free serum histidine concentration for rheumatoid arthritis. *J. Chronic Dis.,* 30:115–127, 1977.

Harris, A., and Delmont, J., 3 Methyl histidine (3MHis) a reliable indicator of protein energy malnutrition (PEM) in esogastric cancer. *J. ACN,* 3, 1984.

Hidesuke, J., Chaihara, K., Abe, H., Minamitani, N., Kodama, H., Kita, T., Fujita, T., and Tatemoto, K., Stimulatory effect of peptide histidine isoleucine amide 1–27 on prolactin release in the rat. *Life Sci.,* 35(6):641–648, 1984.

Hoekstra, W. G., Skeletal and skin lesions of zinc-deficient chickens and swine. *Amer. J. Clin. Nutr.,* 22(9):1268–1277, 1969.

Imamura, I., Watanabe, T., Hase, Y., Sakamoto, Y., Fukuda, Y., Yamamoto, H., Tsuruhara, T., and Wada, H., Effect of food intake on urinary excretions of histamine, N-methylhistamine, imidazole acetic acid and its conjugate(s) in humans and mice. *J. Biochem. Tokyo,* 96(6):1925–1931, 1984.

Ishibashi, T., Donis, O., Fitzpatrick, D., Lee, N.-S., Turetsky, O., and Fisher, H., Effect of age and dietary histidine on histamine metabolism of the growing chick. *Agents & Actions,* 9(5/6):435–444, 1979.

Kulh, D. A., and et al., Alterations in N-acetylation of 3-methylhistidine in endotoxemic parenterally fed rats. *Nutrition,* 14(9), 678–82, September 1998.

Medical World News. How "nonessential" is histidine? 35, November 7, 1969.

Myint, T., and et al., Urinary 1-methylhistidine is a marker of meat consumption in Black and in White California Seventh-day Adventists. *American Journal of Epidemiology,* 152(8), 752–5, October 2000.

Nasset, E. S., Heald, F. P., Calloway, D. H., Margen, S., and Schneeman, P., Amino acids in human blood plasma after single meals of meat, oil, sucrose and whiskey. *J. Nutr.,* 109(4):621–630, 1979.

Nishio, A., Ishiguro, S., Matsumoto, S., and Miyao, N., Histamine content and histidine decarboxylase activity in the spleen of the magnesium-deficient rat: comparison with the skin and peritoneal mast cells. *Japan. J. Pharmacol.,* 36:1–6, 1984.

Pfeiffer, C. C., and Sohler, A., Oral zinc in normal subjects: effect on serum histidine, iron and copper levels. Pamphlet: *Histidine II.* New York: Georg Thieme Verlag, 1980.

Phillips, P., Lim, W., Parkman, P., and Hirshaut, Y., Virus antibody and IgG levels in juvenile rheumatoid arthritis (JRA). *Arthritis & Rheum.* 16(1):126, 1973.

Pickup, M.E., Dixon, S., Lowe, J. R., and Wright, V., Serum histidine in rheumatoid arthritis: changes induced by antirheumatic drug therapy. *J. Rheumatol.,* 7(1):71–76, 1980.

Pinals, R. S., Harris, H. D., Frizzell, J., et al., Treatment of rheumatoid arthritis with histidine—a double-blind trial. *Arthritis & Rheum.* (abst.), 16:126–127, 1973.

Prast, H., and Philippu, A., Does brain histamine contribute to the development of hypertension in spontaneously hypertensive rats. *Naunyn Schmiedebergs Arch Pharmacology,* 343(3), 307–10, March 1991.

Rennie, M. J., Bennegard, K., Eden, E., Emery, P. W., and Lundholm, K., Urinary excretion and efflux from the leg of 3-methylhistidine before and after major surgical operation. *Metabolism,* 33(3):250–256, 1984.

Rocklin, R. E., and Beer, D. J., Histamine and immune modulation. *Advan. Internal. Med.,* 28:225–251, 1983.

Sass, R. L., and Marsh, M. E., Histidinoalanine—a naturally occurring cross-linking amino acid. Posttranslational modifications. *Methods Enzymology,* 106:351–354, 1984.

Snyderman, S. E., Sansaricq, C., Norton, P. M., and Manka, M., The nutritional therapy of histidinemia. *J. Ped.,* 95(11):712–715, 1979.

Steinhauer, H. B., Jackisch, R., and Schollmeyer, P., Modification of prostaglandin generation by L-histidine—possible pathogenic implication in rheumatoid arthritis. *Prostagland. Leuk. Med.,* 13(2):211–216, 1984.

Tyfield, L. A., and Holton, J. B., The effect of high concentrations of histidine on the level of other amino acids in plasma and brain of the mature rat. *J. Neurochem.*, 26:101–105, 1976.

Wang, Z., and et al., Urinary 3-methylhistidine excretion: association with total body skeletal muscle mass by computerized axial tomography. *Journal Parenter Enteral Nutrition*, 22(2), 82–6, March–April 1998.

Woldemussie, E., Eiken, D. L., and Beaven, M. A., Changes in histidine uptake and histamine synthesis during the growth cycle of rat basophilic leukemia (2H3) cells. *J. Pharmacol. Exper. Therap.*, 232(1), 1985.

SECTION NINE
Chapter 21

Abraira, C., DeBartolo, M., Katzen, R., and Lawrence, A. M., Disappearance of glucagonoma rash after surgical resection, but not during dietary normalization of serum amino acids. *Amer. J. Clin. Nutr.*, 39(3):351–355, 1984.

Abumrad, N. N., and Miller, B., The physiologic and nutritional significance of plasma-free amino acid levels. *J. Parenteral & Enteral Nutr.*, 7(2):163–170, 1983.

Aussel, C., et al., Plasma amino acid pattern in burn subjects: influence of septicemia. *Clin. Nutr.*, 3:237–239, 1984.

Bergstrom, J., et al., Free amino acids in muscle tissue and plasma during exercise in man. *Clin. Physiol.*, 5(2):155–160, 1985.

Bjerkenstedt, L., et al., Plasma amino acids in relation to cerebrospinal fluid monamine metabolites in schizophrenic patients and healthy controls. *Brit. J. Psychiatry*, 147:276–282, 1985.

Branchey, M., et al., Association between amino acid alterations and hallucinations in alcoholic patients. *Biol. Psych.*, 20:1167–1173, 1983.

Bremer, H. J., Duran, M., Kamerling, J. P., Przyrembel, H., and Wadman, S. K., eds., *Disturbances of Amino Acid Metabolism: Clinical Chemistry and Diagnosis.* Baltimore, MD: Urban & Schwarzenberg, 1981.

Brenner, U., et al., Free plasma amino acid pattern in gastrointestinal carcinoma: a potential tumor marker? *J. Exper. Clin. Cancer Res.* 4(3):253–258, 1985.

Burger, U., and Burger, D., Nutrition in pediatric patients with cancer or leukemia. *New Aspects Clin. Nutr.*, 631–638, 1983.

Chesney, R. W., et. al., Divergent membrane maturation in rat kidney: exposure by dietary taurine manipulation. *Inter. J. Pediat. Nephrol.*, 6(2):93–100, 1984.

Corman, L. C., The relationship between nutrition, infection, and immunity. *Med. Clin. N. Amer.*, 69(3):519–531, 1985.

Cotton, J. R., et al., Correction of uremic cellular injury with a protein-restricted amino acid-supplemented diet. *Amer. J. Kidney Dis.*, 5(5):233–36, 1985.

Elling, V. D., and Bader, K., Freie Serumaminosauren bei patientinnen mit ovarialkarzinemen. *Zbl. Gynakol.*, 107:1012–1016, 1985.

Eriksson, T., Magnusson, T., Carlsson, A., Hagman, M., and Jagenburg, R., Decrease in plasma amino acids in man after an acute dose of ethanol. *J. Studies Alcohol.*, 44(3):215–221, 1983.

Fisher, H., Essential and nonessential amino acids. *Biomedical Information Corp.*, New York, NY, 1984.

Freund, H. R., et al., Muscle prostaglandin production in the rat: effect of abdominal sepsis and different amino acid formulations. *Arch. Surgery,* 120(9):1037–41, 1985.

Gard, P. R., and Handley, S. L., Human plasma amino acid changes at parturition. *Horm. Metabol. Res.,* 17:112, 1985.

Harvey, S. G., et al., L-cysteine, glycine and dl-threonine in the treatment of hypostatic leg ulceration: a placebo-controlled study. *Pharmatherapeutica,* 4(4):227–230, 1985.

Holst, H., von, Hagenfeldt, L., Increased levels of amino acids in human lumbar and central cerebrospinal fluid after subarachnoid haemorrhage. *Acta Neurochirugica.,* 78(1–2):46–56, 1985.

Kasschau, M. R., and Howard, C. L., Free amino pool of a sea anemone: exposure and recovery after an oil spill. *Bull. Environ. Contam. Toxicol.,* 33:56–62, 1984.

Kennedy, B., et al., Nutrition support of inborn errors of amino acid metabolism. *Int. J. Bio. Medical Computing,* 17:69–76, 1985.

Kluthe, R., Betzler, H., and Vogel, W., Langzeitanalyse des aminosauren und eiwebstoffwechsels nach schwerem polytrauma. *Akt. Ernahr.,* 10:4–13, 1985.

Landel, A. M., et al., Aspects of amino acid and protein metabolism in cancer-bearing states. *Cancer,* 55(1):230–237, 1985.

Ludersdorf, V. R., et al., Konzentration der plasma-aminosauren nach exposition gegenuber organischen losemittelgemischen. *Fortschritte der Medizin,* 103(14):365–366, 1985.

Milakofsky, L., Hare, T. A., Miller, J. M., and Vogel, W. H., Rat plasma levels of amino acids and related compounds during stress. *Life Sci.,* 36:753–761, 1984.

————, Comparison of amino acid levels in rat blood obtained by catheterization and decapitation. *Life Sci.,* 34:1333–1340, 1984.

Moller, S. E., Tryptophan and tyrosine ratios to neutral amino acids in relation to therapeutic response in depressed patients. IVth World Congress of Biological Psychiatry, Philadelphia, PA, September 1985.

Moran, J. R., and Lyerly, A., The effects of severe zinc deficiency on intestinal amino acid losses in the rat. *Life Sci.,* 36:2515–2521, 1985.

Morimoto, Y., et al., Antitumor agent poly (amino acid) conjugates as a drug carrier in cancer chemotherapy. *J. Pharm. Dyn.,* 7:688–698, 1984.

Moss, G., Elevation of postoperative plasma amino acid concentrations by immediate full enteral nutrition. *J. Amer. Col. Nutr.,* 3:335–342, 1984.

Naomi, S., et al., Interrelation between plasma amino acid composition and growth hormone secretion in patients with liver cirrhosis. *Endocrinol. Japan.,* 31(5):557–564, 1984.

Nordenstrom, J., et al., Metabolic utilization of intravenous fat emulsion during total parenteral nutrition. *Ann. Surg.,* 196(2):221–231, 1982.

Norton, J. A., et al., Fasting plasma amino acid levels in cancer patients. *Cancer,* 56(5): 1181–1186, 1985.

Nutrition Reviews, Human protein deficiency—biochemical changes and functional implications. 35(11):294–296, 1977.

Olness, K. N., Nutritional consequences of drugs used in pediatrics. *Clin. Pediatr.,* 24(8): 417–418, 1985.

Pajari, M., Transport of branched-chain amino acids in brain slices of developing and adult rats. *Acta Physiol. Scand.,* 122:415–420, 1984.

Pangborn, J., Building health with amino acids. *Nutrition for Optimal Health Assoc. Conference* in Il. October 6, 1982.

Partsch, G., et al., The effect of D-penicillamine on plasma amino acids in rheumatoid arthritis. *Rheumatol.,* 42:126–129, 1983.

Philpott, W. H., and Kalita, D. K., *Brain Allergies.* New Canaan, CT: Keats Publishing, Inc., 1980, p. 53.

Popov, I. G., Latskevich, A. A., Blood amino acids of the crew members of 211-day space flight. *Kosmicheskaya Biologiya I Aviakosmicheskaya Meditsina,* 18(6):10–14, 1984.

Proietti, R., et al., Plasma free amino acids in trauma: clinical and therapeutic implications. *Resuscitation,* 9:107–11, 1981.

Robert, S., Experimental aminoacidemias. *Handbook of Neurochemistry* (vol. 9), ed. Lajtha, A., New York: Plenum Press, 1986, pp. 203–218.

Rosell, V. L., Threonine requirement of pigs weighing 5 to 15 kg and the effect of excess methionine in diets marginal in threonine. *J. Animal Science,* 60(2):480, 1985.

Schwarcz, R., and Meldrum, B., Excitatory amino acid antagonists provide a therapeutic approach to neurological disorders. *Lancet,* 140, July 20, 1985.

Segawa, K., et al., Amino acid in gastric juice of peptic ulcer patients. *Jap. J. Med.,* 24(1):34–38, 1985.

Snape, W. J., and Yoo, S., Effect of amino acids on isolated colonic smooth muscle from the rabbit. *J. Pharmacol. Exper. Therapeut.,* 235(3):690, 1985.

Tuomanen, E., and Tomasz, A., Protection by D-amino acids against growth inhibition and lysis caused by B-lactam antibiotics. *Antimicrobial Agents & Chemoth.,* September 1984, pp. 414–416.

Turkki, P. R., Chung, R. S., and Gardner, M. J., Riboflavin and vitamin C status of morbidly obese patients before and/or after surgical treatment. *Nutr. Rep. Inter.,* 30(3):709–717, 1984.

Vlasova, T. F., Miroshnikova, E. B., Belozerova, I. N., and Ushakov, A. S., Free amino acids in plasma during preflight training. *Kosmicheskaya Biologiya I Aviakosmicheskaya Meditsina,* 18(6):23–25, 1984.

Walzem, R. L., Clifford, C. K., and Clifford, A. J., Folate deficiency in rats fed amino acid diets. *J. Nutr.,* 113:421–429, 1983.

Wells, I. C., et al., Experimental study of chronic ambulatory peritoneal dialysis. *Clin. Physiol. Biochem.,* 3:8–15, 1985.

Winters, R. W., Heird, W. C., and Dell, R. B., History of parenteral nutrition in pediatrics with emphasis on amino acids. *Federation Proc.,* 43:1407–1411, 1984.

Wunderlich and Kalita, *Nourishing Your Child.* New Canaan, CT: Keats Publishing, 1984, p. 98.

Yu, Y. M., et al., Quantitative aspects of glycine and alanine nitrogen metabolism in postabsorptive young men: effects of level of nitrogen and dispensable amino acid intake. *J. Nutr.,* 115:339–410, 1985.

Index

About the Authors

Eric R. Braverman, M.D., is an integrative physician and Director of the Place for Achieving Total Health (PATH Medical), located in New York City. Dr. Braverman received his B.A. summa cum laude from Brandeis University and his M.D. with honors from New York University Medical School, after which he did his postgraduate work in internal medicine with a Yale Medical School affiliate in Greenwich, Connecticut. Dr. Braverman has published more than eighty research papers and is also coauthor of several books, including *Zinc and Other Micronutrients* (Keats Publishing, 1978), *Male Sexual Fitness* (McGraw-Hill/Contemporary Books, 1991), and *Hypertension and Nutrition.* (McGraw-Hill/Contemporary Books, 1998).

The late **Carl Pfeiffer, M.D., Ph.D.,** pioneered the biochemical basis of behavior and mental illness. He founded the Brain Bio Center in Princeton, New Jersey, in 1973, where he achieved unprecedented success in treating a wide range of mental problems, including schizophrenia, depression, anxiety, and phobia, with diet and nutritional supplements. He is the author of the groundbreaking books *Mental and Elemental Nutrients: A Physician's Guide to Nutrition and Health Care* (Keats Publishing, 1975) and *Nutrition and Mental Illness* (Inner Traditions, 1987). Dr. Pfeiffer also served as chief pharmacologist at Emory University and was director of the New Jersey Neuropsychiatric Clinic.

Kenneth Blum, Ph.D., is world renowned for his work on the role of neurotransmitters in compulsive/addictive behaviors and genetics. The recipient of nearly a dozen patents for treating addictive behavior, he is currently a professor of pharmacology at the University of San Antonio, Texas and the president and CEO of Nutrigenomics, Inc. He has written more than 300 scientific articles and has published in the *Journal of the American Medical Association.* He is the coauthor of several books, including *Folk Medicine and Herbal Healing* (Thomas, Charles C. Publisher, 1981), *Alcohol and the Addictive Brain: New Hope for Alcoholics* (Free Press, 1991), and *Overload: Attention Deficit Disorder and the Addictive Brain* (Andrews McMeel Publishing, 1996). Dr. Blum's work has been featured in major newspapers and on television stations worldwide.

Richard Smayda, D.O., is the Director of Primary Care Medicine at Cape Cod Hospital, in Brewster, Massachusetts. He assisted in the writing of this book and has published extensively on taurine metabolism, his area of expertise.